LEVERAGING THE EDUCATION-HEALTH CONNECTION

LEVERAGING THE EDUCATION–HEALTH CONNECTION

How Educators, Physicians,
and Public Health Professionals
Can Improve Education and
Health Outcomes throughout Life

DAVID A. BIRCH

JOHNS HOPKINS UNIVERSITY PRESS | *Baltimore*

Johns Hopkins University Press
2715 North Charles Street
Baltimore, Maryland 21218
www.press.jhu.edu

Library of Congress Cataloging-in-Publication Data is available.

ISBN 978-1-4214-4695-0 (paperback)
ISBN 978-1-4214-4696-7 (ebook)

A catalog record for this book is available from the British Library.

*Special discounts are available for bulk purchases of this book. For more information,
please contact Special Sales at specialsales@jh.edu.*

CONTENTS

Research clearly supports the premise that healthy children and youth are more successful in school than those dealing with health issues and that adults who attain higher levels of education are more likely to experience better health and well-being in adulthood. Thus, the health of students is an education issue, and access to quality schools and academic success for all children and youth is a public health issue.

Promoting quality education and well-being is not a simple effort. Various community and societal factors have an interdependent influence on both education and health. Thought leaders in education, medicine, public health, and the social sciences recognize that addressing education and health requires broad-based school, family, and community efforts that are well planned, coordinated, and sustained. Throughout my career in education and public health, I have experienced a growing recognition of this need for a broad-based effort.

My professional experiences reflect this increased recognition. At the beginning of my career as a seventh grade health education teacher, close to 50 years ago, I believed that my one-semester course would have a profound, lifelong impact on my students' health-related behaviors. I thought that the health knowledge and skills gained from this one class would be a major life-changer. Over my seven years of public-school teaching, however, I developed a better recognition of the multiple factors that play into students' lifestyles while they are in school and later in adulthood. I recognized that some students entered my classroom with more health knowledge and skills than others. This variation was due to a combination of factors such as the quality of their elementary school health instruction (my course occurred in the first year of junior high school), the influence of their community and home environment on health, and their personal access and their family's access to educational and health-promoting resources, programs, and facilities.

Based on these observations, several conclusions were clear to me. One was that school health instruction was more likely to have an impact on all students if it was taught by qualified teachers in an age-appropriate, sequential manner from elementary school through high school. Episodic, fragmented instruction with a focus on limited topics would not meet the health education needs of students. I also realized that schools needed to go beyond instruction to maximize the promotion of student health. Multiple school programs needed to be part of the effort.

For instance, early in my health education experience, I observed that the food served in the school cafeteria did not reflect what I was teaching students about nutrition. I also became aware that what I taught students about the value of various types of physical activity was not reinforced in their physical education classes. These classes emphasized participation in team sports rather than providing students with instruction and the opportunity to participate in various physical activities that they could continue doing throughout their lives. It soon became clear to me that the counseling and health services programs at the school were understaffed and offered a less-than-optimal range of individual and group programs intended to meet students' physical, mental, emotional, and social health needs. In addition, there were missed opportunities to engage and support parents and family members as partners in children's education.

While these deficits within the school were critical, as I became a more experienced teacher, I recognized that challenges faced by some students and their families outside school posed limitations to academic success and engagement in health-promoting activities. These included inadequate parental resources, limited access to out-of-school organizations that provide learning experiences for students' overall education and well-being, a lack of well-maintained playgrounds and athletic facilities, fewer grocery stores than convenience stores and fast-food restaurants, and community safety concerns. The underlying causes of many of these challenges included racism and other types of institutional bias that fueled discrimination, inequity, and limited opportunity. Together, these community, school, and societal challenges led me to conclude that if we are serious about promoting education and health for school-age children and youth, it will require a broad-based, coordinated school, family, and community commitment with a focus on addressing these injustices.

As my career evolved from public-school teaching to a health education leadership position in a state department of education, and eventually to over 30 years as a university health education faculty member and department chair, an increased recognition emerged within the education and public health sectors on the connection between student health and academic success. The importance of this connection became prominent in the late 1980s through 2000s when the US Centers for Disease Control and Prevention (CDC), Division of Adolescent and School Health, placed emphasis on the Coordinated School Health (CSH) model. The model included eight components intended to provide schools with a coordinated framework to promote student health. This emphasis has continued through the expanded version of CSH—the Whole School, Whole Community, Whole Child (WSCC) model—introduced in 2014 by the CDC and ASCD (formerly the Association for Supervision and Curriculum Development). WSCC focuses on the interdependence between education and health and serves as a framework for schools to address this relationship. The evolution of CSH and WSCC is presented in detail in chapter 6.

Another priority that gained increased recognition in the public health community in the 1990s and early 2000s, and is now an established public health focus, relates to the impact of social determinants on the quality of individuals' lives. These determinants include access to living-wage jobs, the availability of quality housing, food security, community or neighborhood safety, access to facilities for physical activity, accessible public transportation, and an overall sense among residents of a community that values diversity and social justice. Recognition of these factors has led to an increased understanding of the underlying influences of social injustices such as systemic racism and other forms of discrimination and their impact on health, schools, and the ability of children and youth to attain a quality education. Thus, social justice and community well-being are now both public health issues and education issues.

In the early 2000s, increased attention was brought to another aspect of the interdependent education-health relationship—the linkage of higher levels of education to better adult health outcomes. Research indicates that as adults attain higher levels of education, they live longer, experience a higher quality of life, have a reduced risk of chronic diseases such as cardiovascular disease and diabetes, miss less work owing to illness, and have a higher perception of their personal health status (Institute of Medicine, 2015; Kelly & Weitzen, 2010; Marmot, 2015; Zajacova & Lawrence, 2018). Beyond these findings, thought leaders in public health have posited that skills developed through quality education can enable individuals to engage in behaviors that promote their own health and provide support to the health of others (Marmot, 2015; Zimmerman et al., 2015). With the realization that the attainment of higher levels of education leads to better adult health, access to quality education for school-age children and youth gained increased attention as a public health priority.

These research findings and emerging priorities over the course of my career have led me to reconceptualize the promotion of individual and population health. I have moved from a focus on a transformational one-semester seventh grade health education intervention to the realization that having an impact on education and health requires a coordinated, multisectoral, ongoing social movement that focuses on K–12 health-promoting schools, the overall quality of the education that students experience, and the social injustices and other barriers faced by parents and community members that inhibit the ability to promote and support quality education and health for all children and youth.

While numerous well-planned but limited-focus advocacy and support efforts exist, more broad-based, multifocused social movement actions are needed. Advocacy for education is health advocacy, and advocacy for health is education advocacy. Advocacy for social justice is both education and health advocacy. Advocacy efforts must address not only limited-focus education and health policies, programs, and practices but also the larger social justice issues that influence students' ability to learn and communities' opportunities to thrive and support education and health. For example, education and public health advocates can support the provision of healthy food in the local school cafeterias and quality nutrition education and additionally address the state and national political issues that affect the ability of families and community members to provide healthy food for themselves and family members. Applying this to education, health advocates can support evidence-based programs in local schools that are intended to enable all students to reach age- and grade-level learning expectations and also address the state and national political actions that present barriers to parents' efforts to support their children's education and the schools' ability to offer high-quality, meaningful education to all students.

In this book, I propose a community-based coalition as the organizational underpinning for engagement in social movement actions primarily at the local level but also focused on state and national issues. Furthermore, I envision public health professionals, educators, and primary care physicians as logical leaders in this type of movement. These professionals have a common goal in their professional work: overall individual and community well-being. One important aspect of their leadership will be the recruitment and engagement of various sectors of the community, including representatives from local government, other medical specialties, the faith community, the business community, economic development, community development, transportation, parks and recreation, housing, social services, local colleges and universities, and law enforcement. Community leaders and residents are also important participants. With this multisectoral involvement as a framework, the purpose of this book is to provide direction to public health professionals, primary care physicians (pediatricians, family physicians, internal medicine specialists), and education leaders to serve as initiators, leaders, and ongoing partners in coalitions on the local level that promote and support social justice and a health-enhancing family, community, and school environment that results in equal access to high-quality schools for all children and youth.

Knowing that there is an association between education and adult health outcomes is not enough—social movement leaders must be informed and able to contribute to collective action for positive change. To maximize this type of contribution, physicians and public health professionals must understand the potential role of schools in helping students thrive and actively support the policies, processes, and programs that provide a foundation for accessible, meaningful education for all students. Similarly, for educators, only being aware of the role of students' health in influencing academic achievement is not enough. Educators must understand how communities and schools can become centers for the promotion of health for school-age children and youth. In partnership, representatives of these three professions in their role as social movement collaborators must also understand the impact of inequity and social injustices on education and health and be informed advocates in addressing these conditions both in the community and in schools.

The book is organized to provide important information and specific direction for leaders and participants in an education–health–social justice coalition. Chapter 1 presents an overview of the interdependent relationship between education and health and the importance of multisectoral collaboration in the formation and implementation of a community coalition. Social justice and the connection to education and health disparities are the focus of chapter 2. Topics examined in the chapter include equity as it relates to education and health and the specific impact of social injustices related to race and ethnicity, poverty, parental incarceration, immigration, and sexual orientation and identity. Chapter 3 addresses social justice issues related to early childhood, including disparities in school readiness and the importance of high-quality early childhood education and home visiting programs. The chapter also includes background information on adverse childhood experiences. Since education attainment is related to adult health outcomes, high school graduation is the focus of chapter 4. Topics addressed within the chapter include high school graduation challenges within the United States, school connectedness, and the importance of attendance.

Programs, policies, and processes related to high-quality, social justice–

oriented schools are presented in chapter 5. Topics addressed in the chapter include the value of a clear school mission, the limitations of an overemphasis on the results of standardized testing, thoughts on meaningful learning, perspectives on excellence in teaching and leadership, considerations related to the implementation of a restorative justice–based approach to student behavior issues, the importance of school staff being trauma informed, and the impact of inequity in school funding. Chapter 6 is focused on a detailed presentation of the WSCC model. The model was developed collaboratively by the education professional organization ASCD and the CDC. The underlying tenets and components of the model are presented in detail in the chapter. Chapter 7, the concluding chapter in the book, presents specific actions related to both the formation and implementation activities of a multisectoral coalition led by educators, physicians, and public health professionals. Specific topics in the chapter include the rationale for an education-health social movement, considerations for the initiation of a coalition, the development of an action plan, advocacy considerations, and actions related to sustaining a coalition.

I visualize the book serving as a textbook for undergraduate and graduate courses in a variety of disciplines, including public health, medical education, school health, education administration and leadership, social work, school counseling, and school nursing. One of my aspirations is to see interdisciplinary courses that are offered at both the undergraduate and graduate levels for students from relevant disciplines. A course open to education, public health, and medical students would present rich opportunities for interdisciplinary engagement and content application. Beyond the academic setting, the book can serve as a valuable resource for leaders in national, state, and local organizations in education, public health, child health, and community development.

As I was writing this book, current public health and societal issues provided a clear demonstration of the interdependence of education, health, and social justice. The ongoing presence of the COVID-19 pandemic illuminated issues within communities and schools and among community members and public officials. Issues such as misinformation, disinformation, the distrust of science, health and political illiteracy, inadequate school health policies and infrastructures, the lack of individuals' commitment to the overall community, and a lack of caring and responsibility for the well-being of others all surfaced during the pandemic.

In addition to the COVID-19 pandemic, social injustices resulting from racism, anti-Semitism, and other forms of structural discrimination and inequity received extensive attention during my writing. These injustices included police violence that was especially pronounced with regard to police interactions with African American community members; hate crimes perpetuated by community members; mass murders; violent community demonstrations, including an attack on the US Capitol and an attempted assault on the democratic processes that guide elections; and an obvious lack of commitment to diversity, inclusion, and equity among public officials. Specific to schools, most prominent was a mass shooting in an elementary school in Uvalde, Texas. Other education-related injustices also arose. Inaccurate information and, in some cases, obvious racism surfaced among elected and appointed governmental officials, parents, community members, and school board members through opposition to social justice–oriented teaching and learning. Further demonstration of social injustice was the opposition among conservative members of the US Congress to research-based legislative initiatives designed to support education and parenting such as access to early childhood education, the equitable provision of comprehensive health care, family leave, and the extension of the 2021 child tax credit.

It is my belief that the presence of an informed local coalition of education, health, and social justice representatives can serve as a resource to provide support and direction both before and during the presence of crises such as COVID-19 and ongoing social injustices. Communities and schools that are committed to engaging students in meaningful education and nurturing an environment that promotes education, health, and social justice for school-age children and youth, parents and family members, and community members not only will be better prepared to address any crises that may occur but also are more likely to foster children, youth, and adults who understand science; are health literate, politically informed, and compassionate; and act in the best interests of their own well-being and the well-being of others. An education–health–social justice coalition can be a catalyst for this outcome.

This book covers a wide range of content that emanates from three focal points: education, health, and social justice. Because of the wealth of information that exists, I have been educated and challenged: educated through the attainment of a deeper understanding of the interdependence of education, health, and social justice, and challenged to synthesize the plethora of important content into a resource for educators, physicians, public health professionals, and all other stakeholders.

Being able to acknowledge the many individuals who have contributed to my authorship of this book presents an overwhelming task. Throughout my career, I have had mentors and colleagues who have influenced my professional awareness and knowledge and provided inspiration for my work. I have also been influenced and inspired by the opportunity to work and interact with many outstanding students. I will not attempt to identify these individuals but want to call attention to the important influence these mentors, colleagues, and students have had on my professional life.

Beyond those in my immediate personal and professional space, I have been influenced by many thought leaders, researchers, and practitioners through their publications, presentations, and, in some cases, collaborative experiences and personal interactions. Some of them I know professionally; others I only know through their work. Again, I will not attempt to identify these individuals, but many of them are cited as authors of references throughout this book.

I also want to acknowledge individuals who have contributed directly to this book. Two professional colleagues, Kiersten Bond and Megan Campbell, whom I first worked with when they were graduate students, played important roles related to my authorship. Kiersten coordinated the many citations in the book chapters and the development of the overall book reference list. Megan worked with me in the development of the tables and figures and the descriptions of organizations that are included in the appendix. They were a pleasure to work with, and their contributions were of the highest professional quality.

Several Johns Hopkins University Press staff members have provided important direction to my writing. I want to first call attention to Robin Coleman, acquisitions editor, who presented the idea to me of addressing the education–health–social justice relationship in a book format and, throughout the book's development, provided his important thoughts and feedback. I also want to thank Jeremy Horsefield for his expert copyediting. The book's writing is better because of his outstanding work. In addition, staff members Robert Brown, Magdalene Klassen, Adelene Jane Medrano, and Juliana McCarthy contributed to important communication throughout the publication process and the finalization of book components.

Finally, I would like to thank my wonderful wife, Ruthann, for her ongoing understanding during my overwhelming commitment to completing this book. I would not have been able to accomplish this task without her love and support. I am fortunate.

LEVERAGING THE EDUCATION–HEALTH CONNECTION

CHAPTER 1

Health and Education

An Interdependent Relationship

If medical researchers were to discover an elixir that could increase life expectancy, reduce the burden of illness, delay the consequences of aging, and shrink disparities in health, we would celebrate such a remarkable discovery. Robust epidemiological evidence suggests that education is such an elixir.

FREUDENBERG & RUGLIS (2007)

MOST ADULTS place a high value on both education and health. Parents want their children to be successful in school and to be healthy throughout their lives. Employers covet employees who not only have job-specific skills but also possess important life skills such as critical thinking, communication, and problem-solving— as well as the health status to enjoy their work and approach it with commitment and vigor. A community is more likely to thrive when its members are informed, engaged, civic-minded, and physically, mentally, and emotionally able to make contributions that benefit the community. Supporting quality education, promoting health, and advancing social justice benefit community members of all ages.

Education and health are not only important but also interdependent. Research indicates that there is a relationship between the health status and health behaviors of children and adolescents and their success as students. Few would be surprised to learn that students often face academic challenges if they are dealing with stress, physical and emotional abuse, aggression and violence, hunger and malnourishment, physical inactivity, hyperactivity, lack of sleep, safety concerns, pregnancy, vision problems, asthma, dental health issues, or lack of adequate dental and medical care (Basch, 2011; Kolbe, 2019). Research conducted by the US Centers for Disease Control and Prevention (CDC) demonstrates a strong relationship between high school students' healthy behaviors and academic achievement as indicated by grades, standardized test scores, graduation rates, and attendance (CDC, 2021c).

It may also not be surprising that individuals who attain higher levels of education are more likely to become healthier adults. What may be unexpected is that there is a clear distinction in health status among those with varying levels of education. Research indicates that by age 25, US adults who are college graduates can expect to live 9 years longer than those without a high school degree (Institute of Medicine, 2015). Based on an examination of National Center for Health Statistics mortality data for the years 1996 through 2002, Woolf et al. (2007) estimated that an average of 195,619 deaths per year during that time period could have been prevented if adults with a high school education or less had the same mortality rates as adults with at least some level of college education. Relative to another indicator of well-being, individuals with advanced degrees have as many as 12 more quality-adjusted life years compared with those who did not complete high school (Institute of Medicine, 2015).

It is a graded relationship: as the differences between levels of education attainment increase, the health differences also increase. Thus, for example, while there is a health difference between high school graduates and individuals with an undergraduate college degree, the difference is less than that between individuals who graduated from high school and those with advanced or graduate college degrees. Research also indicates that adults with higher levels of education are more likely to rate their health as good than are adults with lesser levels of educational attainment (Zajacova & Lawrence, 2018).

The evidence supporting the reciprocal relationship between education and health illuminates the importance of access for all children to both a health-promoting environment and a high-quality early-childhood, elementary, and secondary education experience. Healthy students are more likely to be academically successful, and children and youth who are exposed to a quality education through high school and attain higher levels of education are more likely to experience better health outcomes in adulthood. Anthony Iton, the senior vice president for Healthy Communities, California Endowment, describes education as the "single most modifiable social determinant of health" (McGill, 2016, p. 1). Thus, the health of school-age children is an important issue for the education sector, and quality education is an important public health issue.

While addressing the education-health linkage is critical, improving the quality of children's health and the accessibility for all children to good schools is a challenging proposition. Education and health are both affected by many of the same complex social justice issues. Educational attainment and health outcomes cannot be separated from social determinants of health such as poverty, the quality of accessible housing, access to living-wage jobs, access to transportation, community resources, community environmental and safety issues, and overall access to opportunity. Factors that influence these determinants include racism, xenophobia, sexism, heterosexism, transphobia, ableism, ageism, and other systemic forms of discrimination. These social injustices influence both the opportunities for individuals, families, and communities to be healthy and the overall quality of education. Any effort designed to maximize the potential of education in improving the health and overall quality of life for all school-age children, both while in school and in their future adult years, must address these multiple social justice issues. It is suggested that "the amelioration of education-associated mortality requires more extensive social change than simply ensuring that all adults complete college or even eliminating educational disparities" (Woolf et al., 2007, p. 681). Marmot (2015) captured the need to address social change, stating that "social injustice is killing on a grand scale" (p. 79).

The overall purpose of this book is to provide direction to public health professionals, primary care physicians (pediatricians, family physicians, internal medicine specialists), and education leaders to serve as initiators, leaders, and ongoing partners in multisector coalitions on the local level that promote and support social justice and a health-enhancing family, community, and school environment that results in equal access to high-quality schools for all children and youth. The intent is that the actions of the coalition will initiate and contribute to a social movement that addresses the multiple complex factors that affect the ability of schools to become centers for students' health and learning and the factors that influence or inhibit the ability of parents, community members, and organizations to be fully engaged as supportive partners. While the primary focus of the coalition is on the local community and school levels, attention must also be paid to laws, policies, and actions at the state, national, and international levels that have an impact on local education and health issues. Positive local action related to education and health is more likely to occur if it is supported at these more distal levels. Thus, a local coalition can be engaged in social movements at multiple levels. Representatives from the education, medical, and public health sectors are identified as potential leaders because of their professional focus on the same ultimate outcome—a healthy, self-fulfilling life for individuals of all ages. Because of this common mission and the strong local, state, and national presence of these professions, the three sectors are logical community partners in initiating and sustaining a coalition to promote equal access to social justice, health, and access to quality educational experiences for all school-age children and youth. This is not to imply that other stakeholder groups and individual community members cannot be involved in these coalition efforts and even play an equal leadership role. Possible participants are organizations and individuals representing local government, other medical specialties, the faith community, the business community, community development, economic development, parks and recreation, housing, social services, transportation, local colleges and universities, and law enforcement, as well as community leaders and residents. All community members and professional groups are possible coalition partners. As with all social movements, it is essential that all actions are community informed and done "with" community members rather than "to" community members.

While the connection between education and health should be of interest to all physicians, the initial focus on the medical sector for this coalition-led social movement is toward family physicians, internal medicine physicians, and pediatricians. These physicians are identified for initial leadership because the scope of their practice involves interaction with a representative cross section of the population and typically addresses a range of health issues. In addition, related professional organizations such as the American Academy of Family Physicians, the American Academy of Pediatrics, and the American College of Physicians have recognized multisector, community-based action as important to their members' work (American Academy of Family Physicians, 2020; American College of Physicians, n.d.; Kuo et al., 2018).

Local education–health–social justice coalitions must be prepared to address issues and challenges that affect both the school and community settings. Communities affect schools, and schools have an impact on communities. In the school setting, coalition actions might include advocating for curriculum or policy change; monitoring the school's commitment to equity, cultural responsiveness, and overall social justice for all students; providing input into the school's health education, health promotion, and health services programs; interviewing school board candidates for their positions on various issues and subsequently providing public support to selected candidates; and maintaining a regular connection with administrators, teachers, staff members, and students.

In the community setting, actions can address social injustices and health issues in the community that affect students' ability to feel safe, supported, and able to learn while in school, as well as factors that prevent parents and family members from being able to support their children's success in school. Other community issues that might warrant coalition attention include a lack of access for all children to meaningful out-of-school activities; local environmental issues that affect children and adults; crime and safety issues; work-related issues, such as minimum wage requirements and access to living-wage jobs; lack of

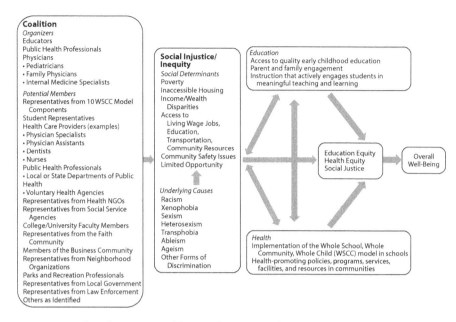

Figure 1.1. The Education–Health–Social Justice Coalition

community resources; and, similar to school board elections, the positions of candidates for city or town council and other elected positions. As noted earlier in the chapter, while the coalition is focused on local community and school issues, state and national policies and laws can also affect local communities and schools—monitoring laws and policies can go beyond the local level. The work of this type of coalition is not time limited. People change, communities change, new challenges and issues surface, and some never go away. Issues related to education, health, and the overall well-being of individuals and communities will persist. The potential members and pathways for action for an education–health–social justice coalition are presented in figure 1.1.

The following considerations provide a foundation for the book and a framework for the activities of an education–health–social justice coalition:

- Healthy students are more likely to be academically successful and attain higher levels of education after high school. Thus, students' health is an education issue.

- Individuals with higher levels of education are more likely to experience healthier adult outcomes than individuals with lower levels of education. Thus, education is a public health issue.
- Inequity and social injustices at the local level and beyond affect education for all students and health for individuals of all ages. Thus, social justice is both an education issue and a public health issue.
- Good schools are based on more than students' standardized test scores. Good schools are social justice oriented and provide a meaningful education that prepares students for a purposeful life in which they promote their own well-being and the well-being of their community.
- All children and youth in a community should have equal access to good schools beginning in early childhood. All students should feel connected to school and view it as safe and supportive. All parents and community members should feel connected to and valued by the schools in their community.
- The community should provide a socially just, health-enhancing, supportive environment for all children, youth, and adults. Residents of socially just communities are more likely to be healthy and better able to be engaged in and provide support to schools and the overall community.
- Educators, physicians, and public health professionals have a professional responsibility to provide expertise and leadership to a multisectoral social movement focused on promoting equal access to quality education for all school-age children.

The remainder of the chapter includes the rationale for a multisectoral approach; examples of collaborative commitment and actions on the part of the education, medical, and public health sectors; considerations on the meaning of personal health and traits of educated individuals; and further information related to the reciprocal relationship between education and health.

Multisectoral Collaboration: Addressing Education, Health, and Social Justice

The United States has a long history of struggles for equity and fairness, yet wealth and power remain concentrated in a very small segment of our society. Now, in the face of growing public awareness and outcry about centuries-long injustices experienced by African Americans, Native Americans, new immigrants and other marginalized groups, our nation urgently needs collaborative multi-sector approaches toward equity and justice.   KEGLER ET AL. (2019)

Collaborative partnerships are an essential means to concomitantly improve both education outcomes and health outcomes among K–12 students.

KOLBE ET AL. (2015)

The importance of a multisectoral approach to address the complex issues affecting education, health, and social justice has received considerable attention from thought leaders representing a range of professions. Involving different sectors to address this complexity brings varied perspectives and experiences, diverse skills, multiple spheres of influence, and shared resources. Michener et al. (2019) capture the importance of collaboration in addressing health issues: "Our communities and the individuals living in them are dying of illnesses we know how to prevent, that have their roots in our communities, and that cannot be effectively treated by any one group alone" (p. 5). DeSalvo et al. (2017) recommend that communities form organizations across multiple sectors that have a shared vision and a long-term road map for promoting health, equity, and resilience. Valles (2018) supports this recommendation: "It is now widely accepted that effective and equitable health promotion requires broad-scoped interdisciplinary and intersectoral efforts" (p. 1).

Bradley and Greene (2013), based on their findings from a systematic literature review of studies addressing the linkage between academic achievement and health, stated that "improving health and increasing academic achievement of children and youth in the U.S. needs to be viewed as a composite goal rather than separate goals that are the responsibilities of different agencies" (p. 528). AASA, the School Superintendents Association (2019), supports the importance of multiagency involvement: "Building partnerships and supporting the education of all students is the responsibility of the entire community. Those partnerships and the contributions made by all stakeholder groups in the community contribute to the educational success and well-being of our children. Communities are responsible for the health, safety, welfare, and education of each child. Schools are but one partner in the community, which includes many domains of public and private agencies" (p. 2).

The medical sector has recognized the importance of collaboration with public health to address social determinants and reach mutual population health goals. Jarris and Sellars (2016) support the importance of this partnership: "Primary care and public health will never reach their shared dream of a healthy nation unless we build robust primary care and public health systems that collaborate and leverage each other's unique contributions to the health of the population" (p. 31). One factor driving physicians' efforts is the realization that social determinants are often key factors that affect the health of their patients. This has led physicians to recognize the need to extend their professional activities to promote the health of not only individuals but also communities (American Academy of Family Physicians, 2020). Kuo et al. (2018) support this recognition: "The prevention of major threats to children's health (such as behavioral health issues) and the control and management of chronic diseases and other problems cannot be managed solely in the pediatric office" (p. 1). Fineberg (2011), in expressing support for physicians' involvement in public health, stated, "The physician who appreciates the role and potential for public health interventions—public health, social campaigns, ordinances and laws, standards and regulations, surveillance, and preparedness—has a deeper understanding of the conditions that preserve health, of the primacy of disease prevention, and the interfaces between personal medical care and community health protection" (p. S149). The importance of the consideration of social determinants is further highlighted in the Robert Wood Johnson Foundation's vision for a Culture of Health that encourages a health care system engaged in multisectoral partnerships that address the life needs of patients and families both within and outside of the health care setting (Witt et al., 2017).

Advocacy has been identified as a specific collaborative action for physicians. The American Medical Association (2001), in its *Declaration of Professional Responsibility: Medicine's Social Contract with Humanity*, presents a commitment that physicians "advocate for social, economic, educational, and political changes that ameliorate suffering and contribute to human wellbeing." Silberberg and Castrucci (2016) view advocacy as a role for primary care physicians in both the school and community settings. Kuo et al. (2018) posit that pediatricians and public health professionals leverage the strengths and expertise of each profession to advance health at the community level. Former US Surgeon General David Satcher and colleagues suggest that pediatricians reach out to educators, social workers, public servants, and politicians to serve as public health advocates for all children within their community (Satcher et al., 2005).

Two edited compilations developed through an initiative of the de Beaumont Foundation in partnership with the CDC and the Duke University Department of Community Medicine, *The Practical Playbook: Public Health and Primary Care Together* (Jarris & Sellars, 2016) and *The Practical Playbook II: Building Multisector Partnerships That Work* (Mattson & Remley, 2019), serve as outstanding resources to provide direction to the initiation and maintenance of partnerships between public health, medicine, and other community members and organizations. These two resources contain multiple chapters that present the rationale for these partnerships and address considerations related to collaborative planning, implementation, and evaluation. The books also include numerous examples of primary care–public health partnerships in communities from across the United States. Another important primary care–public health resource is *Primary Care and Public Health: Exploring Integration to Improve Public Health* (Institute of Medicine, 2012).

The medical sector's commitment to public health has also surfaced in medical education. The American College of Physicians recommends that "social determinants of health and the underlying individual, community, and systemic issues related to health inequities be integrated into medical education at all levels" (Daniel et al., 2018). Mattson and

Remley (2019) suggest that medical training should assist prospective primary care providers in the development of a social justice orientation, a commitment to promote diversity and inclusion within the profession, and skills to work with communities, institutions, and systems to promote health equity and reduce health disparities. Aligned with working in communities, Hollander-Rodriguez and DeVoe (2018) have suggested physician training topics such as skills related to community organizing, collaboration, and teamwork. Both the American Academy of Family Physicians and the American Academy of Pediatrics have specific programs for residents that focus on working with communities to address issues such as health disparities, discrimination, and bias (Mattson & Remley, 2019).

Collaborative action in various projects has occurred between the education and public health sectors. ASCD (formerly the Association for Curriculum Development), an education professional organization, and the CDC collaborated in the development of the Whole School, Whole Community, Whole Child (WSCC) model. The WSCC model presents a framework that provides schools with a coordinated approach to promote both students' health and their academic success (Birch & Videto, 2015). A detailed description of the WSCC model is provided in chapter 6. The Center for School Health and Education of the American Public Health Association (APHA) partners with schools, school-based health centers, community organizations, and other stakeholders to advance equity in school settings to prevent dropout and improve graduation rates for K–12 students. The Center's focus, rooted in social justice, is to help schools create opportunities for all students to achieve their full potential despite social disadvantages (APHA, n.d.). In addition to APHA's collaboration with education, the National Association of Chronic Disease Directors (NACDD) has published several documents focused on public health directors partnering with schools, including *Local Health Departments and School Partnerships: Working Together with Schools* and *The Whole School, Whole Community, Whole Child Model: A Guide to Implementation* (NACDD, 2017a, 2017b). Hahn and Truman (2015), in acknowledging the possible challenges of collaborations between public health and education, emphasize the importance of this relationship: "Such challenges must not deter the public health community from working closely with the education community to investigate and understand this form of social determinant causation, evaluate the wide array of educational program types, and mobilize for action on this powerful force for public health benefits" (p. 673).

While the education, medical, and public health sectors have recognized and demonstrated the importance of multisectoral collaboration, few examples are present of collaborative efforts involving the three sectors together. One example of collaboration between primary care physicians, educators, and public health professionals is the San Diego Healthy Weight Collaborative. As part of this multisector effort in one school district, participants from the three sectors met monthly and developed specific strategies to address obesity among children and their families, which was identified as a major health issue for the school community. The effort included nutritional messages that were incorporated into school wellness programs and family medical visits. In addition, the collaborative advocated for policy change, which resulted in important revisions in the school wellness policy (Serpas et al., 2016). A second example of collaboration involving the education, public health, and medical sectors is the Philadelphia ACE Task Force. The mission of the task force is to provide a venue to address childhood adversity and the related consequences in the Philadelphia metropolitan area. The task force's agenda includes screening for adverse childhood experiences (ACEs), community education regarding ACEs, developing an understanding of ACE interventions available in Philadelphia, and the promotion of local ACE research. The task force's community-based focus includes not only education, medicine, and public health representatives but also representation from federally qualified health centers, the child welfare system, juvenile court, affordable housing advocates, parks and recreation services, and local advocacy groups (Pachter et al., 2017).

As already stated, there is little or no opposition to supporting the development of healthy and well-educated children and youth so that they will become healthy, thriving adults who contribute to society. However, good schools and socially just, healthy, supportive communities that provide direction and support for this outcome do not happen on their own. Community education, mobilization, and advocacy are needed to act on the complex factors that affect education and well-being.

Consider the potential impact on parents, school administrators, and school boards of well-informed and well-organized advocacy efforts on the part of educators, physicians, public health professionals, and other community stakeholders emphasizing the importance of quality education and health promotion in schools. Beyond schools, consider the impact of advocacy by a similar group directed toward appointed and elected community officials related to the development and implementation of policies, practices, and programs designed to address social determinants and social injustices within a community. The education, medical, and public health sectors must be key leaders, partners, and advocates in promoting this collaborative approach.

For these efforts to be effective, advocates, decision-makers, and all stakeholders must have an understanding of the reciprocal relationship between education and health and of what it means to be educated and healthy, recognize that societal injustices affect education and health, realize the importance of meaningful engagement and two-way support between the school and community, and understand the characteristics of quality schools that enhance health and promote meaningful education. In the remainder of this chapter, considerations related to what it means to be healthy, the overall goal and outcomes of education, and further details on the reciprocal relationship between education and health are presented.

What Does It Mean to Be Healthy?

A person's health cannot be seen in isolation but must be placed in the rich contextual web such as the socioeconomic circumstances and other health determinants of where they were conceived, born, bred, and how they shaped and were shaped by their environment and communities.   ARAH (2009)

For multisectoral collaboration to be most effective, all individuals and organizations involved in advocacy must have a clear understanding of and agreement on what it means for an individual and a community to be healthy. This understanding will provide direction to coalition advocacy efforts addressing policies, practices, and programs related to education and health in both the school and community. Bircher and Kuruvilla (2014) emphasize this idea: "A shared understanding of the nature of health and its related determinants could contribute to ongoing collective efforts" (p. 367). Because of different professional preparation, priorities, and experiences, educators, physicians, public health professionals, and other key stakeholders can have different perspectives on the indicators of health. A middle school principal may view health through the lens of student absenteeism due to illness, or school and neighborhood safety; a primary care physician or pediatrician might consider the number of times a patient has experienced illness over the past year or the presence or lack of disease risk factors; and a public health professional might frame a definition based on the leading causes of morbidity and mortality within a specific region or among a subpopulation.

A narrow focus might characterize health by life expectancy or limit it to a focus on behaviors related to physical health with little or no focus on factors related to mental, emotional, social, environmental, and occupational health. Sometimes overlooked from a health perspective might be the quality of family and community life; equity and social injustices that affect the opportunity for accomplishment and enjoyment in life; connectedness to other community members, often referred to as "social capital"; and other issues related to where children, youth, and adults live, learn, work, and spend time. A limited perspective of health can result in a limited approach to maintaining and improving it.

The need to approach health from a more holistic perspective has long been recognized by public health professionals. In 1948, the World Health Organization (WHO) presented the following definition of health: "a state of complete physical, mental, and social well-being and not merely the absence of disease or infirmity" (WHO, 1948, p. 1). This definition was noteworthy when it was first developed because it defined health beyond just the physical dimension by including both mental and social well-being. In addition, it indicates that not being ill or infirm does not mean that a person is healthy. For those reasons, the definition is significant. However, concern about the definition has been expressed because of the inclusion of the term "complete" (Barr, 2019; Valles, 2018). Seldom can individuals claim complete health in all three dimensions—using a strict interpretation of this definition, individuals with minor injuries or illnesses or chronic conditions would not be considered healthy. This concern lends importance to health being considered on an individual basis taking into account factors such as an individual's abilities and disabilities, their family and community environment, and their experiences with physical, emotional, and social conditions.

Other models and definitions have been presented that incorporate an inclusive and comprehensive view of health. These perspectives include various combinations of health dimensions, including physical, mental, emotional, intellectual, spiritual, social, interpersonal, environmental, occupational, financial, and cultural.

One example comes from the integrative health profession. Integrative health encourages individuals, social groups, and communities to develop ways of living that promote meaning, resilience, and well-being across the life course. Based on input from professionals in the field, integrative health was defined as "a state of well-being in body, mind and spirit that reflects aspects of the individual, community and population. It is affected by: (1) individual biological factors and behaviors, social values, and public policy, (2) the physical, social, and economic environments, and (3) an integrative health care system that involves the active participation of the individual and the health care team in applying a broad spectrum of preventive and therapeutic approaches" (Witt et al., 2017, p. 135). Another perspective, the Meikirch Model of Health, was developed in Switzerland to promote coordination within related health, socioeconomic, and environmental initiatives. The Meikirch Model posits that "health is a state of wellbeing emergent from conducive interactions between individuals' potentials, life's demands, and social and environmental determinants" (Bircher & Kuruvilla, 2014, p. 368).

Hales (2017) defined health as "the process of discovering, using, and protecting all the resources within our minds, spirits, families, communities and environment" (p. 2). Going beyond the definition, Hales identified the following "elements" of health:

- A positive, optimistic outlook
- A sense of control over stress and worries; time to relax
- Energy and vitality; freedom from pain or serious illness
- Supportive friends and family and a nurturing intimate relationship with someone you love
- A personally satisfying job or intellectual endeavor
- A clean, healthful environment

When considering a perspective for health, it is important to recognize the role that corporate, environmental, financial, political, and social factors have on the health of individuals and communities. Galea and colleagues calculated the number of deaths attributable to social factors in the United States in the year 2000. Their findings indicated that 245,000 deaths were attributed to low education; 176,000 to racial segregation; 162,000 to low social support; 133,000 to individual-level poverty; 119,000 to income inequality; and 39,000 to area-level poverty (Galea et al., 2011). These findings represent both the magnitude and the complexity of promoting health but also present the urgent need for action to address these social factors.

One other important characteristic of a healthy person deserves attention. A commitment to an individual's health should be more than personal. Healthy people should be engaged not only in promoting and maintaining their own health but also in promoting the health of others. Health-enhancing behaviors are not equally accessible to all individuals. A health-educated person should act in their own best health interests as well as in the interests of others. Plough (2015), in describing actions important to building a "Culture of Health," emphasizes that when individuals develop a community commitment, they engage in actions to improve population health. In essence, communities influence the health of individuals, and individuals have the capacity to influence the overall well-being of the community.

Any effort to improve individual and community health must address health through a physical, mental, emotional, and societal lens. To address this comprehensive perspective and improve community and school efforts to promote well-being, education–health–social justice coalitions must confront the multiple factors that affect both personal and community health.

The Goals of School: What Does It Mean to Be Educated?

Education . . . would enhance your capacity to live an informed life, enable you to learn the values of your culture and society, enable you to participate in the wider community and in the political decisions that affect your life, exercise your freedoms, and claim your rights.   MARMOT (2015)

As with health, community collaborative efforts to improve education must come to agreement on what it means to be educated. Basically, what are the expected education outcomes for students from their experiences in life and through formal education in school? Similar to different views of health, there are different views on or indicators for what it means to be well educated. Some may base it on standardized test scores or years of educational attainment (high school graduate, college graduate, advanced degree), while others view grades or grade point average (GPA), academic awards (graduating with honors, dean's list, etc.), or a person's knowledge around a singular topic as indicators for being well educated. These accomplishments can present some level of the quality of a person's education, but none of these alone should be considered as a definitive indicator.

If education is truly aligned with student outcomes, a common perspective of what it means to be educated should provide direction for a school's policies, programs, and practices. Historically, the purpose of education has often been viewed as preparing students to live well-rounded lives and contribute to society. The 1918 report from the Commission on the Reorganization of Secondary Education presented seven cardinal principles of education: civic education, command of fundamental processes, ethical character, health, worthy home-membership, worthy leadership, and vocation (Commission on the Reorganization of Secondary Education, 1918). In 1938, the Educational Policies Commission, the National Education Association of the United States, and the American Association of School Administrators developed a statement titled *The Purposes of Education in American Democracy* that included student objectives in four areas: civic responsibility, economic responsibility, human relationships, and self-realization (Educational Policies Commission et al., 1938). A third historical example is a 1961 report from the Educational Policies Commission titled *The Central Purpose of American Education*. Regarding the development of the "thinking person," the report states that "objectives can be better achieved as pupils develop (the ability to think) and learn to apply it to all the problems that face them" (Educational Policies Commission of the National Education Association & American Association of School Administrators, 1961, p. 5).

Several education events in the past 30+ years have contributed to a deviation from these well-rounded goals for education. In 2001, one noteworthy event was the passage by the US Congress of the No Child Left Behind Act (NCLB). The law required that all schools test students in grades 3–8 in math and reading and subsequently report test scores. Because the focus was on only two subjects, this led some schools to reduce time spent on subjects such as the arts, civics, history, health education, and physical education. In addition, because the individual school scores were made available to the public, some parents and community members began to see these scores as indicators of the quality of schools and thus view subjects other than math and reading as less important (Ravitch, 2014). Beyond concern about its limited focus, NCLB has been criticized for focusing on school performance but not considering the impact of social determinants on students' ability to succeed on standardized tests.

Many leaders in education have emphasized that test results do not reflect important student learning outcomes such as creativity, critical thinking, problem solving, and the ability to nurture interests and apply knowledge and skills to personal, professional, and community life (Abeles, 2015; Schneider, 2017). In defining achievement, ASCD stated, "A successful learner is knowledgeable, emotionally and physically healthy, civically engaged, prepared for economic self-sufficiency, and prepared for the world beyond formal education" (Valois et al., 2011). Hahn and Truman (2015) presented three foundations for the educated person: basic skills (reading, writing, arithmetic, mathematics, listening and speaking), thinking skills (creative thinking, decision-making, problem-solving, seeing things in the mind's eye, knowing how to learn, reasoning), and personal qualities (responsibility, self-esteem, sociability, self-management, integrity/honesty).

Others have emphasized informed, skilled, and active citizenship as an important outcome of education. Diane Ravitch, a leading education scholar, views the educated person as being able to think critically, listen carefully, consider evidence, and make thoughtful judgments in order to be prepared to assume the rights and responsibilities of living in a democratic society (Ravitch, 2014). Ayers (2004) and Sleeter (2007) have suggested that students' school experiences should promote the development of knowledge, skills, and perspectives that would lead them to become active citizens committed to addressing inequity and social injustices. Former *New York Times* columnist and current Demos Distinguished Senior Fellow Bob Herbert (2014) succinctly described "being educated" as "the capacity of children and teenagers to learn about the myriad wonders of the world, to think critically and independently, and ultimately to become productive citizens and lead rewarding lives" (p. 161).

As society moves forward in a rapidly changing world, individuals and organizations both within and outside of education have proposed knowledge and skills designed to prepare students to make contributions as individuals, professionals, and community members as they move forward into adulthood. While the listings vary, these attributes are sometimes referred to as "21st century skills" or "deeper learning." The following list represents some of the more common skills or deeper learning outcomes:

- Civic literacy
- Collaboration
- Communication
- Creativity
- Critical thinking

- Cultural competency
- Ethics
- Global awareness
- Learning how to learn
- Problem-solving
- Reflection

Clearly education involves more than competency in reading and math. It will be important that all stakeholders understand the need for a broad approach to education designed to address the needs of the whole person and diverse communities. One positive step is a shift at the federal level away from NCLB toward a somewhat more comprehensive approach toward student assessment. In December 2015, the Every Student Succeeds Act (ESSA) was passed by the US Congress and signed by President Barrack Obama. It is a replacement for NCLB. While ESSA still requires annual testing in grades 3–8, as well as once in high school for math and reading/language arts and once in elementary, middle, and high school for science, many view it as an improvement over NCLB because it requires states to identify a criterion beyond test scores for the assessment of school performance, such as attendance, graduation rates, student engagement, school climate, and college or career readiness. In addition, ESSA encourages states to offer students a "well-rounded" education through instruction in a variety of different subjects, including art, music, health education, geography, history, and physical education. ESSA also includes a requirement that a portion of block grants that states provide to local school districts be used to support safe and healthy students (American School Health Association, 2018; Klein, 2019a, 2019b).

Similar to a clear perspective on what it means to be healthy, education–health–social justice coalitions should have a common perspective on the desired outcomes achieved by students as a result of their school experience. Test scores and other indicators of academic achievement are important; however, students should also leave school with the ability to promote not only their own well-being and life goals but also the well-being and quality of life of other individuals and their overall community. Education, health, and social justice advocacy efforts support these outcomes.

The Healthy, Educated Person

Based on the preceding considerations, how does "healthy and educated" translate to real life for young people and adults? How can schools prepare students for appropriate education and health outcomes? The following examples present behaviors that could be considered as characteristic of a healthy, educated person; note that these behaviors reflect an emphasis on knowledge acquisition, critical thinking, a commitment to community engagement and social justice, and the application of knowledge and skills to maintain and improve quality of life for themselves and their communities:

- Tyler and Leslie, a couple with two children in the local school system, prepare for their attendance at a forum for school board candidates. Prior to the forum, they review the candidates' positions on key issues related to education and health and prepare the questions they will ask of the candidates.
- Dylan, a college student just beginning a difficult semester, plans a tentative weekly schedule that will include adequate time for study and assignments, physical activity, healthy meal preparation, and social time with friends.
- Amari, who just turned 18 in August, looks forward to voting for the first time in the upcoming election in November. Amari appreciates the middle and high school courses that presented the opportunity to analyze the positive and negative aspects of US history and provided information about current political issues through active engagement in learning, including meaningful class discussion with other students.
- Bailey and Kiran engage in a daily walk after dinner through the neighborhood with their elementary-school-age children. Once a week, at the end of the walk, the entire family goes to the local library and selects books for personal reading.

- Morgan and Alex have lived in the community for close to 30 years. Now that both are retired, they have initiated planning on how they can provide financial support to political candidates and nongovernmental agencies. They would like to focus on donating to candidates and agencies committed to addressing social justice issues in the community that affect education and health.
- Abdul, a middle school student, plans an afterschool schedule for weekdays that includes time for outside physical activity, homework, and nonschool screen time. After discussing the schedule with his parents, together they agree on a proposed daily time allocation.
- McKinley is a member of a community committee that schedules and facilitates monthly discussions at the local public library. Recent discussions have addressed racial profiling and police violence, the community's public transportation system, the school history curriculum, gun violence and mass shootings, and local parks and recreation facilities and activities.
- Ali is a retiree who is active in the community and just registered for continuing education courses at the local community college. One course focuses on injury prevention for older adults, and another focuses on healthy meal preparation.
- Leigh, a pediatrician with an interest in the education and health needs of children, develops a platform for candidacy for the school board in the local community. Leigh's platform includes a review of the school system's core values, expected student outcomes, parent and family engagement, and the promotion of student and staff well-being.

These scenarios present individuals who have the knowledge, skills, and dispositions to demonstrate a commitment to personal and community well-being. Advocates should have expectations that schools prepare students to apply these education, health, and social outcomes in school and throughout life. Preparation for these outcomes should be reflected through a school's philosophy, expectations, policies, programs, and practices.

Better Health Leads to Academic Success

The more health risks students have, the more likely they will be academically challenged.   DILLEY (2009)

Both health behaviors and health conditions are associated with students' academic performance. Health conditions such as asthma, chronic illness, sensory perception problems (hearing and vision), hunger, experiencing aggression and violence, safety concerns, and ongoing stress have been linked to academic challenges for school-age children and youth. In addition, students' perception of a lack of feeling welcomed, supported, valued, connected, and engaged appears to be related to academic achievement issues (Basch, 2011; Slade, 2015).

There is strong national evidence of the relationship between health behaviors and students' self-reported grades. Based on data from the 2019 CDC National Youth Risk Behavior Survey (YRBS), numerous associations between self-reported grades and health risk behaviors of US high school students were identified. The YRBS is conducted every two years by the CDC among students in public and private schools throughout the United States. The students participating in the study are representative of ninth through twelfth grade students throughout the country (CDC, 2020). The following findings do not indicate cause and effect; rather, they denote associations between selected health behaviors and students' self-reported grades.

Alcohol use and binge drinking are linked to lower grades among the high school students who participated in the study.

- 12% of students with mostly A grades reported that they drank alcohol for the first time (other than a few sips) before the age of 13, compared to 26% of students with mostly D and F grades (CDC, 2021a).
- 27% of students with mostly A grades reported that they currently drink alcohol (at least one drink of alcohol on at least one day during the 30 days before the survey), compared to 40% of students with mostly D and F grades (CDC, 2021a).
- 13% of students with mostly A grades reported binge drinking

(four or more drinks of alcohol in a row for females or five or more in a row for males, within a couple of hours, on at least one day during the 30 days before the survey), compared to 23% of students with mostly D and F grades (CDC, 2021a).

The use of electronic vapor products, cigarettes, cigars, and smokeless tobacco was lower among students with higher grades.

- 26% of students with mostly A grades reported using electronic vapor products, including e-cigarettes, e-cigars, vape pipes, e-hookahs, hookah pens, and mods (such as JUUL, Vuse, Market Ten, and blu), on at least one day during the 30 days before the survey, compared to 52% of students with mostly D and F grades (CDC, 2021f).
- 4% of students with mostly A grades smoked cigarettes on at least one day during the 30 days before the survey, compared to 19% of students with mostly D and F grades (CDC, 2021f).
- 4% of US high school students with mostly A grades currently smoked cigars (cigars, cigarillos, or little cigars) on at least one day during the 30 days before the survey, compared to 16% of students with mostly D and F grades (CDC, 2021f).
- 2% of US high school students with mostly A grades used smokeless tobacco (chewing tobacco, snuff, dip, snus, or dissolvable tobacco products [such as Copenhagen, Grizzly, Skoal, or Camel Snus]), not counting any electronic vapor products, on at least one day during the 30 days before the survey, compared to 12% of students with mostly D and F grades (CDC, 2021f).

Students participating in the study who reported higher levels of physical activity had higher grades in comparison to students engaged in less activity.

- 24% of students with mostly A grades were physically active for at least 60 minutes per day on five or more days per week on all seven days before the survey, compared to 20% of students with mostly D and F grades (CDC, 2021e).

- 41% of US high school students with mostly A grades played video games or used a computer for three or more hours per day (for something that was not school work on an average school day), compared to 54% of students with mostly D and F grades (CDC, 2021e).
- 15% of US high school students with mostly A grades watched television for three or more hours per day (on an average school day), compared to 28% of students with mostly D and F grades (CDC, 2021e).

Healthier dietary behaviors were present among students with higher grades.

- 42% of students with mostly A grades ate breakfast on all seven days before the survey, compared to 20% of students with mostly D and F grades (CDC, 2021b).
- 62% of students with mostly A grades ate fruit or drank 100% fruit juices one or more times per day (during the seven days before the survey), compared to 54% of students with mostly D and F grades (CDC, 2021b).
- 66% of students with mostly A grades ate vegetables (excluding french fries, fried potatoes, or potato chips) one or more times per day during the seven days before the survey, compared to 52% of students with mostly D and F grades (CDC, 2021b).
- 41% of students with mostly A grades did not drink a can, bottle, or glass of soda during the seven days before the survey, compared to 21% of students with mostly D and F grades (CDC, 2021b).

The YRBS results demonstrate significant associations between students' alcohol behaviors, physical activity/sedentary behaviors, dietary behaviors, and tobacco product use behaviors and grades. Regarding these four categories of health behaviors, students with mostly A grades are more likely to engage in positive behaviors than those with mostly D and F grades. It is not known whether academic success leads to engagement in health-promoting behaviors or engaging in health-promoting behaviors leads to better grades. However, based on these findings, it is evident that pointed efforts to improve both education and health are important to the overall well-being of high school students (CDC, 2021d).

Additional research supports the relationship between health behaviors and academic achievement. Bradley and Greene (2013) conducted a systematic literature review of publications from 1985 through 2011 that focused on studies that examined the relationships between six health risk behaviors and at least one of the following educational outcomes: GPA, grades in specific subjects, performance on standardized tests, years of schooling completed, high school graduation or passing the General Educational Development test, and grade level retention. A total of 122 articles met the criteria for inclusion in the review. The six health risk behaviors were (1) violence, (2) tobacco use, (3) alcohol and other drug use, (4) sexual behaviors contributing to unintended pregnancy and sexually transmitted diseases, (5) inadequate physical activity, and (6) unhealthy dietary behaviors. Findings from this literature review indicated statistically significant relationships between all six of the high-risk behaviors and academic achievement. Approximately 96% of the 122 studies reported that higher levels of involvement by school-age children in health risk behaviors were linked to decreased academic achievement. Based on the findings, Bradley and Greene (2013) concluded that the study presents clear evidence of the linkage between health-related behaviors and academic achievement. In addition, they emphasized the long-term impact of these behaviors, the societal consequences, and the need for education and health leaders to address this relationship for the benefit of all citizens.

A study conducted in the state of Washington by the State Board of Health, the State Office of the Superintendent of Public Instruction, and the State Department of Health focused on the relationship between 13 health risk behaviors and conditions experienced by Washington students and selected academic indicators. The findings of this study clearly indicated that students who reported experiencing any of the health risk factors were at increased academic risk compared to students who were not subject to any of the risk factors. The research also indicated that even if a student had experience related to one risk factor they were at increased academic risk, and that the more health risk factors linked to a student, the more likely that the student was academically challenged (Dilley, 2009). Cabrera et al. (2018) analyzed data from two surveys of Minnesota high school students. Each sample included approximately 80,000 students. The findings indicated that students' healthy behavior choices are positively associated with academic performance, commitment to learning, and education aspirations. The CDC has reported that participation in school breakfast programs is associated with better grades and higher standardized test scores, reduced absenteeism, and improved cognitive performance, while hunger due to insufficient food intake is related to lower grades and increased absenteeism. In addition, the CDC has presented linkages between school-related physical activity (physical education, recess, classroom physical activity breaks) and better classroom behavior, better grades, and higher standardized test scores (CDC, 2014).

Basch (2011) focused on the relationship between health and learning. Through multiple articles, Basch presented the impact of conditions such as vision problems, asthma, teen pregnancy, aggression and violence, and lack of breakfast on the achievement of urban minority youth. Based on the summary and synthesis of research presented in the articles, Basch emphasized that health-related issues play a major role in limiting the motivation and ability of urban minority youth to succeed academically. Beyond academic success, these health issues affect the quality of their lives and the ability to contribute and lead productive lives in a democratic society (Basch, 2011).

Many health and social issues experienced by students lead to absence from school, which, when chronic (defined as missing 10% of school days for any reason), often leads to academic problems. Tooth decay, asthma, behavioral health issues, and students' perceptions of school to be a physically or emotionally safe environment are among the leading health reasons for absence (The Colorado Education Initiative, 2015, p. 5). The Robert Wood Johnson Foundation reports that more than 10% of kindergartners and first graders are chronically absent from school. Obviously, this early absenteeism places these students at academic risk at the beginning of their elementary school experience. Chronically absent students in preschool, kindergarten, and first grade are less likely to read at grade level when they reach third grade. These students who are reading behind grade level at this point are four times more likely to drop out of high school than those reading at grade level. At the high school level, students who are chronically absent for any year between grades 8 and 12 are seven times more likely to drop out compared to other students (Basch, 2011; Robert Wood Johnson Foundation, 2016). School attendance, including the impact of chronic absenteeism, is examined in more detail in chapter 4.

Academic Success Leads to Better Adult Health

Health and education are symbiotic. What affects one affects the other. The healthy child learns better just as the educated child leads a healthier life.

ASCD (2015)

As presented earlier, clear evidence exists that higher levels of educational attainment are related to better adult health outcomes. Zimmerman and Woolf (2014) indicate that decades of research in the developing world have indicated that educational status is a prominent determinant of health outcomes and that differences have increased over the past 30–40 years. Clear recognition of the linkage between education and health outcomes is demonstrated by the inclusion of education objectives in Healthy People 2030, a plan developed by the US Office of Disease Prevention and Health to improve health and well-being by 2030. The education-related health objectives are presented in table 1.1. While most evidence is based on educational attainment (levels/years of completed education), the quality of education also needs to be a consideration. Marmot (2015) believes that more than just time spent in a classroom is important—benefits such as knowledge, skills, and control over a person's life can result from education and have an impact on health. Mirowsky and Ross (2003) indicate that skills developed through education will help students gain a greater sense of personal agency and engage in a health-promoting lifestyle. Zimmerman and Woolf (2014)

TABLE 1.1. Healthy People 2030: Selected Education-Related Objectives

Increase the proportion of children who are developmentally ready for school.

Increase the proportion of children who participate in high-quality early childhood programs.

Increase the proportion of fourth graders with reading skills at or above the proficient level.

Increase the proportion of fourth graders with math skills at or above the proficient level.

Increase the proportion of eighth graders with reading skills at or above the proficient level.

Increase the proportion of eighth graders with math skills at or above the proficient level.

Increase the proportion of high schoolers who graduate within four years.

SOURCE: Healthy People 2030. (n.d.). *Education access and quality objectives.* US. Department of Health and Human Services. https://health.gov/healthypeople/objectives-and-data/browse -objectives/education-access-and-quality

identify character development and skills such as critical thinking and problem-solving as other educational outcomes for consideration. Zimmerman et al. (2015) posit that the health benefits of education can have an impact on the individual level (knowledge, skills, and the ability to apply both), the community level (access and support to health promotion and protection), and the societal level (cultural factors, public policy, laws). Thus, in addition to levels of educational attainment, consideration must be given to the quality and focus of education. Better education at all levels of schooling has the potential to increase the likelihood of engagement in behaviors that support an individual's own health and the health of others.

A wide range of research findings substantiate the education-health linkage:

- US adults at age 25 with a college degree can expect to live 9 years longer than those who did not graduate from high school (Institute of Medicine, 2015).
- Individuals with advanced degrees have as many as 12 additional quality-adjusted life years compared to those who have not completed high school. To put this into context with another health

risk behavior, the difference in quality-adjusted life years between 30-year smokers and nonsmokers is 6 years (Institute of Medicine, 2015).

- Adults with higher levels of education have a reduced risk of heart disease and diabetes, have a decreased likelihood of reporting either fair or poor health, and experience fewer lost days of work related to illness (Kelly & Weitzen, 2010; Marmot, 2015; Zajacova & Lawrence, 2018).
- Individuals who attended college are more likely to receive physical and dental exams, a flu shot, and a cholesterol test (Eide & Showalter, 2011).
- In a national study of COVID-19 vaccinations, lack of a high school diploma was one of the two strongest predictors of both vaccine hesitancy and not being fully vaccinated (Khairat et al., 2022).

Various reasons might account for this relationship. Higher income can lead to better health outcomes for adults because of a higher likelihood of living in healthier, safe neighborhoods and having easier access to better personal and public transportation, healthier foods, physical activity, and medical care. Individuals with higher levels of education are more likely to have jobs with better working conditions that offer benefits such as health insurance, paid leave, and retirement plans (Egerter et al., 2011). These jobs are often more in line with their personal aspirations and lead to higher job satisfaction. Hummer and Hernandez (2013) suggest that individuals with higher levels of education are also more likely to benefit from having friends, neighbors, and coworkers with higher levels of education who can provide health-related support when needed.

Beyond adults' personal health, benefits also exist related to education level and the health of family members. Brown et al. (2014), in a study of 337,846 married men and women (168,923 couples), found that an individual married to a person with higher levels of education is less likely to report being in fair or poor health in comparison to an individual married to a person with a lower level of education. Children of mothers who have not graduated from high school are nearly twice as likely to die in the first year of life as compared to babies born to mothers who have graduated from college (Egerter et al., 2011). Additional research has indicated higher levels of health for children whose parents are college graduates (Egerter et al., 2011) and increased life expectancy for less educated spouses of higher-educated spouses (Montez et al., 2009). It is also notable that children's academic achievement is related to their parents' education levels. Children with parents with lower levels of education are less likely to experience school success than children with parents with higher levels of education. The likelihood progressively decreases from children whose parents have professional or doctoral degrees to children whose parents have not graduated from high school (Egerter et al., 2011). Thus, children with parents who have attained higher levels of education are more likely to experience academic success, attain higher levels of education, and experience better adult health outcomes.

In this chapter, evidence has been presented that shows the existence of an interdependent relationship between education and health. Healthy children and adolescents at all grade levels are more likely to be academically successful than peers who are experiencing health issues or engaging more frequently in unhealthy behaviors. In turn, individuals who attain higher levels of education are more likely to have better health outcomes in adulthood. Because of this reciprocal relationship, access to quality education for all school-age children and youth should be a priority not simply for the education, medicine, and public health sectors but for all community members. However, equal opportunity for access to quality education and health for all school-age children and youth is not a reality in the United States. Social injustices have a profound effect on both education and health. Confronting social injustices must be an integral component of efforts to provide equal access to quality education for all children and youth and address the education-health reciprocal relationship so that it has a positive impact on individuals and communities.

The remaining chapters in the book are intended to provide information and direction to support multisector coalition and social movement actions to promote access to health and quality education for all school-age children and youth. Chapter 2 presents background information related to various social injustices that present barriers to equity and access. Considerations related to early childhood health and learning, including brain development, ACEs, early childhood education, and parental support, are addressed in chapter 3. Issues that directly affect academic success and education attainment are addressed in chapter 4, including students' connectedness to school, attendance (including chronic absenteeism), and dropout prevention. Chapters 5 and 6 present background related to school quality. Chapter 5 identifies characteristics that are evident in a quality school, while chapter 6 presents the WSCC model. The WSCC model provides a broad-based coordinated approach to promoting both education and health and a framework for addressing the education and health needs of the whole child. Chapter 7 provides direction for the initiation and maintenance of a community coalition that serves as the focal point for a community-wide social movement designed to promote equal access for all children to quality education and health and increased opportunities for a healthy, self-fulfilling adulthood.

CHAPTER 2

Education and Health Disparities

The Connection to Social Justice

We need to devote ourselves to achieving social justice, which requires valuing all individuals and populations equally, recognizing and rectifying historical injustices and providing resources according to need.   JONES (2016)

NDIVIDUAL DECISIONS and behaviors related to education and health have many external influences. Family, community, and societal factors, often described as social determinants, affect decisions and behaviors related to education, health, and overall quality of life. Children and youth who come from financially secure, supportive families and communities that value health and social justice are more likely to be healthy and academically successful than children who do not benefit from these conditions. Because their academic success will often lead to higher levels of educational attainment, these individuals will experience an increased likelihood of higher levels of health during adulthood.

Public health professionals have recognized the impact of social determinants on population health outcomes, especially in regard to health differences between the most and least advantaged populations in the United States (Galea, 2018). Healthy People 2030 (HP 2030), a plan developed by the US Office of Disease Prevention and Health, includes data-driven objectives developed to improve health and well-being by the end of the current decade. HP 2030 has defined social determinants of health as "conditions in the environments where people are born, live, learn, work, play, worship, and age that affect a wide range of health, functioning, and quality-of-life outcomes and risks." Within HP 2030, social determinants of health are grouped into five domains: economic stability, education access and quality, health care access and quality, neighborhood and built environment, and social and community context (Office of Disease Prevention and Health Promotion, n.d.).

Consideration has also been given to the impact of social determinants on teaching, learning, and education attainment. Many of the same overarching factors that have been identified as social determinants of health have also been linked to education (Gorski, 2018). Social determinants can have both a direct effect on students' ability to learn and an impact on schools' practices, policies, and resources. These factors can then affect the overall quality of schools and children's ability to maximize their educational experience and to attain higher levels in their education.

It is important to recognize that the factors identified as social determinants of both education and health are affected by underlying social injustices such as systemic racism, xenophobia, sexism, homophobia, transphobia, ableism, ageism, and other types of population-based discrimination. These biases can result in limited or no access to important life resources such as health care, meaningful employment that provides a living wage, affordable housing, healthy food, environmental health, transportation, community safety, and educational enrichment opportunities for both children and adults. Jones et al. (2009), in referring to the social determinants of health, emphasize that the contexts of the determinants are not randomly distributed but "are instead shaped by historical injustices and by contemporary structural factors that perpetuate historical injustices" (p. 2).

Thus, addressing social determinants and social injustices is essential in improving both education and health. Prominent thought leaders in education have reinforced the importance of social action. Diane Ravitch (2014) captures the need to address determinants: "If we are serious about significantly narrowing the achievement gap between black and white students, Hispanic and white students, and poor and affluent students, then we need to think in terms of long-term, comprehensive strategies. These strategies must address the problems of poverty, unemployment, racial isolation and mass incarceration" (p. 61). Linda Darling-Hammond (2010) emphasizes that to provide quality education to all children, there must be access to food, adequate housing, and health care, along with a supportive early learning environment and equitably funded schools. David Berliner (2013) posits that jobs that provide families with living wages are the best method for improving schools in the United States.

Leaders in medicine and public health have also emphasized the importance of addressing social determinants and social justice issues in order to enhance both education and health. Allensworth et al. (2011) identified factors such as lack of access to health care, inadequate community infrastructure, and poverty as social determinants that can be addressed by both the education and health sectors to promote better education and health outcomes for both children and adults. In a 2015 Institute of Medicine report, childhood nutrition, parental and maternal health, stress, immigrant status, gender, and socioeconomic status (SES) were identified as factors that affect both education and health (Institute of Medicine, 2015). In an address to the International Union of Health Promotion and Education, Navarro (2009) stated, "We have plenty of evidence that programs aimed at changing individual behavior have limited effectiveness. And understandably so. Instead, we need to broaden health strategies to include political, economic, social, and cultural interventions that touch on the social (as distinct from the individual) determinants of health" (p. 15).

In reviewing social determinants and injustices that influence education and health, it is important to realize that these influences are usually interdependent rather than separate, mutually exclusive factors. The combination of influencing factors can create unique types of privilege or oppression for individuals or groups (Eager, 2019). The connection and complexity of this interaction is referred to as intersectionality. The term gained prominence in the early 1990s after development by several civil rights activists and legal scholars. Intersectionality refers to the overlapping, complex, and synergistic impact of multiple forms of discrimination experienced by individuals or groups. Johns et al. (2019) describe intersectionality as the perspective that individuals have multiple social identities (e.g., ability status, ethnicity, gender, racial, sexual orientation, and SES) that mutually shape their experience of the world, social relationships, and understanding of themselves. Love (2019b) suggests that individuals' complex identities, including culture, language, race, gender, sexuality, ability, religion, and spirituality, cannot be addressed in isolation from one another. Runyan (2018) emphasizes that "forms of oppression are not just additive, as if they were wholly separate layers of domination" (para. 6).

Recognizing and understanding the complex nature of intersectionality is essential in addressing social determinants of education and health. Intersectionality requires that individuals and organizations embrace and celebrate individuals' multiple social identities (National Association for the Education of Young Children, 2019). When considering the need to address social determinants or social injustices to improve education or health, seldom can one factor be addressed by itself or as a simple combination of individual factors. Eager (2019) suggests that viewing individuals through a single lens provides a limited picture of a person's lived experiences. Love (2019b) presents intersectionality as a "necessary analytic tool to explain the complexities and the realities of discrimination and of power or the lack thereof, and how they intersect with identities" (p. 3). For example, the oppression related to poverty experienced by Black high school students may involve some similar but also different forms of discrimination and barriers compared to those faced by white students living in poverty. Because of the synergistic nature of these factors, Black and white students may experience a different mix of oppressive factors that result in differences in challenges and lack of opportunity. The planning, development, implementation, and evaluation phases of efforts designed to improve the impact of education and promote and maintain health for all children, youth, and adults must take into account the various intersectional spaces that can be experienced by individuals.

Social determinants of education and health, along with the underlying social injustices, have led to distinct disparities in access to quality education and health outcomes among various population groups in the United States. As noted in chapter 1, the overall purpose of this book is to provide direction to public health professionals, primary care physicians (pediatricians, family physicians, internal medicine specialists), and education leaders to serve as initiators, leaders, and ongoing partners in multisector coalitions on the local level that promote and support social justice and a health-enhancing family, community, and school environment that results in equal access to high-quality schools for all children and youth. Education–health–social justice advocates must have an understanding of education and health disparities and an understanding of equity as an important principle in addressing social injustices and the resulting disparities. The intent of this chapter is to present an overview of the concept of equity as a social justice strategy and provide background information on education and health disparities.

Equity: An Essential Principle in Addressing Education and Health Disparities

Equity exists when race and income are no longer the most reliable predictors of student success and systems work to ensure that each child receives what they need when they need it, to develop to their full academic and social potential. We envision a world where every student, regardless of background, enjoys an education that propels them toward the opportunity-rich life they deserve.

SOUTHERN EDUCATION FOUNDATION (n.d.)

There is no path to equity that does not include a direct confrontation with inequity. GORSKI (2017)

Children have unique assets and face different challenges regarding their health and the optimization of their school experience. Parents, families, communities, and schools possess varied assets and face a range of challenges related to the provision of support to children, youth, and adults. Because of these individualized situations, schools and communities have distinct needs regarding levels and types of support and resources. Providing the exact same support and resources to each child, parent and family, school, and community will not address the different challenges and gaps faced by these individuals and groups. To address these distinct situations, stakeholders must have an understanding of and strong commitment to equity.

Equality and equity are sometimes confused. Equality refers to everyone—or all programs, institutions, or communities—receiving the same levels of support and resources and is based on the assumption that everyone benefits when levels of support and resources are the same (Breny, 2020). Equity represents being fair and attempting to meet the needs and unique challenges faced by all individuals and groups. However, fair is not always equal. Providing the same amount of funding to both a community health agency or school serving an affluent community that historically has received strong financial support and a school or community agency that has historically been underfunded and affected by systemic racism, lack of living-wage jobs, a dearth of affordable housing, and other challenges represents "equality." However, identifying the needs and challenges of the school or agency in the latter example and providing a higher level of funding to ameliorate these conditions represents "equity."

While numerous definitions of equity exist, most clearly emphasize the principle of meeting unique individual and collective needs. Focusing on young children, the National Association for the Education of Young Children (2019) defined equity as "the state that would be achieved if individuals fared the same way in society regardless of race, gender, class, language, disability or any other social or cultural characteristic. In practice, equity means all children and families receive necessary supports in a timely fashion so they can develop their full intellectual, social, and physical potential" (p. 17). Lehner (2017) describes equity for children in a simple but functional manner: "Ensuring equity means treating children according to their needs, not merely treating all children equally" (p. 21). Health equity is defined by the Centers for Disease Control and Prevention (CDC) as "when everyone has the opportunity to be as healthy as possible" (CDC, 2022).

An equity-oriented approach to supporting education is characterized by an allocation of resources and funding to schools, families, and communities to ensure the same educational opportunities for all children and youth. Health equity enables all individuals to have the same opportunity to make health-promoting decisions and engage in healthy behaviors. It also provides all communities with the capacity to provide support so that all community members have access to optimal health and overall well-being.

Equity is intended to counteract past and current systemic racism and other systemic discrimination emanating from the uneven distribution of power and privilege in social, political, economic, and educational structures (National Association for the Education of Young Children, 2019). Ultimately, equity will decrease or eliminate education and health disparities that result from systemic racism and other forms of discrimination, community injustices, inadequate family and community resources, and challenged schools and school systems.

Equity is not always an easy concept or movement to sell to professionals or the public. Many do not perceive an opportunity gap and view equal allocation of support and resources as fair. Advocates for equity must educate professionals, parents and family members, community members, and all other stakeholders about historical inequity, the opportunity gap, and the distinction between equality and equity. Love (2021) posits that equity efforts are an attempt to overcome a history of violence, trauma, and racial and economic inequities. Regarding equity in schools, Milner (2015) emphasized, "In short, educators are either fighting for equitable education for all students or they are fighting against it. There is no neutral space in this work" (p. 11). This emphasis is applicable to all who believe in equity. Dugan (2021), in suggesting that "equity requires an unwavering commitment to a journey" (p. 35), presented the following important considerations for educators to work toward equity (while these considerations are intended for educators, the underlying concepts are applicable to any individual or group addressing equity):

- Acknowledge that our systems, practices, and narratives are designed to perpetuate disparities in outcomes for Black and brown students—thus, there is no path to equity without a consistent anti-racist approach.

- Deliberately identify barriers that predict success or failure and actively disrupt them.
- Consistently examine personal identity, bias, and both personal and collective contributions to the creation and/or reproduction of inequitable practices.
- (Re)allocate (tools, time, money, people, support) to ensure that every child gets what they need to thrive socially, emotionally, and intellectually.
- Cultivate the unique gifts, talents, and interests that every person possesses.

Adding to these considerations, the National Association for the Education of Young Children (2019) presented recommendations for promoting equity that are important to all education and health stakeholders:

- Build awareness and understanding of your culture, personal beliefs, values, and biases.
- Recognize the power and benefits of diversity and inclusivity.
- Take responsibility for biased actions, even if unintended, and actively work to repair the harm.
- Acknowledge and seek to understand structural inequities and their impact over time.
- View your commitment to cultural responsiveness as an ongoing process.
- Create meaningful, ongoing opportunities for multiple voices with diverse perspectives to engage in leadership and decision-making.

What might equity look like in practice? Visualize a hypothetical school district with five elementary schools. Three of the schools are in affluent neighborhoods. Because of parental connections and an active parent organization, these three schools have raised considerable private funding to enhance teaching and learning. The other two schools are in neighborhoods that have historically faced challenges related to employment, businesses closing, safety, and lack of access to healthy foods and public spaces for physical activity. For very understandable reasons, these schools have not been able to raise the same level of private funding. Over many years, one local foundation has allocated an equal amount of money to each of the five elementary schools (equality). With changes to the foundation's board of directors over time, more emphasis has been placed on a social justice–oriented funding approach. Working with the representatives from all five schools, the foundation now provides annual funding based on need. To implement this change, the board identified criteria based on each school's assets and needs and made decisions for different allocations to each school based on these criteria (equity). One important underlying element of the board's new funding direction is a commitment to have all elementary schools in the district provide the same opportunity for academic success to all students.

Equal opportunity is more likely to be present regarding education and health when an equity-based approach is used in the allocation of funding and resources. To implement a social justice–oriented allocation approach, Gorski (2018) recommends four abilities for cultivating "equity literacy": the ability to recognize biases and inequities, the ability to respond to biases and inequities, the ability to redress biases and inequities so they do not continue to reappear, and the ability to create and sustain a bias-free and equitable environment. Leaders in social movements promoting equal access to education and health for all must demonstrate these abilities.

Health Disparities: A Product of Discrimination and Inequity

We must do the necessary and deliberate work of confronting and eradicating the unjust systems that perpetuate trauma for too many of us because of the color of our skin, our zip code, our gender, our health status, and other aspects of our identities.   SIMMONS (2020)

In his book *Healthier: Fifty Thoughts on the Foundations of Population Health*, Galea (2018) poses this question: "What are the health indicators that matter? Do we judge progress by the aggregate improvements in health outcomes or by the degree to which these improvements are equally distributed within and across populations?" (p. 21). This question deserves careful consideration by educators, public health professionals, physicians, and all those who place value on well-being. It is, and has been, especially timely in the United States because of the country's ongoing history of health disparities. Numerous definitions have been presented for health disparities. In general, health disparities are preventable, unjust differences in health status and health risks between populations and between groups within populations. HP 2030 defines health disparities as "a particular type of health difference that is closely linked with social, economic, and/or environmental disadvantage. Health disparities adversely affect groups of people who have systematically experienced greater obstacles to health based on their racial or ethnic group; religion; socioeconomic status; gender; age; mental health; cognitive, sensory, or physical disability; sexual orientation or gender identity; geographic location; or other characteristics historically linked to discrimination or exclusion" (Office of Disease Prevention and Health Promotion, 2021, para. 3). These differences in health may be indicated through variances among groups in incidence, prevalence, mortality, burden of disease, and other adverse health conditions (National Academies of Sciences, Engineering, and Medicine, 2017). Distinctions among groups regarding access to health care and health screening are also indicators of health disparities.

While the public health recognition of health disparities has a long history, the challenge of this public health issue has not lessened. According to US Census Bureau projections, the 2020 life expectancy at birth for Blacks was 77.0 years, specifically 79.8 years for women and 74.0 years for men. For non-Hispanic whites, the projected life expectancy was 80.6 years, with 82.7 years for women and 78.4 years for men. Death rates from cardiovascular disease (including stroke), cancer, asthma, influenza and pneumonia, diabetes, HIV/AIDS, and homicide are higher for Blacks/African Americans than for whites (Office of Minority Health, 2021).

Infant mortality rates are another indicator of the overall health of a population. The rate reflects the number of infants in a population who die before their first birthday per 1,000 live births. In 2019, the infant mortality rates among racial and ethnic groups were clustered into two groups. Rates in the higher group included non-Hispanic Black (10.8), Native Hawaiian and other Pacific Islander (9.4), and American Indian/Alaska Native (8.2). Rates in the lower group included Hispanic (4.9), non-Hispanic white (4.6), and Asian (3.6) (CDC, 2021).

Numerous indicators affirm the presence of health disparities among children. Children of color have higher rates of asthma and obesity and are more likely to live in neighborhoods that have greater access to fast-food restaurants and convenience stores and fewer accessible venues for engaging in physical activity (Barr, 2019). Findings from the CDC Youth Risk Behavior Surveillance System (YRBSS), a national system of surveys that collects health behavior information from high school students, identify further health disparities among students. These findings indicate that lesbian, gay, and bisexual (LGB) students experienced more violence victimization and reported more suicide risk behaviors than heterosexual youths (Johns et al., 2019); non-Hispanic Black and Hispanic students were less likely to use pregnancy prevention methods than non-Hispanic white students (Szucs et al., 2020); female students, LGB students, and students not sure of their sexual identity reported the highest prevalence estimates of dating violence and bullying victimization (Basile et al., 2020); sexual minority youths, those who identified as LGB, and those who had sexual contact with the same or with both sexes reported higher levels of suicidal ideation, suicide plans, attempts, and attempts requiring medical treatment (Ivey-Stephenson et al., 2020); and the prevalence of not always wearing a seat belt was higher among students who were younger, were Black, or had lower grades. In addition, riding with a drinking driver was higher among Hispanic students or students with lower grades, and driving after drinking alcohol was higher among students who were older, were male, were Hispanic, or had lower grades (Yellman et al., 2020).

Access to and quality of health care is another type of health disparity. Though the Affordable Care Act (ACA) health coverage increased overall access, people of color and low-income individuals continue to have lower rates of coverage. In 2017, actions related to coverage implemented by the Trump administration and immigration policy changes increased fears among immigrant families participating in Medicaid and the Children's Health Insurance Program (CHIP). These fears appear to have decreased previous coverage gains under ACA, especially among Hispanic individuals who were at increased risk of having no coverage. In addition to coverage issues, adults of color, in comparison to white adults, report higher distrust between the provider and patient and a higher likelihood of refusal for the provision of certain screenings, treatments, and pain medications (Ndugga & Artiga, 2021).

Poverty presents an increased likelihood of individuals experiencing a range of health issues from childhood through adulthood. Children living in poverty have higher rates of asthma, obesity, depression, antisocial behavioral problems, and death from unintentional injuries than children not living in poverty (Coller & Kuo, 2016). Other childhood health issues associated with poverty include impaired physical development, structural changes in brain development, toxic stress from continual coping with challenge and inequity, mental health problems, food insecurity, lack of access to quality health care, and increased exposure to unsafe neighborhood conditions, violence, and environmental toxins (Coller & Kuo, 2016; National Academies of Sciences, Engineering, and Medicine, 2019). In addition, children who are poor are more likely than children who are not poor to develop problems related to certain aspects of social and emotional competence such as communication, respecting others, managing emotions, working cooperatively, seeking and providing help, decision-making, and problem-solving (Wilson-Simmons et al., 2017). Children who grew up in poverty are more likely, as adults, to be unemployed, receive public assistance, be involved in crime, and abuse drugs and alcohol (Coller & Kuo, 2016).

Emphasis in this book has been placed on the association between levels of education attainment and adult health outcomes. Disparities exist regarding educational attainment. The following listings, based on National Center for Education Statistics data, present rates of high school completion and bachelor's degree attainment among adults 25 years and older in the United States (National Center for Education Statistics, 2021a). Since these disparities relate to educational attainment, which is clearly linked to adult health outcomes, they can be considered both education and health disparities.

High School Completion or Higher, by Ethnicity

- American Indian / Alaska Native, 88.6%
- Asian, 91.7%
- Black, 90%
- Hispanic, 74.3%
- Pacific Islander, 93.1%
- White, 95.1%
- Two or more races, 93.3

Bachelor's Degree Attainment

- American Indian / Alaska Native, 19.7%
- Asian, 61.7%
- Black, 27.9%
- Hispanic, 20.8%
- Pacific Islander, 29.4%
- White, 41.3%
- Two or more races, 35.2%

A few observations related to these data are noteworthy. Regarding high school graduation, all race and ethnicity groups are in a range from 88.6% to 95.1% except for the Hispanic rate, which is considerably lower at 74.3%. With the Hispanic population increasing across the United States, communities and schools must be aware of this disparity as policies and programs are implemented to move all students toward high school graduation. The data regarding bachelor's degree attainment present a different picture from that of high school graduation. Completion rates range from 19.7% to 61.7%, with no obvious clusters within that span. Of special notice is the 61.7% completion rate for Asian adults. While much more needs to be learned about this phenomenon, Fishman (2020), in an analysis of two nationally represented studies, found that both internal pressure and parental pressure for higher levels of education played a role in this higher level of attainment. Interestingly, Fishman found that the levels of parental pressure were similar among parents with both higher and lower levels of education.

As with most education and health challenges, social injustices undergird health disparities. Few schools and communities are not facing significant issues related to health disparities. The presence of systemic racism and all other forms of discrimination must be addressed directly. Educators, public health professionals, physicians, and community members must not only recognize the presence of health disparities but also identify equitable actions for addressing these differences. Beyond actual professional practice, all social justice–oriented professionals, community members, and other stakeholders must advocate for equity, anti-racism, and other anti-discriminatory actions within their spheres of influence to provide all children and adults an equal opportunity for positive health outcomes and well-being.

At the beginning of this chapter, the following questions posed by Galea were presented: "What are the health indicators that matter? Do we judge progress by the aggregate improvements in health outcomes or by the degree to which these improvements are equally distributed within and across populations?" Galea (2018) provides direction with his own response to his two questions: "I would argue that in public health, we ought to be firmly on the side of minimizing disparities and ensuring that no one gets left behind as we move collectively in the direction of greater health for all. Doing so requires analysis, advocacy, and a willingness to engage with a range of strategies that can advance our ideas. Adopting a social welfare approach is an example of this thinking in action" (p. 21).

While Galea's response appears to be directed toward public health professionals, it is germane to anyone who believes in equal opportunity for health for all. We cannot move forward for the well-being of all children, youth, adults, and communities without a commitment to social justice, equity, and action.

Education Disparities: Challenges to Quality Education for All Children and Youth

When schools mirror our society's hate, educational justice becomes out of our reach. LOVE (2019a)

In the United States, there are clear differences among minoritized students regarding educational opportunity, experiences, quality, and outcomes. For many reasons, schools are not positive experiences for students of color; students whose families are dealing with socioeconomic issues; students from immigrant families; lesbian, gay, bisexual, and transgender students; and students affected by other social factors such as parental incarceration. In this section, background information is presented on these issues, along with recommendations for schools to become positive forces in addressing these issues.

Race and Ethnicity

Children of different racial and ethnic backgrounds experience educational differences. For example, the results from the 2019 National Assessment of Educational Progress standardized exams represent two clusters of scores in reading and math at both the fourth grade and eighth grade levels. The reading scores at the fourth grade level for Asian / Pacific Islander, white students, and students from two or more races range from 226 to 237, while those for American Indian / Alaska Native, Black, and Hispanic students range from 204 to 209. The scores are clustered in a similar manner for reading among eighth grade students. While not as pronounced for the math scores, similar clusters appear for the same groups of students in both the fourth and eighth grade math scores. The fourth grade math scores for Asian / Pacific Islander, white students, and students from two or more races range from 244 to 266, while those for American Indian / Alaska Native, Black, and Hispanic students range from 224 to 231. Math scores for the eighth grade students are clustered in a similar manner (The Nation's Report Card, n.d.-a, n.d.-b). As emphasized throughout this book, standardized test scores present a limited perspective on students' ability to succeed in school and beyond. Many thought leaders in education have characterized these differences as opportunity gaps rather than achievement gaps (Viadero, 2020). Note also that test scores do not account for important student characteristics such as aspirations, leadership, commitment, creativity, artistic ability, and critical thinking. These characteristics are important to overall satisfaction and success throughout life. Beyond standardized test scores, disparities exist between white students and students of color pertaining to graduation rates, college enrollment, enrollment in Advanced Placement courses, and disciplinary referrals (Khalifa, 2018). These disparities will be examined in more detail later in the chapter.

Inequality regarding access to adequately funded school is one type of "opportunity gap." Students of color often attend schools that receive less financial support. Based on a Pew Research Center analysis of US Department of Education data, findings indicated that during the 2018–19 school year, 42% of Black students, 56% of Hispanic students, and 79% of white students attended elementary and secondary schools in which 50% or more of the enrollment of the school consisted of students from their own ethnicity or race (Schaeffer, 2021). Unfortunately, equitable funding is not always present to support these students. In schools that have the largest populations of minority students, approximately $1,800 less per student is allocated in comparison to those schools that serve majority populations (Stoltzfus, 2019). Many students of color attend aging urban schools that are often extremely underfunded and lack up-to-date resources (Hall, 2019). Underfunding is not just a problem among urban schools. Many rural and small-town schools, as well as an increasing number of suburban schools, also face funding challenges. Regardless of location, less funding leads to important differences in resources between "have" and "have not" schools. Beyond the issue of funding, schools that lack a diverse student body inhibit the opportunity for students to interact and learn from others who have different life experiences and perspectives.

Another factor that affects students of color is teacher preparation. Students of color and low-income students are more likely than other students to be taught by teachers without appropriate certification, with lesser experience, and who are less likely to have advanced degrees (Cardichon et al., 2020). In addition, there is a higher rate of teacher turnover in high-poverty schools (Ingersoll et al., 2018).

Not only can teacher preparation and experience present challenges, but the lack of access to advanced courses presents limitations on the richness of educational experiences and opportunities for college admission. A 2020 report from the Education Trust, based on data from the

2015–16 US Department of Education's Civil Rights Data Collection and the Common Core of Data, indicates that while Black and Latino students succeed in courses such as Algebra I and Advanced Placement courses at the same rate as other students, enrollment for students of color was not at the same representative proportions as for other students. Regarding enrollment in algebra, 16% of students of color were enrolled in Algebra I, while the enrollment rate for other students was 48%. Students of color were also underrepresented in Advanced Placement courses in comparison to white students (Patrick et al., 2020). Several underlying factors were identified for the disparities described in the Education Trust Report. These include resource inequities, educator bias, assessment and grading bias, lack of teacher diversity, lack of equal access to early childhood learning opportunities, and lack of communication with families regarding course and program opportunities for students (Patrick et al., 2020).

A focal point of this book is the linkage between educational attainment and adult health outcomes. Racial and ethnic disparities are present in high school graduation rates. Pertaining to 2018–19 high school graduation rates, Asian / Pacific Islander students (93%) and white students (89%) were above the 86% national average. However, Hispanic (82%), Black (80%), and American Indian / Alaska Native students (74%) were below the national average. State percentages ranged from 51% to 94% for American Indian / Alaska Native students; 83%–97%, Asian students; 67%–90%, Black students; 60%–91%, Hispanic students; and 79%–95%, white students (National Center for Education Statistics, 2021b).

There are also differences in US out-of-school suspension rates. In 2013–14, the suspension rate for Black students was 13.7%, while it was 6.7% for American Indian / Alaska Native students, 5.3% for students of two or more races, 4.5% for both Hispanic and Pacific Islander students, 3.4% for white students, and 1.1% for Asian students (National Center for Education Statistics, 2019).

Beyond these differences, many students of color must deal with internalized, interpersonal, and institutional racism as part of their school experience. Internalized racism has been defined as "the private racial beliefs held by and within individuals," interpersonal racism has been defined as "private beliefs becoming public when racist individuals interact with others," while institutional racism is "racial inequity within institutions and systems of power such as places of employment, government agencies, and social services" (Annie E. Casey Foundation, 2014, p. 5). These experiences of discrimination may be expressed or reinforced through the attitudes, beliefs, and actions of teachers, staff, and students; lessened expectations emanating from teachers' perceptions of students' lower levels of academic ability; disparities in discipline; and culturally inappropriate school policies and actions (Benson et al., 2020).

These different experiences with racism take a toll. Patricia Williams, a legal scholar, introduced the term "spirit murdering" to describe the emotional and social impact on students—the loss of humanity and dignity, and the accompanying psychological and spiritual damage. This can be traumatic to children because it takes away a sense of protection, safety, nurturance, and acceptance, all important to school success (Love, 2019b). Obviously, this trauma can affect students' connectedness to school and their academic success.

Some school districts are taking steps to address inequalities in educational outcomes among students. One action taken by districts located in Jefferson County, Kentucky; Oakland, California; Orange County, North Carolina; Portland, Oregon; and Washoe County, Nevada, among others, is the creation of a position with focused responsibility for overseeing diversity and inclusion within the district. The individuals in these positions address educational inequities in the districts, often focusing on racial, economic, and gender gaps in academic performance and the schools' role in perpetuating these disparities (Samuels, 2019).

Reducing school segregation is another challenge related to diversity and inclusion in schools. As previously indicated, schools with higher percentages of students of color are more likely to have fewer resources and less experienced and less qualified teachers. Schools with diverse student bodies and diversity among faculty members present opportunities for students, families, and teachers to interact and learn among individuals who are from different ethnic and racial backgrounds, have varying educational and socioeconomic levels, and live in different neighborhoods or communities. George Theoharis, a Syracuse University education professor, states, "The best way to understand a diverse world is to live it" (Varlas, 2017, p. 5).

Segregation can also take place within individual schools that have diverse student bodies. Thus, true integration goes beyond just paying attention to school demographics. Focus must also be placed on supporting accessible integration within the school culture and equal educational opportunities for all students, including advanced course work, access to educational materials and support, mentoring, and academic and post–high school advising.

School segregation and disparities in financial support, teacher quality, disciplinary approaches and policies, and graduation rates present major challenges to the likelihood of children of color becoming healthy, fulfilled adults. These challenges must be eliminated so that all schools can become sites for meaningful teaching and learning. Meaningful learning goes beyond promoting student mastery in subjects such as math, science, language arts, and technology. The school experience should help students develop skills related to critical thinking, problem-solving, community involvement, and healthful living. Schools must also provide students with opportunities to examine responsibilities and develop competencies related to the promotion of a society that values justice, equity, and equality. Phelan and Teitel (2019) list academics, belonging, commitment to dismantling racism and oppression, and diversity as the "ABCDs of Diverse and Equitable Schools."

Disparities in opportunity, resources, and achievement must be addressed by all schools. In chapter 5, detailed descriptions are provided of equitable and social justice–oriented schools, leadership, and teaching, along with other actions that are related to addressing disparities. The following actions are recommended for coalition and social movement advocacy related to educational equity and equal opportunity for all students:

- Support efforts to provide and enhance early childhood development and education for all children. These efforts can focus on parental support, including home visiting programs, and access to and no cost for early childhood education (ECE). ECE should be viewed as an essential component of a child's total education. These issues are addressed in detail in chapter 3.

• Address the inequity of funding for public schools. Funding should be provided in an equitable manner with particular attention provided to schools that, over time, have been underfunded and lacking in resources. Funding inequity, both public and private, is addressed in chapter 5.

• Schools should have diverse leadership and faculty members whose demographic characteristics reflect the student population. Teachers should have appropriate professional preparation and certification in their teaching areas and receive the support needed to be successful. All schools should have the financial capacity to keep highly qualified, experienced, successful teachers.

• All parents, family members, and caregivers should have equal access to supporting their children's education, including involvement in decision-making. Invitational schools consider logistics related to culturally appropriate communication and parents' and family members' transportation and work schedules when attempting to engage families. Detailed information related to family engagement is presented in chapter 6.

• All school districts should have a full-time position devoted to equity, diversity, and inclusion. Through this level of leadership, social justice should be a consideration in all policies, programs, and teaching and learning practices in all school districts and individual schools.

• Monitor racial and ethnic enrollment in advanced courses to assure representativeness among students. Several underlying factors have been identified related to enrollment disparities in college preparation courses. These include resource inequities, educator bias, assessment and grading bias, lack of teacher diversity, lack of equal access to early childhood learning opportunities, and lack of communication with families regarding course and program opportunities for students (Khalifa, 2018). School districts must be attentive to these factors as they strive to provide equivalent academic and postgraduation opportunities for all students.

- Opportunities should be presented for students, school staff, and community members to engage in open discussion regarding race and ethnicity, opportunity, and other pertinent social justice issues. Students should have the opportunity to engage in active learning related to the history of social injustices in the United States, including racism and all forms of systemic discrimination, the concept of privilege, and racism versus anti-racism. Engaged instruction should include opportunities to discuss and analyze current social justice issues. School staff members should address these topics through professional development, in faculty meetings, in curriculum development processes, and when other opportunities arise. Community forums can be periodically organized to discuss these topics with parents, family members, and community residents.

Poverty

As I consider these realities, what stands out most about the barriers low-income families face, is that none of them, not a single one, has anything to do with students' intellectual capabilities or desire to learn. . . . If anything, they reflect just the opposite: the level of society's commitment—our commitment—to fulfill the promise of equal educational opportunity.   GORSKI (2018)

The United States is faced with a major challenge in regard to children living in poverty. In 2019, over 10 million children, 14.4% of all children in the United States, lived in poverty. The poverty rate for children is higher than that for adults of all ages. The poverty level in the United States, as defined by the federal government, varies according to the number of adults and children in a family. For example, in 2019, the poverty line for a family of four was an annual income of $26,172. A family with income below that figure was considered to be living in poverty. Extreme poverty was defined by an annual income for a family of four of $13,086 or less (Children's Defense Fund, 2021). Children's poverty differs by race and ethnicity. Among children of color, 20.5% live in poverty, which accounts for 71% of all children living in poverty. American Indian / Alaska Native children (20.6%), Black children (26.5%), and Hispanic children (20.8%) had poverty rates above the national average (19%) and higher than those of Asian, Native Hawaiian, and other Pacific Islander children (7.7%) and white children (8.3%) (Children's Defense Fund, 2021).

Poverty is a global issue—and the United States does not fare well in comparison to other industrialized nations. A 2020 United Nations Children's Fund Office of Research—Innocenti (UNICEF Innocenti) report indicates that of the 41 Organisation for Economic Co-operation and Development and European Union countries, described in the report as "the world's richest countries," the United States had the fourth-highest percentage of children living in poverty. Noteworthy as well, of the 41 countries, based on cash, services, and tax breaks, the United States ranked 38th in funding provided to families (UNICEF Innocenti, 2020). Thus, in comparison to similar countries, the United States has a high number of children living in poverty but low levels of family support.

Numerous factors related to poverty have an impact on learning. Disparities exist in early childhood regarding language development. Fernald found differences in vocabulary and language processing efficiency at as early as 18 months between infants from higher- and lower-SES families. At 24 months their findings indicated a six-month difference between SES groups in processing skills critical to language development (Fernald et al., 2013). Hart and Risley (1995), in a prominent study of children in 42 families from age 7 months to 3 years, found that lower-income children heard considerably fewer words by age 3 than children living in upper-income situations.

Students living in poverty often face factors in their schools that add to the challenges of living in poverty and make academic success less likely. Schools with a large percentage of students living in poverty, which are often schools with a high percentage of minority students, are more likely to have beginning teachers as faculty members and have a higher percentage of uncertified teachers than schools in areas with more financial resources. In addition, in attempts to address the need to improve standardized test scores of students living in poverty, schools sometime focus on low-level math and literacy skills at the expense of art, music, health education, and physical education, as well as instruction focused on higher-order thinking skills (Gorski, 2018). Research indicates that engagement in these subjects and instruction that emphasizes higher-level teaching and learning can contribute to the improvement of academic outcomes of low-income students (Banks, 2018). This limited teaching and learning approach for students living in poverty is not new. Haberman (1991) labeled the focus on non-research-based teaching that does not address critical thinking or skill development and application as "The Pedagogy of Poverty" (p. 290). This instructional discrepancy has even carried over into the use of technology. Studies indicate that in low-poverty schools technology is most often used to promote the development of creative or critical thinking, whereas in high-poverty schools it is more often used for rote learning (Gorski, 2018). School attendance can also be a challenge in schools with a high percentage of students living in poverty. According to a UCLA study, students in schools with high poverty levels lose about 22 days of instruction, compared to 12 days missed by students in schools with lower poverty levels (Carter, 2016).

Some education-specific challenges are directly affected by inequity in school funding. Differences in tax bases (an important source of funding in local US school districts) and the wealth of communities in which schools are located create considerable discrepancies in per-student funding between low-poverty and high-poverty school districts (Milner, 2015). This inequity can result in insufficient instructional resources, inexperienced and lesser-qualified teachers, limited student access to technology, large numbers of students in individual classes, limited health and social services for students, and inadequate opportunities for enrichment and other extracurricular activities.

Related to resources outside of school, children in poverty lack certain opportunities that enhance school-based learning. These include limited access to community and family experiences such as high-quality ECE; home-based technology; afterschool and summer enrichment programs in areas such as art, music, dance, drama, and sports; library and museum visits; travel; and private tutoring programs (Gorski, 2018; Ravitch, 2014). In a study of access to print resources in local libraries and bookstores, in two urban neighborhoods, one lower income and one upper income, Neuman and Celano (2012) found considerable differences in the quality and number of print resources available to young children and their parents. Beyond access to resources, children living in poverty are sometimes faced with frequent movement among schools because of family relocation related to financial issues or housing availability (Gorski, 2018). Children living in "deep poverty" are often in family situations where challenges might include having, at best, one meal per day, or the ongoing challenge of finding shelter or lodging (Herbert, 2014).

Regarding shelter, one of the most damaging outcomes of poverty for school-age children and youth is homelessness. The McKinney-Vento Homeless Assistance Act of 1987 defines a student experiencing homelessness as one who lacks fixed, regular, and adequate nighttime residence. This includes students who

- share housing with others as a result of loss of housing, economic hardship, or a similar reason;
- stay in hotels, motels, trailer parks, or camping grounds owing to a lack of alternative, adequate housing;
- stay in emergency or transitional shelters;
- are abandoned in hospitals;
- stay in public or private places not designed for humans to live; and
- stay in cars, parks, bus or train stations, abandoned buildings, or substandard housing (National Center for Homeless Education, 2021).

Homelessness among school-age children presents numerous challenges to US schools. During the 2019–20 school year, 1,280,886 students, equaling 2.5% of all public school students, experienced homelessness. Of these students, 78% lived with others, 11.9% lived in shelters, 7% lived in hotels or motels, and 4% lived in unsheltered situations (National Center for Homeless Education, 2021). Being homeless presents a number of possible challenges for teaching and learning. Students who are homeless may have to move often and change schools, which can create a lack of connection to other students, teachers, and their schools. In addition, these students often experience hunger and fatigue from a lack of sleep. Directly related to academic success, students experiencing homelessness may not have internet access, necessary school supplies, or a place to study. Associated with these challenges, students dealing with homelessness are more likely to be chronically absent, more likely to receive lower grades, and less likely to graduate than students who are not homeless (Goodwin, 2018).

It is not surprising that living in poverty affects childrens' ability to learn and achieve academic success. The ultimate impact for many of these children is an adulthood with lower levels of educational attainment, well-being, hope and optimism, and overall quality of life.

Addressing child poverty has not only the potential for improved child and adult education and health outcomes but also financial benefits. The National Academies of Sciences, Engineering, and Medicine (2019) examined the financial impact of child poverty. Based on their findings, it was estimated that the cost to the US economy of child poverty was $800 billion to $1.1 trillion in 2018. However, it was also estimated that outlays for new programs designed to reduce child poverty would come with a cost that is much less than the cost of child poverty. Conversely, if individual or multiple existing programs were eliminated, child poverty would increase (National Academies of Sciences, Engineering, and Medicine, 2019).

As with all social problems, addressing poverty must begin with comprehensive efforts to eliminate or minimize the underlying causes. Education and health advocates must consider the following actions as part of any action agenda to move toward the elimination of poverty and the promotion of equal opportunity for all children:

- The "big picture" counts—poverty and factors such as systemic racism and other types of discrimination, the income/wealth gap, and access to living-wage jobs are interdependent and must be addressed at the national, state, and local levels through laws, policies, processes, and programs. Education, health, and social justice advocacy is essential in addressing systemic issues at all levels. Confronting these challenges not only addresses the issue of poverty but also has the potential of increasing access to quality education for all children. Berliner et al. (2014), in emphasizing the importance of addressing poverty, provide guidance to advocates by suggesting that calling for school reform without confronting economic and social reforms is an example of foolishness.

- To directly address equal access to quality education for all students, engage in advocacy for education policies that require the provision of free ECE for all students; support for parents; equitable funding of public schools; social justice–oriented schools; the hiring of, and support for, well-prepared, certified, passionate teachers; quality instruction that actively engages students in meaningful learning; and schools that engage all parents and family members and provide a safe, supportive environment (see chaps. 3, 5, and 6 for more details).

- Education enrichment should be equally accessible to all students. Advocates should support access to afterschool and summer enrichment programs for all children and youth. Students living in poverty often face financial challenges to engagement in programs and may also lack transportation and have conflicting work or family responsibilities. Research demonstrates the loss in learning experienced by low-income students during the summer months. As this loss builds up over an accumulation of summers for younger students, it can account for major academic achievement deficits in later grades. These differences can affect course placements, academic achievement, and graduation rates.

- All schools should be sensitive to the presence of students experiencing homelessness. The National Center for Homeless Education has developed a one-page document with an inventory of possible signs to help schools identify homeless students. The signs are organized into various categories that include student's lack of educational continuity (attendance at many different schools, missing records, inability to pay fees, etc.); poor health and nutrition; transportation and attendance problems; poor hygiene; incomplete or missing homework; social and behavioral concerns; and the parent's, guardian's, or student's reluctance to provide information related to a current address, name of last school, as well as other comments or nonresponses (National Center for Homeless Education, 2021).

Important considerations for schools to respond in a meaningful manner for students experiencing homelessness include the provision of professional development for all teachers and school staff members, identifying one person with coordination responsibilities for the school's responses to meeting the needs of students and families dealing with homelessness, the provision of comprehensive health and social services or supportive referrals to community providers, connecting students with education enhancement programs in the community (libraries, museums, opportunities with involvement in various arts, engagement in physical activity and sports programs, etc.), and pointed efforts to connect and engage students with the school community both within and outside of the regular school day.

• Support schools in the provision of professional development for school administrators and teachers to gain an understanding of the strong influence of poverty on students' academic success and education attainment. This understanding should encompass the underlying causes of poverty, the racial and ethnic disparities among children affected by poverty, the presence of students experiencing homelessness, the educational challenges faced by children and families, and appropriate school and community strategies for addressing challenges and moving toward equitable opportunity for all children.

Parental Incarceration

Parents who are incarcerated do not live in isolation. They are fathers, mothers, partners, caregivers, breadwinners, and community members, and their kids inevitably end up sharing the sentences.

ADAPTED FROM THE ANNIE E. CASEY FOUNDATION (2016)

Since the 1970s, a dramatic increase in the number of individuals who have been incarcerated in the United States has led to public health and social justice concerns. A Vera Institute of Justice report indicates that in 1980 approximately 500,000 people were incarcerated in US jails and prisons. While the overall number has dropped from the highest point in 2008, 1.8 million individuals were incarcerated in local jails and state and federal prisons in June 2020 (Kang-Brown et al., 2021). While the United States represents 5% of the world population, it accounts for close to 25% of those incarcerated worldwide (Vera Institute of Justice, n.d.). The World Prison Brief reported that in 2018 the United States imprisoned 639 per 100,000 residents, which is the highest rate in the world. El Salvador has the second-highest rate at 564 per 100,000. The US figure is noticeably different in comparison to those of England and Wales (131 per 100,000), France (93 per 100,000), and Germany (69 per 100,000) (Gramlich, 2021). This large number of imprisoned individuals impacts many sectors of our society, including the children of incarcerated parents and their likelihood of academic success. Approximately 2.7 million children have a parent serving a jail or prison sentence in the United States, while 5.2 million have had a parent incarcerated at some time during their lifetime (Ghandnoosh et al., 2021).

While the focus of this section is on parental incarceration and its impact on children, it is important to recognize that the incarceration of children and youth, while decreasing over the past 20 years, is still an issue of concern in the United States. Youth.gov reports that in 2019 36,479 youth were detained in residential placement. Children and youth of color are disproportionately affected in these placements. For every 100,000 non-Hispanic Black youth, 315 were detained in a residential placement facility, compared to 92 Hispanic youth and 72 non-Hispanic white youth (youth.gov, n.d.). There is an important interdependence between children and youth and their academic performance in both school and residential placement facilities. Regarding school performance, nearly half of those who are detained have achievement levels below grade level, and many have high levels of truancy and grade retention. However, incarcerated boys between ages 12 and 18 who demonstrate high academic performance while in residential detention are two times less likely to engage in repeated involvement with the juvenile justice system than peers with lower performance. In addition, youth with above-average academic performance while detained are more likely to return to school than lower-performing peers (youth.gov, n.d.).

Unfortunately, schools sometimes serve as the site for teenagers' first encounter with the juvenile justice system. This dilemma is often referred to as the "school-to-prison pipeline." The policies and practices that contribute to these situations, along with considerations for alternative school discipline approaches, are addressed in chapter 5.

Numerous reasons have been presented by thought leaders and in various reports for the extremely high rate of adult incarceration in the United States. Factors that have been identified as contributing causes include increased arrests and excessive sentences for drug crimes resulting from the 1980s "War on Drugs" (Foreman, 2017), inadequate treatment programs for those incarcerated who are dealing with mental health issues and substance abuse disorders (Bazelon, 2019), mandatory sentences for certain offenses (Alexander, 2010), a bail system that penalizes individuals who are unable to pay for bail with incarceration (Yates, 2018), and the influence of the prison industrial complex (Klein & Lima, 2021). Underlying the overwhelmingly high rate of incarceration in the United States are racism and other forms of systemic discrimination that result in barriers to education, employment, medical care, and housing.

One of the harshest realities of the staggering rate of incarceration in the United States is the dramatic racial discrepancy. Alexander (2010) reports that the United States has imprisoned a larger percentage of the Black population than South Africa did during the height of apartheid. In 2018, Blacks represented 12% of the total US population yet were 33% of the sentenced prison population; Hispanics, 16% of the total population while 23% of the prison population; and whites, 63% of the total population while 30% of the prison population. From another perspective, 2,272 Black men per 100,000 were incarcerated, in comparison to 1,018 Hispanic men and 392 white men per 100,000 (Gramlich, 2021). Based on 2018 data, 20% of Native American children, 13% of Black children, 6% of Latinx children, and 6% of white children experienced parental incarceration at some time in their lives (Ghandnoosh et al., 2021).

Parental incarceration has been associated with health outcomes faced by their children that jeopardize opportunities for academic success. These health issues include migraines, asthma, high cholesterol, depression, anxiety, and post-traumatic stress disorder (Morsy & Rothstein, 2016). In addition, children of incarcerated parents have a greater likelihood of exposure to family economic issues, housing instability (including homelessness), and stigmatization (Turney & Goodsell, 2018). These situations are often exacerbated because children of incarcerated parents are more likely to live in challenged neighborhoods that have a lesser capacity to provide family support services (Annie E. Casey Foundation, 2016).

Specific to academic outcomes, parental incarceration has been found to be a risk factor for grade retention (Turney & Haskins, 2014) and not graduating from high school (Huynh-Hohnbaum et al., 2015). Based on a survey of eighth, ninth, and eleventh grade students in Minnesota public schools, Shlafer et al. (2017) found that parental incarceration was significantly associated with lower odds of getting A and B grades and a higher likelihood of receiving school disciplinary action. These youth also reported lower levels of school connectedness and school engagement.

The impact of parental incarceration can extend beyond childhood. Children of an incarcerated parent face an increased possibility of health and social issues that can affect them during adulthood. These adult outcomes include mental health issues, substance abuse, social isolation, and involvement with the criminal justice system, including incarceration (Gifford et al., 2019). It should be noted that in abusive situations separation from an incarcerated parent can be a positive event for children (Wakefield & Wildeman, 2014).

Advocates for better schools and healthier children, adults, and communities must monitor and, in appropriate situations, act on issues related to incarceration and its societal impact. Some positive actions have been implemented. Several states have initiated incarceration reform through the identification of less costly alternatives for nonviolent offenders (Annie E. Casey Foundation, 2016; Wakefield & Wildeman, 2014). Thus far, the most consequential action is the passage in December 2018 by the US Congress of the First Step Act (FSA). This new federal law enacts sentencing reform along with federal government actions to support the implementation of the new law. These supportive actions include the Bureau of Prisons establishing partnerships with businesses to provide employment opportunities for individuals released from prison; the expansion of educational opportunities for those incarcerated; and, in collaboration with the Salvation Army, assistance with housing after release (Root & Rebound & #cut50, 2019). Based on the implementation of FSA, in July 2019 over 3,100 federal prison inmates were released as a result of a recalculation of their good conduct time. In addition, 1,691 incarcerated individuals received a sentence reduction based on a retroactive application of the Fair Sentencing Act to 2010 (US Department of Justice, 2020).

The FSA is one step in addressing the incarceration situation in the United States. The following considerations are additional components of meaningful reform:

- The underlying causes of criminal behavior must be identified, analyzed, and addressed. As Wakefield and Wildeman (2014) argued, "The prison is not the place to solve problems that have very little to do with crime" (p. 164). Examples of problems related to criminal activity that have the potential to be decreased through prevention, treatment, education, and policy include mental illness, drug addiction, lack of access to living-wage jobs, housing instability, and racism and other forms of systemic discrimination. These problems must be addressed through systematic, science-based approaches at the individual and community levels.

- The FSA has been a first step in the examination of selected federal incarceration policies and practices and the effectiveness of current sentencing approaches in the United States. Note that the FSA does not apply to state policies and prisons. Moving forward, imprisonment, probation, and parole related to nonviolent crime must be examined for their value (or lack thereof) to public safety and potential rehabilitation. The point is not to eliminate punishment but to consider it in the context of financial and nonfinancial costs and overall benefits to the community. Another issue often related to sentencing includes the excessive cost of bail. This cost is often prohibitive to low-income defendants and can result in pretrial detention, often lasting several months. Sally Yates (2018), former US deputy attorney general and acting attorney general, addressed this issue by stating, "Poverty is not a crime and we must ensure that we have one system of justice that applies to all" (p. A17). Education–health–social justice advocates must support continued consideration of criminal justice reform, including action at both the state and federal levels.

• Incarceration must be considered first as a method of rehabilitation rather than punishment. Just being imprisoned is punishment—during this time of punishment, rehabilitation must be a priority. Rehabilitation can include addressing mental health issues and addiction, education and job training, regular family visits that include children or other methods of regular contact, individual and family counseling to prepare for reentry to society and meaningful family reunification, and future life planning. The nature of reentry to community and family life will have an impact on children and their overall quality of life, including their educational success and health. Gerson (2018) emphasizes this concept: "The children of prisoners are at high risk of future incarceration themselves. Writing off prisoners as worthless and hopeless has the effect of writing off many of their sons and daughters. It is moral malpractice with generational consequences" (p. A4).

• Schools, in partnership with the criminal justice system and community agencies, can play an important role in providing education and support to address the needs of incarcerated children and their parents and caregivers. These efforts must be characterized by a caring and stigma-free environment. School administrators and teachers can be provided with professional development related to issues faced by children and families and gain an understanding of specific strategies to address these issues. Examples of school efforts include Atlanta's ForeverFamily program, which offers afterschool and leadership programs for children and teens with incarcerated parents, and Syracuse's Center for Community Alternatives, which offers mentoring and support groups for students in the local public school system whose parents are incarcerated (Annie E. Casey Foundation, 2016).

Immigration

Embracing immigrant children and cultivating their full potential is the educational challenge of our generation. The stakes are high: Their future is our future.   SUÁREZ-OROZCO & SUÁREZ-OROZCO (2015)

The United States has a long history of immigration. Early in the twentieth century, many immigrants, primarily of white ancestry, entered the United States from southern and eastern Europe. Their children entered US schools, which, at that point in time, placed emphasis on helping immigrant students succeed academically and become acclimated to life in the United States. Over time, these educational efforts assisted many students in becoming part of the US social and political cultures and achieving varying levels of economic success (Crosnoe & Turley, 2011).

The United States is now in a period of a new large-scale wave of immigration. The US foreign-born population was 44.8 million people in 2018 (Budiman, 2020). Many of the immigrants are US citizens, some are lawfully present noncitizens, and some are undocumented residents. In contrast to earlier immigration, the current generation of immigrants and their children are more diverse by race, ethnicity, and country of origin. Regarding country of origin, 25% of US immigrants are from Mexico. The next-highest countries of origin are China (6%), India (6%), the Philippines (4%), and El Salvador (3%) (Budiman, 2020). While it can be anticipated that large-scale immigration to the United States will continue, current national and world events present a level of uncertainty to the nature of its immediate future.

One in four children in the United States, a total of 18.2 million, live with an immigrant parent. While some children immigrated from other countries, many were born in the United States to immigrant parents and, because of place of birth, are US citizens. In 2019, 90% of the children from immigrant families were US citizens (Annie E. Casey Foundation, 2021). Between 2015 and 2019, the following percentages of children and youth by ethnicity lived in immigrant families: 77% for Asian / Pacific Islander, 51% for Latino, 21% for two or more races, 14% for Black, 11% for American Indian, and 6% for non-Hispanic white. In 2019, 5.1 million US students were English language learners (National Center for Education Statistics, 2022). The parents of immigrant children represent varying socioeconomic and education levels and multiple cultural backgrounds. While parental economic situations and educational levels differ, between 2015 and 2019 44% of immigrant children and youth lived in low-income households and 12% lived in high-poverty areas (Budiman, 2020). In regard to education attainment, 22% of immigrants did not complete high school, in comparison to 8% of US residents. Pertaining to higher education, academic achievement is almost identical—32% of foreign-born individuals earned a bachelor's degree or above, while 33% of US-born individuals reached the level of bachelor's degree or above.

Similar to nonimmigrant children, life experiences within the family, school, and community environment can affect the health behaviors and health status of immigrant children and support or jeopardize their opportunities for academic success. While many families voluntarily came to the United States, a subset of immigrants, refugees, are displaced from their countries of origin and come to the United States because of violence or persecution (Dorsainvil, 2021). For some immigrant children, their life experiences in their countries of origin and their actual immigration experience occurred in dangerous, unhealthy, and otherwise challenging environments. In addition, during their immigration or before, these children might have had an interruption in their formal education (Potochnick, 2018).

While some children living in immigrant families speak English and come from highly educated, financially secure families, others face challenges such as lack of fluency in the English language, low levels of health literacy, family poverty, and challenged neighborhoods and schools. Some may have to work to contribute to the family income (Case, 2019). Unfortunately, immigrant children may also experience bias, discrimination, and a hostile political climate, which complicate their opportunities for an optimal transition (Kugler, 2018). Others face challenges related to family relocation and school disruption because of parents' migrant farm work (Cardoza, 2019). All of these factors influence the nature of the acculturation experience of immigrants, present challenges to academic success for school-age children, and affect the ability of immigrant families to thrive in their new place of residency. The lack of English language fluency can present difficult teaching and learning challenges. In 2019, 91% of fourth graders who were English language learners scored below proficiency in reading, in comparison to 62% of English-speaking fourth graders (Annie E. Casey Foundation, 2019). While parents born outside of the United States have high education attainment expectations for their children—91% expect their children to get a college degree, compared to 72% of US-born parents (Zill, 2020)—a range of challenges are present that can affect parental support for academic success. Parents of immigrant families may have limited English language fluency, low levels of formal education, limited time with children due to employment demands, and financial issues that present limitations for acquiring educational resources for their children.

Despite these unique challenges, many children of immigrants have demonstrated successes in their school experiences. Data from the 2016 US Department of Education's National Household Education Survey indicate that students from immigrant families are more likely to earn "mostly A grades" than students from nonimmigrant families (51% vs. 48%), less likely to have parents contacted for learning problems, and less likely to be suspended from school (Zill, 2020).

The successful transition and long-term well-being of immigrant children, youth, and their families is an important responsibility of both communities and schools. Parents who thrive will be able to provide support to their children in their school experiences and be active, contributing community members. Children who succeed in school will be more likely to become healthy adults, successful professionals, and contributing members of their communities. Maximum support should be provided to all members of the immigrant community regardless of immigration status. The US Supreme Court, in 1982, ruled that every child in the United States has a right to a free public K–12 education (*Plyler v. Doe*, 457 U.S. 202 [1982]). In November 2017, the International Society of Social Pediatrics and Child Health passed the Budapest Declaration—On the Rights, Health, and Well-Being of Children and Youth on the Move (Oberg, 2018). While the declaration is focused on children and health, the emphasis within the document on the inclusion of all members of the immigrant community and the holistic nature of responses provides a model for action-related educational efforts in schools for children from immigrant families.

The following are recommendations for communities and schools to provide optimal support for students and families:

- Know the immigrant community. It is important to realize not only that there are differences within the immigrant community by country of origin but also that there are differences among immigrants from the same country. These differences may be related to socioeconomic and education level, pre-immigration experiences, exposure to discrimination, and the immigration experience itself. For some, immigration may have been low in or free of trauma. For others, it may have involved long, dangerous travel; violence; lack of shelter; food insecurity; detention; or other forms of trauma. School programs will be more meaningful when based on the experiences and needs of students, parents, and family members. Both quantitative data and qualitative data are necessary to develop an informed understanding of the community.

- Maintain a school environment that is invitational to students, parents, and family members and committed to students' health and academic success. Invitational schools implement policies, programs, and practices that meet the needs of all students and engage parents and family members as active partners in teaching and learning. Case (2019) suggests that schools value both the cultural and linguistic resources of families and support the linkage between their original culture and the US culture. Parent and family engagement is supported through the use of interpreters, documents and online resources presented in multiple languages, parent education programs, the development of familiarity with the local community, and addressing issues related to scheduling of and transportation to school events (parent engagement is addressed in detail in chap. 6).

- Schools can serve as a bridge for students and parents to community resources. Parents and students from immigrant families may not be aware of the health and social services available in the school and local community. Even with awareness of programs, immigrant families may be reluctant to take advantage of these resources because of fear of deportation or threats to efforts for future citizenship (Bovell-

Ammon et al., 2019). Schools and community agencies need to inform families of services, perform culturally appropriate outreach, and provide referrals.

Dealing with immigration in a positive, supportive manner will produce benefits for all community members—both immigrants and non-immigrants. On the national level, the United States must present an invitational and safe environment to current and prospective immigrants. This requires citizens, institutions, and political leaders who are committed to diversity and committed to the provision of a culture that provides an environment, resources, and social and material support to promote a successful transition to the United States. Well-adjusted parents and families are more likely to have children who are safe, comfortable, and academically successful in schools.

LGBTQ+

I love learning but most days I just hate school. I can't deal with the comments and the inability for people to just be kind to LGBTQIA students.

KOSCIW ET AL. (2020)

Lesbian, gay, bisexual, transgender, and questioning/queer (LGBTQ+) students face school challenges based on bias and discrimination that have a high likelihood of affecting personal health, safety, and academic achievement. These challenges include victimization from bullying and physical assault; verbal, electronic, and sexual harassment; stigma-based stress; and various forms of discrimination (Johns et al., 2019; Kosciw et al., 2020).

Data related to the well-being and educational experiences of LGBTQ+ students are captured every two years through the National School Climate Survey from the Gay, Lesbian & Straight Education Network (GLSEN), which is a national organization that focuses on safe and affirming schools for all students regardless of their sexual orientation, gender identity, and gender expression. The biennial survey assesses topics such as school safety, anti-LGBTQ remarks in school, harassment and assault at school, the presence of discriminatory school policies and practices, the effects of the school climate on LGBTQ students' academic outcomes and mental health, and the availability of school resources and support. The survey is conducted online through outreach efforts to national, regional, and state LGBTQ youth organizations and advertising on social networking sites. The 2019 survey was conducted during the 2018–19 school year (Kosciw et al., 2020).

The findings from the 2019 study identify challenges faced by the 16,713 LGBTQ students who participated in the survey. The students ranged in age from 13 to 21, with an average age of 15.5. The students were in grades 6–12, with approximately 65% from grades 9, 10, and 11. Regarding race and ethnicity, 69.2% of the students were white; 14.6%, Hispanic or Latinx, any race; 8.6%, multiracial; 3.1%, Asian American, Pacific Islander, and Native Hawaiian; 2.6%, African American or Black; 1.3%, Arab American; and 0.5%, Native American, American Indian, or Alaska Native. Representation from students came from all 50 states, along with the District of Columbia, Puerto Rico, American Samoa, and Guam (Kosciw et al., 2020). The following findings are from the 2019 survey:

- 59.1% of the students felt unsafe because of their sexual orientation, 42.5% because of their gender expression, and 37.4% because of their gender.
- 96.9% of the students heard the term "gay" used in a negative way (75.6% heard this often or frequently), 95.2% heard other types of homophobic remarks, 91.8% heard negative remarks about gender expression, and 87.4% heard negative remarks about transgender persons.
- 68.7% of students experienced verbal harassment (called names or threatened).
- 25.7% of students experienced physical harassment (e.g., pushed or shoved), while 11% reported being physically assaulted (e.g., punched, kicked, injured with a weapon).
- 44.9% of the students experienced electronic harassment in the past year (via text messages or postings on social media).
- 58.3% of the students were sexually harassed (e.g., unwanted touching or sexual remarks).

- 59.1% of the students reported personally experiencing LGBTQ-related discriminatory policies or practices at school. Examples include being prevented from using bathrooms aligned with their gender identity (28.4%), prevented from using chosen names/pronouns (22.8%), and prohibited from discussing or writing about LGBTQ topics in school assignments (16.9%).
- 19.4% of the students were taught positive representation of LGBTQ people, history, or events in their schools; 17% were taught negative content.
- 32.7% of LGBTQ students missed at least one entire day of school in the past month because they felt unsafe or uncomfortable; 8.6% missed four or more days in the past month.
- 97.7% of LGBTQ students could identify at least one staff member supportive of LGBTQ students at the school; 66.3% could identify at least six supportive staff members.

In almost all of these examples, schools are indicated to be sites for trauma for LGBTQ students. Exposure to these discrimination-based challenges has been shown to be associated with school issues such as increased absenteeism, decreased intention to engage in postsecondary education, and lower academic performance. The following findings from the 2019 GLSEN study illuminate these outcomes:

- LGBTQ students who experienced higher levels of victimization because of either their sexual orientation or gender expression were close to three times as likely to have missed school in the past month than those LGBTQ students who experienced lower levels. Regarding grade point average (GPA), those students who experienced higher levels of victimization had lower GPAs and were twice as likely to report that they did not plan to engage in any postsecondary education (e.g., college or trade school).
- LGBTQ students who experienced LGBTQ-related discrimination at school were more than three times as likely to have missed school in the past month than students who had not experienced discrimination.

Schools exist for all students. Communities and school districts must move forward to make schools invitational, safe, and supportive for all students, including LGBTQ+ students. The following recommendations are presented for schools in regard to a comprehensive approach to supporting LGBTQ+ students in a comprehensive manner:

- An anti-bullying policy. Anti-bullying policies provide a framework for a safe and supportive environment for all students, identify protections based on personal characteristics such as sexual orientation and gender identity/expression, and convey a message that bullying, harassment, and assault are not acceptable and will not be tolerated. GLSEN strongly recommends a comprehensive policy in which "enumeration" is a clear component. Enumeration refers to a specific listing of all examples of LGBTQ+ and other student bullying to inform administrators, teachers, and students of all possible types of harassment or assault. These specific examples are intended to protect not simply the most vulnerable of students, including LGBTQ+ students, but all who might be subject to bullying. In addition, a comprehensive policy should include specific procedures for reporting violations to school authorities. The 2019 GLSEN report indicates that in schools with comprehensive policies students are less likely to be subject to verbal harassment such as homophobic remarks, more likely to report that staff intervene when hearing anti-LGBTQ remarks, more likely to report victimization incidents to school staff, and more likely to rate the school staff's response as effective (Kosciw et al., 2020). GLSEN has developed a Model District Anti-Bullying & Harassment Policy that details the importance of enumeration and includes model language, commentary, and resources (Kosciw et al., 2020)

- Supportive school staff members / LGBTQ+ Safe Zones. Based on the 2019 GLSEN research, LGBTQ students who identified higher numbers of supportive staff in their schools were less likely to feel unsafe, less likely to miss school, had higher GPAs, and expressed higher postsecondary educational aspirations. In addition, these students felt a greater connectedness to their school. The 2019 GLSEN report clearly presents the benefits of having several LGBTQ-supportive staff at school rather than only a few. Safe Zones are designated spaces that are intended to publicly identify teachers, counselors, administrators, or staff members who are LGBTQ+ friendly and are open to discussion or the provision of support. This designation is typically demonstrated through the presence of Safe Zone stickers on office or classroom doors or other visible locations. The 2019 GLSEN findings indicated that students who reported a higher number of Safe Zones also reported a higher number of supportive faculty members. The findings related to Safe Zones and supportive staff members bring attention to the importance of professional development for all staff on recognizing and responding to the needs of LGBTQ+ students (Kosciw et al., 2020). While emphasizing the importance of Safe Zones and recognizing the positive impact on the school experience their presence has brought, Sadowski (2017) raised an intriguing question for consideration—if certain areas of schools are designated as "Safe Zones" and specific individuals designated as "LGBTQ friendly," what does this imply about the remaining areas of the school and other administrators, faculty members, and staff? The point is obvious—the entire school should be a Safe Zone for all students, and all administrators, faculty members, and staff should be friendly for all students.

- Gay-straight alliances (GSAs) or similar clubs. GSAs are extracurricular organizations that include gay, lesbian, bisexual, transgender and other gender expansive, queer, questioning, and straight students. These organizations can supply mutual sources of support and socialization, provide a safe environment for all students, and serve as a resource for school educational programs addressing LGBTQ+ issues. Many GSAs engage in advocacy designed to improve the school experiences of all students and the overall school environment. Engagement in GSA advocacy activities is associated with involved students reporting an ability to accomplish goals and a greater sense of purpose, agency, and empowerment. In addition, some GSAs have developed collaborative relationships with other student groups dealing with discrimination (race, gender, etc.) in order to focus on intersectional aspects of oppression (Poteat, 2017; Sadowski, 2017). Findings from the 2019 GLSEN National School Climate Survey indicated that in comparison to LGBTQ students who did not have a GSA in their school, LGBTQ students attending schools with GSAs were less likely to hear homophobic or negative remarks, less likely to feel unsafe because of their sexual orientation, less likely to experience victimization, less likely to miss school because of safety or discomfort concerns, and more likely to report that school staff intervened when hearing homophobic remarks (Kosciw et al., 2020). Porta et al. (2017) analyzed 466 comments about GSAs from interviews conducted with 66 LGBTQ youth in Minnesota, Massachusetts, and British Columbia ages 14–19. Three themes emerged from the analysis: (1) the GSAs provided the youth with a sense of community based on their sense of emotional connection, support and belonging, opportunities for leadership, and fulfillment of needs; (2) the GSAs provided a pathway to outside resources, including supportive adults and informal social locations; and (3) the GSAs represented safety. The study authors recommend that schools, relative to the implementation of GSAs, provide an adult adviser, meeting space, and financial support and resources comparable to other student organizations (Porta et al., 2017).

- An inclusive curriculum and inclusive instruction. Many subjects within the overall school curriculum can provide an opportunity for instruction about LGBTQ+ history, current and past leaders, political issues, and personal and population-based health topics, including sexual health. Pertaining to exposure to coverage of LGBTQ people, history, or events in school lessons, 66.8% of the students in the 2019 GLSEN study reported that their classes did not address these topics. Only 8.2% received LGBTQ-inclusive sex education that included positive representations of LGB, transgender, and nonbinary identities and topics (Kosciw et al., 2020). A review of state school-based sexuality policies found that 22 states mentioned LGBTQ as subject topics. Nine of the states mandate inclusive education, six mandate discriminatory education, and five mandate neutral education. Two states recommend inclusive education but do not mandate it (Garg & Volerman, 2021). Without education on LGBTQ+ topics many students (both straight and LGBTQ+) will not develop the comfort level, knowledge, and skills needed to maximize access to the highest quality of life for everyone in society.

- An inclusive commitment for all LGBTQ+ students. Even in schools that are committed to supporting all students, some students within the LGBTQ+ space may be overlooked. With the increasing visibility of the needs of transgender students, many schools are recognizing the importance of providing support to gender expansive students who demonstrate a range of gender identities and expression. Gender expansive children and youth do not conform to the culture's expectations for boys or girls and express behaviors and personal traits in ways that some may view as gender atypical. Transgender students are within the gender expansive grouping, but not all children and youth who are within the grouping are transgender (Murchison et al., 2016). Relative to health risks, transgender youth are at a higher risk than cisgender youth for violence victimization, substance use, and sexual risk behaviors. Approximately 1 in 50 youth in the United States identifies as transgender (Johns et al., 2019). Research indicates that close to half of all male and nearly a third of all female transgender adolescents reported attempting suicide (Toomey et al., 2018). A guide for schools in meeting the needs of transgender students titled *Schools in Transition: A Guide for Supporting Transgender Students in K–12 Schools* was published under the aegis of the American Civil Liberties Union, Gender Spectrum, the Human Rights Campaign Foundation, the National Center for Lesbian Rights, and the National Education Association. This comprehensive resource provides direction to schools in topics such as student records; names and pronouns; dress codes; sex-separated facilities, activities, and programs; restrooms and lockers; sports teams; physical education classes; homecoming, prom, and other school traditions; discrimination, harassment, and bullying; and working with parents (Orr et al., 2015).
- Professional development. In order to maximize the development and enforcement of policy, the initiation and implementation of GSAs, Safe Zones, and the implementation of an inclusive curriculum, school administrators, teachers, and staff must be committed to providing

support and meeting needs for LGBTQ+ students. Evidence suggests that professional development focused on LGBTQ+ students' school experiences can increase the likelihood that educators and school staff members will act to improve school programs and the school environment (Greytak et al., 2016; Johns et al., 2019). Shattuck et al. (2020) conducted 75 interviews and 32 focus groups with professionals in 18 New Mexico high schools. Their findings indicate that professional development promoted the interview and focus group participants' reflection and critical thinking related to LGBTQ students' issues faced in school; enhanced the participants' awareness of the issues faced by LGBTQ students and their comfort level in discussing these issues; promoted a deeper understanding of the social, political, and economic influences on LGBTQ issues; and increased the recognition of the need for support specific to the needs of LGBTQ students.

It is essential that public health agencies, physicians, and schools partner with LGBTQ+ students, their families, and community agencies to provide a safe, supportive, and inclusive environment in schools and communities. One important method of partnering with LBGTQ+ students (and all other students) is to provide them with a voice within the school. In order to better understand their perspectives, schools should intentionally include LGBTQ+ students' input in the evaluation of the school environment, policies, practices, curriculum, and instruction, along with inviting them to be members of school committees. There are also national organizations that can serve as informed partners and resource providers. These organizations include the Children's Defense Fund, GLSEN, GSA Network, PFLAG, the Safe Schools Coalition, Trans Student Educational Resources, Trans Youth Family Allies, the Trevor Project, and Welcoming Schools.

Children, adults, and communities will not reach their full potential in education and health until social injustice is minimized and eventually eliminated. Addressing racism and all other biases and discrimination must be in the forefront of all advocacy efforts focusing on access to quality education and overall community well-being.

CHAPTER 3

Early Childhood

May all children everywhere have the opportunity for a strong start and may all who have parenting responsibilities have the time, money, resources, support, and equal opportunity to practice positive, enjoyable parenting.

ADAPTED FROM THE DOCUMENTARY SERIES *The Raising of America* (2015)

ARLY CHILDHOOD is the beginning of the pathway that will eventually lead a young child into elementary school, middle school, high school, and then adulthood. Home life, beginning after birth, is an important influence on a child's health, safety, support, and learning. Beyond the home, social and community factors are also influential in a young child's development. These factors are interdependent and have both an immediate impact on very young children and a continuing effect on their overall health, early learning, and readiness for school. Early life influences can also have an impact on education attainment, health, social outcomes, and employment in adulthood. These important considerations are linked to the position statement of the National Association for the Education of Young Children (NAEYC), *Advancing Equity in Early Childhood Education* (NAEYC, 2019). The statement includes the following 10 "Principles of Child Development and Learning":

1. Early childhood (birth through age 8) is a uniquely valuable and vulnerable time in the human life cycle.

2. Each individual—child, family member, and early educator—is unique.
3. Each individual belongs to multiple social and cultural groups.
4. Learning is a social process profoundly shaped by culture, social interaction, and language.
5. Language and communication are essential to the learning process.
6. Families are the primary context for children's development and learning.
7. Learning, emotions, and memory are inextricably interconnected in brain processing networks.
8. Toxic stress and anxiety can undermine learning.
9. Children's learning is facilitated when teaching practices, curricula, and learning environments build on children's strengths and are developmentally, culturally, and linguistically appropriate for each child.
10. Reflective practice is required to achieve equitable learning opportunities.

Life influences at all ages are complex and interactive. Shaping these influences to promote the best possible outcomes in early childhood requires comprehensive, coordinated, cross-sector actions. It is beyond the responsibility of one person, one family, one profession, or one organization. It requires personal, family, local, state, national, and, in some cases, global actions. Potential partners with parents and family members in this coordinated approach come from the early childhood, K–12, public health, and medical sectors, along with other possible community partners such as the business community, juvenile justice, social work, law enforcement, parks and recreation, public libraries, and colleges and universities. In addition, elected and nonelected policy makers are logical partners.

The ability to experience a caring, supportive, healthy early childhood is a positive not only for children and their families but also for the community and society at large. Young children who start kindergarten healthy and ready to learn are more likely to be successful throughout their elementary, middle, and high school experiences and more likely to contribute to society as healthy productive citizens. Numerous state governmental agencies and various children's organizations have identified indicators of children's readiness for kindergarten. While these listings vary somewhat, common overarching areas include cognitive development, social and emotional development, language development, mathematical development, sensory development, and health and physical development. The various organizations also include a range of specific skills and dispositions for the overarching areas (Alabama Partnership for Children, n.d.; Better Beginnings, 2017; Healthychildren.org, 2019). During the child's growth and development, the skills and dispositions are interactive. For example, oral language acquisition demonstrates the connection between cognitive and social and emotional development. From a cognitive development perspective, language acquisition depends on the ability to differentiate sounds and the capacity to link meaning to specific words. However, the development of language acquisition will also depend on social and emotional skills related to concentration such as paying attention and engaging in meaningful conversation (National Scientific Council on the Developing Child, 2007).

Brain Development

All cognitive, emotional, and social capabilities and physical and mental well-being develop through a lifelong process that is deeply embedded in the function of the brain as well as in the cardiovascular, immune, neuroendocrine, and metabolic regulatory systems. These capacities are highly interrelated through multiple biological systems that are woven together like strands of a rope. Together, these strands comprise the foundations of success in school and later in the workplace and community.   CENTER ON THE DEVELOPING CHILD (n.d.)

Brain development is malleable, and the brain grows and develops in response to experiences and relationships (Darling-Hammond & Cook-Harvey, 2018). While brain development occurs throughout life, most "brain building" occurs between birth and age 8 (Bergen et al., 2020). Influencing the positive development of both cognitive and noncognitive skills should begin at birth and continue through infancy and early childhood. Parental actions that support positive development include providing infants with opportunities to move, touch, and be touched; responding to babbling, facial expressions, words, gestures, and cries; reading to and with children throughout early childhood; modeling positive behaviors; engaging in empathetic back-and-forth conversations; and providing a warm, nurturing environment and opportunities for social interactions, relationships, and physical activity (Bergen et al., 2020; Putnam, 2015).

Darling-Hammond and Cook-Harvey (2018) stress the importance of positive interactions with your children: "The brain's capacity develops most fully when children and youth feel emotionally and physically safe; when they feel connected, supported, engaged, and challenged; and when they have robust opportunities to learn—with rich materials and experiences that allow them to inquire into the world around them— and equally robust support for learning" (p. v).

Information continues to increase regarding the linkage between early childhood experiences and brain development and future life outcomes (Bergen et al., 2020). Brain development begins before birth and continues through adulthood. As the brain develops in early childhood, synapses or connections between neurons are formed. Synapses are first developed for very basic skills. Synapses related to more complex skills build on these early connections. The connections that are used and protected become strong and established and provide an important foundation for building more advanced cognitive, social, and emotional skills. Thus, a child's experiences early in life provide the foundation for behavior and continued learning beyond early childhood. Both animal research and human research have indicated that nurturing care such as physical contact and consistent, ongoing interaction early in life positively affects synapses related to social and emotional functioning. Infants who experience warm nurturing care and interactions with parents and caregivers are more likely to accept positive relationships in later life and act accordingly. Conversely, infants who experience fear, humiliation, or physical attack are more likely to anticipate threatening relationships with others and act accordingly (Kuo et al., 2016; Putnam, 2015).

Based on the current understanding of brain development, significant stress experienced by young children is now viewed as a risk factor for the initiation of at-risk health behaviors and difficulties in learning, as well as a catalyst for chronic stress-related diseases in adulthood. Thus, the important overall principle for consideration is that a child's early experiences and environment affect early brain development, and this early development has an impact on school performance, as well as health and behavior in adulthood (Putnam, 2015).

Another important aspect of early childhood development is the effect of a child's environment and experiences on gene expression, known as epigenetics. Positive learning experiences and safe, supportive environments activate positive genetic expression that results in a capacity for effective learning and positive social, emotional, and physical health. Sustained stressful experiences can result in gene expression that may lead to long-term problems in cognitive, social, and emotional development and impairments to health that can continue into adulthood (Center on the Developing Child, n.d.).

It is also important to emphasize that as a child gets older and pathways or circuits mature, it becomes more difficult for the brain to change. The brain's ability to change, or its "plasticity," is at its highest point in early childhood and decreases with age. Attempts to remediate brain pathways that did not develop properly are more difficult as age increases (Crosnoe et al., 2015; Putnam, 2015).

Disparities in Early Childhood and School Readiness

The longer society waits to intervene in the life cycle of a disadvantaged child, the more costly it is to remediate disadvantage.   HECKMAN (2008)

Not all parents, families, and communities have an equal capacity for providing a nurturing, supportive, and education-rich early childhood. Potential barriers can include financial stress, work demands, inability to secure resources that enhance the child home experience (books, educational toys, games, etc.), family issues, an unsafe or nonsupportive neighborhood or community, and a lack of awareness or skills to engage children in positive developmental and educational activities.

Researchers have identified the following outcomes related to school readiness that are linked to these parenting challenges:

- Based on the use of magnetic resonance imagery of the emotion regulatory section of the brains of study participants at age 24, Kim et al. (2013) found that participants who experienced poverty at age 9 had a lower level of ability in regulating emotions in comparison to participants who did not experience poverty during childhood.
- D'Angiulli et al. (2008), in a study based on an examination of brain waves of children from upper and lower socioeconomic backgrounds, found that the students from the lower socioeconomic group had more difficulty concentrating on a simple task than those from the higher socioeconomic group.
- Regarding language development in children, disparities in vocabulary and language processing efficiency were found to exist between infants from higher and lower socioeconomic groups at as early as 18 months. At 24 months, there was a six-month difference between the groups in processing skills that are important to language development (Fernald et al., 2013). Research suggests that children in low socioeconomic groups are exposed to fewer vocabulary words during early childhood (Golinkoff et al., 2019).

Children who are exposed to negative life experiences and a lack of positive interaction and support, even in early childhood, are at an increased risk for having less-than-optimal life outcomes in their K–12 school experience and in adulthood. For example, childhood trauma and adolescent trauma are related to a greater likelihood of repeating a grade in school, lower resilience, increased risk for learning and behavioral issues, suicidal ideation, and the early initiation of sexual activity and pregnancy (Soleimanpour et al., 2017). Harmful outcomes can also extend into adulthood. Children exposed over time to toxic stress emanating from threats such as extreme poverty, parental addiction, family violence, physical and emotional abuse, unstable and unsafe environments, discrimination, and marginalization have challenges related to concentrating, controlling impulsive behavior, and following directions. These children also face an increased chance of experiencing decreased productivity and chronic health conditions throughout adulthood (Ellis & Dietz, 2017; Putnam, 2015). Adverse childhood experiences (ACEs), which will be addressed in more detail later in the chapter, demonstrate that these situations are harmful in a graded manner. As the number of adverse experiences that children are exposed to increases, the harmful effects increase (Ellis & Dietz, 2017; Felitti et al., 1998).

Ethnic, racial, and socioeconomic differences are related to disparities in school readiness. Many children from families living in poverty and living with racism and other systemic forms of discrimination begin kindergarten with lower levels of school readiness than more advantaged children. Fernald et al. (2013) found significant differences in vocabulary and language development at 18 and 24 months of age between children in high and low socioeconomic groups. Bassok et al. (2016) analyzed two national data sets of young children from 1998 to 2010 and concluded that during this period the school readiness gap between high- and low-income children decreased, but a large difference was still present. Reardon and Portilla (2016) examined school readiness in students in kindergarten in 1998, 2006, and 2010 and found differences between socioeconomic levels, between white and Hispanic students, and between white and Black students. Levels of school readiness were found to be more advanced in higher socioeconomic students compared to students from lower socioeconomic levels, and more advanced among white students in comparison to Black and Hispanic students. These disadvantages often affect students' performance not only in kindergarten but also in subsequent school years, including middle and high school.

Social injustices such as racism, sexism, and other forms of systemic discrimination can present challenges to families and children. These challenges include parents' lack of access to living-wage jobs and, in some cases, the need to hold down two jobs or work frequent overtime hours; a lack of affordable housing; inadequate community resources, health care, and social services; and a lack of transportation and affordable childcare. Additional barriers, also present because of systemic discrimination, can include unsupportive public policies, unsafe neighborhoods, and environmental injustices. These situations can result in young children having less time to interact with their parents in meaningful discussion; young children having exposure to a smaller number of words, resulting in a more limited vocabulary; parents and children having access to fewer educational resources in the home, including books and educational games; and parents and children having less time for engaging together in recreational activities and educational visits to children's museums and libraries.

Carefully considered action must be taken to address the factors that create inequality in opportunity. Bruner (2017) describes the interdependence of race, place, and poverty through an analysis of the year 2000 US census tract data. From the analysis, four key findings are described that are critical considerations in addressing early childhood disparities: (1) poor neighborhoods have high numbers of young children; (2) poor neighborhoods are home to a disproportionate number of children of color; (3) differences in income, wealth, education, and social structure are profound; and (4) all states have these disparities, but there are differences among states regarding the composition of their poor neighborhoods. To promote a healthier early childhood environment, Bruner (2017) identified needs within challenged neighborhoods that warrant action and leadership, including more parks, playgrounds, and family- and child-friendly locations to promote healthy social and emotional development, as well as increased support for families and communities.

Interventions have been developed to address the challenges of early childhood. Family-based programs can help parents and family members decrease or prevent disruptive behavioral issues and promote social competence and academic performance (Biglan et al., 2017). Ellis and Dietz (2017) describe the Building Community Resilience Model (BCR) as an initiative that engages community members in collaboration with the public health, social welfare, education, human services, juvenile justice, and public safety sectors in the provision of support to children and families to address the causes of toxic stress and childhood adversity that can affect young children and families. BCR considers community resilience as an essential factor in improving public health and an important program outcome. Important to building and sustaining community resilience is the presence of buffers within the community and families to protect individuals from the accumulation of stress due to ACEs. One important focus of the BCR collaboration is connecting community organizations (a church health ministry or trusted food pantry, for example) with larger systems (including health care, education, business, law enforcement). An important outcome of this collaboration was addressing gaps and leveraging assets to promote health, create stronger community and organizational linkages, and increase social supports for families and individuals (Ellis & Dietz, 2017).

The UCLA Center for Healthier Children, Families, and Communities (n.d.-a) works with pediatricians, public health experts, psychologists, economists, lawyers, and policy experts, in conjunction with local families, communities, and businesses, to develop programs to improve children's health; increase the efficiency, effectiveness, and access of health and social services; and assist communities in becoming healthier environments. One of the center's programs, Transforming Early Childhood Community Systems (TECCS), is a partnership between the center and United Way Worldwide. TECCS works with communities around the country to determine the school readiness of young children using the Early Development Instrument (EDI; UCLA Center for Healthier Children, Families, and Communities, n.d.-b). The instrument measures five areas of early childhood development that relate to school readiness: physical health and well-being, social well-being, emotional maturity, language and cognitive skills, and communication skills and general knowledge. The EDI is used to inform local communities about methods to improve early childhood services and systems. The communities are provided with maps that show neighborhood-level data and EDI results that indicate the percentage of young children vulnerable within each of the five developmental domains that measure school readiness. The information is used to provide direction to local strategic planning and systems improvement efforts. The community school readiness mapping process is repeated on a regular basis to determine progress and identify challenges (UCLA Center for Healthier Children, Families, and Communities, n.d.-c).

Adverse Childhood Experiences

Pediatric practitioners are well positioned to transform the way society responds to children exposed to significant ACEs, but they cannot resolve this public health crisis alone. Collective action is required to prevent, screen, and heal the toxic effects of early adversity. Together, we can help children thrive.

HARRIS ET AL. (2017)

As emphasized in this chapter, negative childhood experiences have the potential to affect children's lives in childhood and through adulthood. Children exposed to toxic stress in the home such as physical, psychological, or sexual abuse; neglect; family socioeconomic challenges; parental incarceration or death; and parent or caregiver alcohol or substance abuse face difficult challenges to their growth and development. Beyond the home, children's maturation might be affected by community issues such as systemic racism and other systemic discrimination, violence, and lack of support services. Unfortunately, children are not limited to exposure to only one type of negative experience. Many children have exposures to multiple types of adverse experiences. Note that while childhood trauma, or ACEs, is presented in a chapter focusing on early childhood, ACEs can occur from early childhood through the late teen years. Providing support and services in early childhood to children who have experienced ACEs and their families is of utmost importance. Jimenez et al. (2016) conducted a secondary data analysis of 1,007 children from the national Fragile Families and Child Wellbeing Study. Findings indicated a strong association between children who had experienced ACEs in early childhood (by age 5) and below-average academic and literacy skills and behavior problems.

Research over the past 20 years that has examined the impact of these experiences has brought the term "ACEs" to the attention of educators, physicians, public health professionals, and various social service professionals. A landmark study conducted by a research team led by Vincent

Fellitti of the Kaiser Permanente Medical Group, Department of Preventive Medicine, found a graded relationship between the number of childhood exposures to abuse and household dysfunction and engagement in multiple risk behaviors for some of the leading causes of death among adults. The data from the study, published in 1998 in the *Journal of the American Medical Association*, were based on responses to a standardized questionnaire that was completed by adults who were Kaiser Health Plan members who had recently completed a standardized medical evaluation. The medical evaluation included a physical examination and a review of lab tests, demographic and biopsychosocial information, previous medical diagnoses, and family medical history. One week after completing the medical evaluation, participants were mailed the ACE Study questionnaire, which included questions about childhood exposure to forms of household dysfunction. A total of 9,508 individuals participated in the study, representing a response rate of 70.5%. The study questionnaire included items to assess adverse experiences that occurred during the participants' childhood (up to age 18). Additional information for data analysis, including disease history for study respondents, was accessible to the research team from the Health Appraisal Clinic (Felitti et al., 1998).

The questionnaire used in the study included questions in seven categories of ACEs related to abuse and household dysfunction. Three categories related to abuse: psychological (two questions), physical (two questions), and sexual (four questions). Four categories related to household dysfunction: substance abuse (two questions), mental illness (two questions), mother treated violently (four questions), and criminal behavior in household (one question). Each of the questions required a "yes" or "no" response. Respondents were classified as exposed to a category if one "yes" response was provided to a question in that category (Felitti et al., 1998).

The analysis included an assessment of the relationship between respondents' exposure during the first 18 years of life to abuses in the seven categories and their personal connection during adulthood to 10 health risk factors: smoking, severe obesity, physical inactivity, depressed mood, suicide attempts, alcoholism, drug abuse, parenteral drug abuse, a high lifetime number of sexual partners (50 or more), and a history of having a sexually transmitted disease. In addition, the relationship between exposure to the ACE categories and adult disease conditions such as ischemic heart disease, cancer, stroke, chronic bronchitis, emphysema (COPD), diabetes, hepatitis or jaundice, and any skeletal fractures (as a proxy for unintentional injury) was included in the analyses (Felitti et al., 1998).

The researchers used the seven categories of adverse experiences as the basis for the analyses. The number of exposures was the sum of the categories with an exposure (a "yes" response to one or more questions in a category equated to an exposure for that category). Thus, the range for the number of exposures was 0 to 7. The prevalence for exposures to the seven categories ranged from 3.4% for "criminal behavior in the household" to 25.6% for "substance abuse." Overall, 52% of the respondents had one or more exposures to ACE categories, while 6.2% had four or more exposures. The majority of individuals who were exposed to one category of adverse experiences were also exposed to at least one other. The findings verified the linkage between ACEs and health risk factors. Of the individuals in the study who were not exposed to any of the adverse experience categories, 56% did not have a personal connection to any of the 10 health risk factors. In contrast, only 14% of the individuals who were exposed to four or more of the adverse experience categories did not have a personal connection with any of the 10 risk factors. Regarding the relationship between adverse experiences and disease conditions, individuals with four or more exposures to adverse experiences were more likely to exhibit the presence of each of the disease conditions than those with no exposure (Felitti et al., 1998).

The researchers found a strong dose-response relationship between the number of childhood exposures to adverse experience categories and each of the 10 health risk factors. Essentially, as the number of exposures increased, there was a greater likelihood of connection to each risk factor. In addition, a dose-response relationship was also found between the number of exposures to adverse experience categories and all of the disease conditions except for a history of stroke and diabetes. Thus, as the number of exposures increased, the likelihood of exhibiting the disease connections increased. The researchers describe the exposure to ACEs as having a strong and cumulative effect on adult health status (Felitti et al., 1998).

Recent research reinforces the ongoing extent of the problem of ACEs and builds on the work of Felitti et al. (1998). Data from the 2018–19 National Survey of Children's Health indicate that among all children up to age 17, 60.2% were not exposed to any ACEs, 21.6% were exposed to at least one ACE, and 18.2% were exposed to two or more out of a total of nine ACEs (Child and Adolescent Health Measurement Initiative, n.d.-b). The proportion of children in each of the 50 states and the District of Columbia exposed to no ACEs ranged from 48.1% to 65.6%; children with exposure to one ACE, from 16.7% to 26.4%; and children with exposure to two or more ACEs, from 14.3% to 29% (Child and Adolescent Health Measurement Initiative, n.d.-a).

Regarding exposure to ACEs by age, 73.1% of children ages 0–5 were not exposed to any ACEs, 18.1% were exposed to one ACE, and 8.8% were exposed to two or more ACEs. As children got older, exposure to ACEs increased. For those children ages 6–11, 58.5% were not exposed to any ACEs, 21.8% were exposed to one ACE, and 19.7% were exposed to two or more ACEs. In the 12–17 age range, 49.8% were not exposed to any ACEs, 24.7% were exposed to one ACE, and 25.5% were exposed to two or more ACEs (Child and Adolescent Health Measurement Initiative, n.d.-c).

Accounting for race and ethnicity, 79.3% of Asian, non-Hispanic children; 63.7% of white, non-Hispanic children; 58.2% of Hispanic children; and 46.7% of Black, non-Hispanic children were not exposed to any ACEs, while 14.7% of Asian, non-Hispanic children; 19.9% of white, non-Hispanic children; 23% of Hispanic children; and 27.9% of Black, non-Hispanic children were exposed to one ACE. Children exposed to two or more ACEs included 6% of Asian, non-Hispanic children; 16.3% of white, non-Hispanic children; 18.9% of Hispanic children; and 25.4% of Black, non-Hispanic children (Child and Adolescent Health Measurement Initiative, n.d.-d).

Additional research confirms the relationship between number of exposures to ACEs and the increased likelihood of adult health issues.

In a meta-analysis based on 23 studies (10 conducted in the United States) that examined risk factors in individuals with exposure to ACEs compared to individuals without exposure to ACEs, the researchers found that the number of risk factors was higher for individuals exposed to two or more ACEs compared to those exposed to one ACE. A similar finding was applicable regarding the relation between exposure to ACEs and six disease factors or causes of ill health (anxiety, depression, cancer, cardiovascular disease, diabetes, and respiratory disease). Based on the findings from the meta-analysis, the researchers estimated the annual costs of ACEs in North America to be $748 billion (Bellis et al., 2019).

Because of the research-based linkage between early life experiences and brain development and the connection to learning, adult diseases, and social disorders, many professionals, including educators, neuroscientists, physicians, public health professionals, and social service providers, have focused their attention on early childhood. In response to the multisector nature of this professional interest and activity, the Johns Hopkins University, Bloomberg School of Public Health, Child and Adolescent Health Measurement Initiative, in collaboration with Academy Health, undertook the development of a field-building, research, policy, and practice agenda to address ACEs and promote child and family well-being (Bethell et al., 2017; Davis et al., 2017). The agenda was developed over a four-year period using deliberate processes that engaged over 500 individuals. One of the products linked to the agenda is a special 2017 issue of *Academic Pediatrics* focused on ACEs. This issue includes multiple commentaries and research articles. The articles present the critical roles for Medicaid and private sector health plans, children's hospitals, primary care providers, and all children's health services as partners with families and communities. In addition, the issue identifies efforts to address the effects of current and accumulated individual, intergenerational, systems-level, and community-level ACEs.

As research and practice related to ACEs move forward, the identification of trauma experiences has changed from the original listing in the Felitti study. Venet and Duane (2021) warn of the possible limitations of the original listing and suggest the consideration of historical, generational, and cultural factors in understanding trauma. One example of the revision of the original listing is the National Survey of Children's Health (NSCH), funded and directed by the Health Resources and Services Administration. Since 2011, the NSCH has incorporated items related to familial death, neighborhood violence, economic hardship, and unfair treatment based on race or ethnicity (National Conference of State Legislatures, 2021). Supporting the consideration of unfair treatment based on race and ethnicity, Geller (2021), based on an analysis of the national Fragile Families and Child Wellbeing Study, recommends the designation of police aggression as an ACE. The factors noted by Venet and Duane and those incorporated into the NSCH bring attention to the importance of community involvement in research and practice related to ACEs.

Pachter et al. (2017) reported on a community-wide initiative to address ACEs in Philadelphia that added a local perspective to the adverse experiences examined in the Felitti study. The leadership group of the Philadelphia ACE Task Force convened a research committee to provide direction to the project's data collection. Based on qualitative research conducted in predominantly Black neighborhoods in Philadelphia, additional ACEs were identified, including witnessing violence, experiencing racism/discrimination, living in unsafe and unsupportive neighborhoods, experiencing bullying, and being in foster care.

Low socioeconomic status, limited educational attainment, disrupted social networks, mental health issues, and substance use problems are factors that present challenges to parents in the provision of a supportive, nurturing environment for children. Woods-Jaeger et al. (2018) conducted in-depth interviews with 11 low-income parents with histories of ACEs in order to better understand the parents' perception of the impact of ACEs on parenting, to highlight the protective factors that buffer any negative impact, and to elicit the parents' recommendations on supports and services that would reduce the number and severity of ACEs and promote resilience among their children. Three themes were identified from the interviews: the recognition of the intergenerational cycle of ACEs, the parents' aspirations to make their children's lives better, and descriptions of how the parents provide nurturing and support, as well as related barriers to such action. The parents also presented recommendations for addressing ACEs, including increasing community awareness of the presence of ACEs locally, building a supportive community, and providing parenting education, support, and mental health services (Woods-Jaeger et al., 2018).

Early Childhood Education

Tonight, I propose working with states to make high-quality preschool available to every single child in America. . . . Every dollar we invest in high-quality early education can save more than seven dollars later on.

PRESIDENT BARRACK OBAMA, 2013 State of the Union Address

Early childhood education (ECE) has gained increased recognition as an essential part of a child's total educational experience. Parents, leaders in education, and other stakeholders are increasingly viewing ECE as early education rather than childcare (Neuman, 2014; Wechsler et al., 2018). Residents in cities such as Seattle, Cincinnati, San Antonio, Denver, and Philadelphia have voted for tax increases to support ECE programs (Iasevoli, 2019). While public awareness and enrollment in programs increased in the 2000s, many children still do not participate in ECE.

ECE programs in the United States are a combination of federally funded programs, state-funded programs, locally funded programs, and, in some cases, programs with funding from a combination of these sources. Beyond these public programs, many children are in private programs, which are often a mixture of childcare and ECE. According to data from the US National Center for Education Statistics, 68% of 4-year-old children and 40% of 3-year-old children were enrolled in preschool programs that provided educational experiences in 2018. Approximately 55% of 3- and 4-year-olds attended full-day programs (National Center for Education Statistics, 2021).

There are a number of reasons why quality ECE is important:

- Children begin learning at birth. As described earlier, knowledge about brain development has grown considerably over the past

20 years. Important brain building occurs between birth and age 8. Both cognitive (educational) and noncognitive (social) skills develop during this early period in life (Bergen et al., 2020).

- Children are more likely to be successful in elementary school and beyond when they are ready for kindergarten. ECE helps children develop both cognitive and noncognitive skills that are important for learning and success in school. The level of readiness a child has upon entering kindergarten has been shown to be influential throughout their entire school experience. A higher level of education increases the likelihood of high school graduation and can have positive effects on the quality of life in adulthood (Hahn et al., 2016).
- Early childhood educators can be partners with parents in helping their children develop cognitive and noncognitive skills both at home and while in school. This partnership can be important for all parents, but especially for those facing socioeconomic challenges, discrimination, job-related time conflicts, community challenges, and other life issues (Crosnoe et al., 2015).
- ECE makes economic sense. Evaluation of ECE shows that quality programs more than cover their costs through educational attainment and decreased social costs. Many education leaders emphasize that government investment in quality ECE will bring both short-term and long-term educational, economic, and social benefits. Crosnoe et al. (2015) emphasize that funding spent on early childhood will be more cost efficient than funding spent on later interventions for older children, adolescents, or adults.
- ECE has a role in addressing discrimination at the systemic, interpersonal, and educational levels that affects program leaders, educators, and students. NAEYC recommends that ECE leaders and educators address both the systemic inequities based on the uneven distribution of power and privilege that can have an impact on ECE programs and those at the interpersonal level that can surface in daily relationships and interactions (NAEYC, 2019). NAEYC (2019) has presented the following goal related to addressing inequity in ECE: "to nurture a more diverse and

inclusive generation of young children who thrive through their experiences of equitable learning opportunities in early learning programs" (p. 4). NAEYC believes that through the creation of "a caring, equitable community of engaged learners" children will develop comfort and joy regarding human diversity, develop caring relationships with children from different backgrounds, recognize injustice, and act against discrimination either individually or with others (NAEYC, 2019).

Research indicates that children benefit from quality ECE. Quality ECE programs implement and provide support for activities that promote learning in early childhood. Learning occurs among children through interaction with caring adults, by engaging in "hands-on" play and experiences, by connecting new ideas and skills to what children already know, and by exploring the world around them (NAEYC, n.d.). In quality ECE programs, teachers will implement activities that promote learning in these areas, and teachers and other staff will educate and support parents in using these strategies at home.

Wechsler et al. (2018) have presented specific characteristics describing quality ECE programs:

- Rely on pedagogy and curricula that address the social-emotional and physical, as well as cognitive, dimensions of children's experiences.
- Prepare teachers to use engaging materials; to talk with, not at, children; and to design classrooms that pique children's curiosity to make sense of the world around them.
- Provide teachers with on-point mentoring and coaching for their entire careers in the field.
- Attend to children with diverse needs, including English language learners and youngsters with special needs.
- Engage families, children's primary educators, as partners in the education of their offspring.
- Provide sufficient classroom time for real learning to occur.
- Keep class sizes small and student-teacher ratios low.

- Use evaluation instruments that relate to the whole child, measure structural factors like the resources in the classroom, and assess how teachers interact with their students.

NAEYC (2019) has presented the following recommendations intended to promote a caring, equitable community of engaged learners in ECE programs:

- Uphold the unique value of each child and family.
- Recognize each child's unique strengths and support the full inclusion of all children—given differences in culture, family structure, language, racial identity, gender, abilities and disabilities, religious beliefs, or economic class.
- Develop trusting relationships with children and nurture relationships among them while building on their knowledge and skills.
- Consider the developmental, cultural, and linguistic appropriateness of the learning environment and teaching practices for each child.
- Involve children, families, and the community in the design and implementation of learning activities.
- Actively promote children's agency.
- Scaffold children's learning to achieve meaningful goals.
- Design and implement learning activities using language(s) that children understand.
- Recognize and be prepared to provide different levels of support to different children depending on what they need.
- Consider how your own biases (implicit and explicit) may be contributing to your interactions and the messages you are sending children.
- Use multitiered systems of support.

A third perspective on quality programs comes from the National Institute for Early Education Research (NIEER). This organization prepares an annual report that tracks state-funded preschool access, resources, and quality. To assess quality, NIEER has identified 10 minimum quality standards, with each standard containing both a policy and a related benchmark (Friedman-Krauss et al., 2021):

1. Policy: early learning and development standards. Benchmark: comprehensive, aligned, supported, culturally sensitive.
2. Policy: curriculum supports. Benchmark: approval process and supports.
3. Policy: teacher degree. Benchmark: bachelor's degree.
4. Policy: teacher specialized training. Benchmark: specializing in pre-K.
5. Policy: assistant teacher degree. Benchmark: child development assistant or equivalent.
6. Policy: staff professional development. Benchmark: for teachers and assistants, at least 15 hours per year, individual professional development plans, coaching.
7. Policy: maximum class size. Benchmark: 20 or lower.
8. Policy: staff-to-child ratio. Benchmark: 1:10 or better.
9. Policy: screening and referral. Benchmark: vision, hearing, and health screenings and referrals.
10. Policy: continuous quality improvement system. Benchmark: structured classroom observations; data used for program improvement.

Research demonstrates the educational, social, and financial value of high-quality ECE. The Perry and Abecedarian program evaluations are two prominent longitudinal studies that illuminate the value of high-quality ECE (Wechsler et al., 2018). The Perry program, implemented from 1961 to 1967 in Ypsilanti, Michigan, involved students randomly assigned to either an experimental group that received a high-quality program or a non-preschool control group. The intervention consisted of a 2.5-hour program on weekdays during the school year and included weekly home visits by teachers (Heckman et al., 2010). Findings from the longitudinal study that followed the Perry children until they were over 50 years old showed that, in comparison to the control group, the individuals in the experimental group scored higher on standardized tests, were less likely to experience special education placement or experience grade retention, had a higher high school graduation rate, had higher lifetime earnings at age 40 (about $150,000 higher on average), and, as adults, were less likely to be convicted of a crime (Lamy, 2013). Regarding the economic impact of the study, while there is some variation in different reports, evidence clearly indicates that the program provided a very positive return on investment. Lamy (2013) reports the lifetime return on a dollar invested in the project as 17:1, while Heckman et al. (2010) report that the range of estimated return is $7–$12 for every dollar invested. An important intergenerational outcome of the Perry Project is the impact on several hundred children whose parents were the original students in the program. While the participants in the project, as adults, did better than the students not in the Perry Project (the control group) regarding school suspension, drug issues, employment, high school graduation, and levels of college experience, the participants' children did even better than their parents related to these outcomes (Heckman & Karapakula, 2019).

The evaluation of the North Carolina–based Abecedarian Project, initiated in 1972, also involved experimental and control groups. The full-day, year-round program emphasized language development and social skills (Campbell et al., 2012). The Abecedarian children, at age 30, showed results similar to the Perry children in adulthood. The Abecedarian children in the experimental group had higher scores on standardized tests throughout their school years, were less likely to experience grade retention and special education placement, and were more likely to earn college degrees. Females in the experimental group were less likely to become teenage parents than females in the control group (Campbell et al., 2012; Lamy, 2013). The lifetime cost return for the Abecedarian program was less than the Perry Project at a rate of 3:1. For both programs, the return was calculated on increased adult earnings, increased income and sales tax revenues, reduced use of safety net programs, and savings to the criminal justice system from a reduction in crime (Lamy, 2013).

Head Start is an ECE program that has been funded by the federal government since its inception in the 1960s. The program offers activities and services that support cognitive and noncognitive development to promote school readiness for children from low-income families. The program promotes school readiness through an instructional focus on social skills, emotional well-being, language and literacy skills, mathematics, and science. The learning experiences incorporate the cultural and language heritage of children and families in relevant ways. Children's health is addressed through health and safety learning experiences, health screenings, and the provision of nutritious meals. Families are connected with medical, dental, and mental health services for their children. Head Start programs emphasize the engagement of parents and key family members as active partners in the well-being of children and their families. Most Head Start programs are offered through nonprofit organizations, schools, and community organizations (Office of Head Start, 2020). An additional program, Early Head Start, was established in 1994 to focus on parents and their children under the age of 3. This version of Head Start focuses on nurturing positive, healthy attachments between parents and caregivers and their children (Elango et al., 2016).

The Head Start Impact Study (HSIS) is recognized as an important national evaluation of Head Start programs. The randomized controlled trial was conducted from 2000 to 2008 and included 3- and 4-year-old Head Start applicants from 383 Head Start Centers in 84 program agencies across 23 states. The applicants were randomly assigned to either a treatment group with access to one year of Head Start or a control group without access to Head Start. The children and their parents were followed to the end of their third grade year to assess the impact of one year of Head Start at age 3 or 4 on children's cognitive, social-emotional, and health development and parenting practices (Lee et al. 2021).

The initial HSIS reports indicate that Head Start had beneficial impacts on multiple cognitive, social-emotional, health, and parental outcomes for the study participants at the end of Head Start, though follow-up studies indicated that the positive impact on cognitive skills dissipated early in elementary school (Montialoux, 2016). Further analyses of the HSIS data have identified important short-term and long-term benefits for children who were Head Start participants. These benefits include higher standardized test scores, decreased grade retention, increased high school graduation rates, and a lesser likelihood of teen births (Hahn et al., 2016; Kay & Pennucci, 2014). Additional findings also indicate improved longer-term education; improved health and social outcomes, including a higher likelihood of a college degree or professional license or certification; and higher adult measures for social, emotional, and behavioral development (Bauer & Schanzenback, 2016).

Lee et al. (2021), based on a systematic review of previous HSIS studies, found important differences among subgroups of students related to Head Start impact. Subgroup analyses indicate that children who had lower cognitive skills at baseline, were dual language learners, and had parents with lower levels of education experienced beneficial impacts across multiple outcomes. These outcomes were long-lasting, with some being sustained through third grade (Lee et al., 2021). Thus, Head Start appears to be beneficial over time for these students facing potential barriers to learning.

Beyond the Abecedarian, Perry, and Head Start evaluation studies, additional research supports the value and positive impact of ECE for children facing challenges. Ravitch (2014), in addressing the inequality in wealth and opportunity that presents a challenge to outcomes for young children, states that "researchers have concluded that it [ECE] is more successful in narrowing the gap than most other interventions" (p. 230). Hahn et al. (2016) reported on a meta-analysis of 59 studies conducted by Kay and Pennucci (2014) that examined the impact of ECE programs on children ages 3–4 from primarily low-income or racial and ethnic minority populations. Findings from the analysis showed increases in standardized test scores and high school graduation rates among children in the intervention group in comparison to those in the control group. In addition, the analysis showed decreases in grade retention and special education assignment for children in the intervention group in comparison to those in the control group. Regarding social outcomes, the findings showed an increase in emotional self-regulation and emotional development and a decrease in teen births and crime for the children in the intervention group. Karoly and Auger (2016), in a

RAND Corporation report described by the authors as a "compilation and critical assessment of the most rigorous evidence regarding the effects of publicly-funded preschool programs in the U.S. at the national, state, and local levels," found that the children in the programs experienced improved school readiness, lowered grade retention and special education placement, and increased graduation rates. The positive impact of the programs was highest for disadvantaged children. The study was based on the evaluation of 15 programs—1 national program (Head Start), 11 state-funded programs, and 3 district-level programs. All 15 studies utilized either random assignment or quasi-experimental design.

Research supports early childhood education and development (ECED) as a vehicle for promoting health among young children. Recognizing the importance of the education-health relationship, some ECE programs have included the provision of on-site health and social services for students and/or family members. These services can include primary care; well-child assessments; dental, hearing, and vision screening; medication management; nutrition services; parent education; and assistance to families in accessing health and social services. Friedman-Krauss et al. (2019) identified three evidence-based pathways for children's health in ECED programs. The first pathway, "Direct Effects of ECED on Child Physical and Mental Health," includes health promotion actions such as the provision of nutritious meals, opportunities for physical activity, and dental care for children in ECE programs. Focusing on parents, the second pathway, "Indirect Effects on Child's Health through Parents," refers to parent education focused on parenting skills, home visits, and health and substance abuse prevention and treatment. The third pathway, "Effects on Child Development That Lead to Improved Physical and Mental Health," is focused on educational activities that promote children's cognitive and social-emotional skills. The development of these skills increases the likelihood of academic success in elementary, middle, and high school and increases the opportunity for further education attainment. As emphasized, the attainment of higher levels of education is associated with improved adult health outcomes.

Going beyond the education, health, and social benefits, research supports the positive financial impact of quality ECE for disadvantaged children. In the late 1960s, Chicago Public Schools opened four Child-Parent Education Centers in high-poverty neighborhoods. The programs were originally offered to children 3–4 years old, and soon after opening, they expanded to include children up to third grade. Over time, children in these programs showed many of the same benefits as indicated in previous studies—higher high school graduation rates, lower rates of crime, and higher levels of economic well-being. Based on these results, cost-benefit analysis has shown that for every dollar invested there is a return of over $10 (Reynolds, 2017). García et al. (2016) posit that for each dollar spent on quality ECE for disadvantaged children, there is a return on investment of 13% per year.

Home Visiting Programs

Half a century of program evaluation research has demonstrated repeatedly that effective early childhood services can improve life outcomes for children facing adversity, produce important benefits for society, and generate positive returns on investments.   CENTER ON THE DEVELOPING CHILD (n.d.)

One method of parent education and support for new and expectant parents is home visiting programs (HVPs). HVPs link a support person—a trained nurse, a social worker, or an early childhood specialist—with new or expectant parents. The intent of the programs is to set the foundation for positive health and developmental trajectories for parents and children. The programs sometimes vary in terms of target populations, content, and the ages served, with some requiring enrollment prenatally and others enrolling children in infancy or later in early childhood. Most programs begin with a needs assessment and consist of weekly or monthly visits (Sandstrom, 2019).

Typically, HVPs provide screening, case management, family support or counseling, and parental skills training. Specific activities can include the following:

- Teaching positive parenting skills and parent-child interaction.
- Promoting early learning in the home, with an emphasis on

strong communication between parents and children that stimulate early language development.

- Screening for and responding to risk factors (e.g., depression, substance abuse, family violence, and food insecurity).
- Screening children for developmental delays and facilitating early diagnosis and intervention for autism and other developmental disabilities.
- Identifying and addressing health care needs (e.g., enrolling in Medicaid and finding a primary care physician).
- Assessing the safety of the home environment and advising parents on childproofing, such as locking up poisonous products.
- Educating pregnant women on the importance of prenatal care, nutrition, and exercise; the effects of smoking and secondhand smoke; and signs of labor.
- Supporting timely well-child visits, as well as postpartum visits with a health care provider for mothers.
- Educating parents on safe sleep, breastfeeding, immunizations, basic care (swaddling, diapering, and bathing), and how to handle sleep deprivation and stress.
- Educating parents on child development, responsive caregiving, and positive discipline practices.
- Supporting positive parent-child interactions and healthy attachment.
- Linking families to other resources to meet basic needs (e.g., housing, nutrition, education, and employment).
- Coaching parents to achieve their personal goals to better support their families (Sandstrom, 2019).

Programs receive a combination of federal, state, and foundation funding (Supplee, 2016). Based on specific criteria, the Home Visiting Evidence of Effectiveness (HomVEE) sponsored by the US Department of Health and Human Services (HHS) identified 20 home visiting models as evidence based. These programs are approved for implementation under the HHS Health, Resources and Services Administration, Maternal, Infant, and Early Childhood Home Visiting Programs. The programs have been implemented in all 50 states, the District of Columbia, 5 US territories, and 25 tribal communities. Approximately 53% of US counties have implemented evidence-based home visiting services (Sandstrom, 2019). In 2018, evidence-based HVPs were delivered by over 3,000 local agencies (National Home Visiting Resource Center, 2019). Most HVPs are intended for poor and high-risk families, while others reach out to all families within a community (Supplee, 2016).

The University of Texas Child and Family Research Partnership has identified five research-based benefits from HVPs: moms and babies are healthier, children are better prepared for school, children are safer, families are more self-sufficient, and the programs save money (Child and Family Research Partnership, 2015). HomVEE has identified the following research findings from program implementation:

- A statewide quasi-experimental study of the Kentucky HANDS program that compared participants to eligible nonparticipants found lower rates of newborn deaths (0% vs. 2%), preterm babies (11% vs. 14%), and low-birthweight babies (7% vs. 12%).
- A randomized controlled trial found that first-time pregnant women receiving nurse home visiting were less likely to have pregnancy-induced hypertension (13% vs. 20%), more likely to attempt breastfeeding (26% vs. 16%), and more likely to delay having a second baby within two years postpartum (47% vs. 36%).
- Families randomly assigned to the Family Connects nurse HVP had 50% less infant emergency medical care between birth and age 12 months than control families.
- Children participating in the Healthy Families America program had lower rates of substantiated child abuse and neglect up to two years after enrollment, compared to children in a control group.
- At 12 months postpartum, compared to control group participants, mothers who received home visits through Child FIRST demonstrated fewer depressive symptoms and lower rates of clinically concerning problems on the Parenting Stress Index

(38.1% vs. 57.6%). Child FIRST employs mental health clinicians to provide behavioral therapy to high-risk families.

- In a long-term follow-up of the Nurse-Family Partnership, an analysis of administrative records found that 1.6% of children in the control group had died before their twentieth birthday due to preventable causes (e.g., homicide) as opposed to none of the children in the treatment group (Sandstrom, 2019).

Additional research supports HVPs. The Nurse-Family Partnership is an evidence-based HVP that uses trained nurses to implement regularly scheduled visits with first-time mothers beginning early in the pregnancy and continuing through the child's second birthday. Research from random control trials shows that the programs have resulted in reductions in child abuse and neglect, less behavioral and intellectual problems and language delays among the children, less emergency room visits for injuries and poisonings, increased employment among mothers, and fewer arrests among mothers and also among children at age 15 (Nurse-Family Partnership, 2021).

Moving toward the Best Start Possible for All Children

The charge to society is to blend the skepticism of a scientist, the passion of an advocate, the pragmatism of a policy maker, the creativity of a practitioner, and the devotion of a parent—and to use existing knowledge to ensure both a decent quality of life for all of our children and a promising future for the nation.

NATIONAL RESEARCH COUNCIL ET AL. (2000)

Early childhood is the beginning of the pathway for children to progress to adulthood. It is the foundation for learning, academic success, and physical, mental, emotional, and social health and well-being throughout life. Like all stages of life, early childhood is affected by family, community, and social factors. Research and practice provide direction to parents, educators, physicians, public health professionals, decision-makers, and stakeholders to act individually and collectively to support and positively influence children during this important time of life. The following recommendations are presented to support and guide meaningful actions:

Address social injustices. As emphasized throughout this book, social injustice has an impact on both education and health. The current lives and future potential of young children can be affected by racism and other forms of systemic discrimination, poverty, lack of parental education and resources, inadequate community support and resources, and a lack of caring and empathy for all children. Advocacy for the well-being of young children will not be complete if it does not include a focus on addressing social injustices. Focusing on quality early childhood programs or the prevention of ACEs is obviously important for addressing the needs of younger children, but it is more likely to be effective if coupled with advocacy directed toward community social injustices such as racism, xenophobia, the lack of living-wage jobs, inadequate public transportation, safety and access to educational resources, and recreation. A quality early childhood program is more likely to have a greater positive impact on children if parents and community members are not affected by the challenges of injustice. Harris et al. (2017) capture the importance of promoting social justice: "Effective intervention has a powerful potential to arrest the pathway between early adversity and negative health outcomes, improving the health and well-being of children. Sustaining widespread impact, however, will require collective action by multiple sectors, with an understanding that children's health is a reflection of their socioecological realities" (p. S14).

Promote equitable access to quality ECE for all 3- and 4-year-old children as an essential component of formal education. Research clearly indicates the positive benefits of ECE. Children who have participated in high-quality ECE programs have a greater likelihood of higher standardized test scores and graduating from high school, higher lifetime earnings at age 40, a lesser likelihood of criminal involvement, and, for females, a lower rate of teen pregnancy

(Lamy, 2013). While the funding sources and current proportion of 3- and 4-year-olds in ECE programs vary by state, the national percentage is below that of many other countries (Morgan, 2019). An equitable system of funding needs to be developed involving federal, state, and local agencies so that no child in the United States is denied enrollment in a quality ECE program because of affordability.

One important consideration in moving toward universal ECE is a change in the mindset of many US citizens and decision-makers. Unlike in some other countries, many individuals in the United States do not recognize ECE as an essential component of a child's total education. In the United States, traditionally, formal education has been viewed as beginning at kindergarten. However, as research increasingly documents the life impact of ECE, this perception must change. ECE for all 3- and 4-year-old children should be viewed not as an add-on or a childcare experience but instead as an essential phase of a child's formal education. The overall essential educational experience should no longer be viewed as K–12 but as pre-K–12.

Conduct advocacy and public education campaigns. Decision-makers and all stakeholders need to be knowledgeable regarding the linkage between positive early childhood experiences and later school success and overall well-being throughout life.

Research not only demonstrates the effectiveness of a supportive, nurturing environment; positive parent interactions; and quality ECE regarding brain development, academic success, and health throughout the elementary, middle, and high school years but also supports the relationship of these factors to economic, social, and overall well-being during adulthood. Decision-makers need to develop an appreciation of the relationship between both adverse and positive early childhood experiences and the impact on school readiness, long-term school success, and positive adult health and social outcomes. It is important for these individuals to understand that investing in ECE pays long-term financial dividends—it is a meaningful and financially wise investment. The National Scientific Council, based at the Center on the Developing Child, Harvard University, recommends that policy makers view child development as a foundation for community and economic development, as children who experience positive early childhood development become essential to a prosperous and sustainable society. The council further emphasizes that supporting ECE programs is likely to be more effective and less costly than addressing issues later in life (National Scientific Council on the Developing Child, 2007).

Provide support to parents. Few would argue with the importance of parenting. Insight related to parenting is not inherited and sometimes not observed or experienced. Meaningful support enables parents to educate and support children and guide them to learning, health, and overall well-being. The following actions will provide support to improve the early childhood experiences of young children:

- Parent education. Parent education programs can help parents develop an understanding of appropriate stages of child development, the basics of brain development, the consequences of ACEs, methods of providing nurture and support to young children, activities and resources for promoting cognitive and noncognitive skills in the home environment, the importance of readiness for kindergarten, and the characteristics of a high-quality ECE program. Promoting the development of knowledge and skills in these areas will support parents in optimizing early life experiences for their children.
- HVPs. HVPs are an evidence-based strategy of supporting expectant and new parents. The programs provide screening, case management, family support, counseling, and parent skill training. Research has indicated that the programs improve the health of mothers and children, promote children's safety, improve school readiness, increase family self-sufficiency, and are positive investments for public and private funding. While programs are present across the United States, not all parents and families have access. Advocacy for the funding and provi-

sion of HVPs for all expectant and new parents is a meaningful, research-based method for parental and family support.

- Living-wage jobs that support employees in their role as parents. A common need related to many education and health issues is access to living-wage jobs. Without adequate income, parents may be forced to work two jobs or work overtime and thus lose time with their children that could be used for interaction and nurturing, reading with children, and the provision of other educational experiences. In addition, limited income can limit access to resources such as books, educational toys, and admission to children's learning centers. Another work-related consideration is paid family leave and medical and sick leave for employees. Paid family leave can be an important factor in helping parents provide a supportive, nurturing environment for children. There is no national standard in the United States for paid family leave. Some states, local jurisdictions, and private employers have expanded access for employees. The federal Family and Medical Leave Act (FMLA) requires public and private employers with 50 or more employees to provide unpaid family leave (Kaiser Family Foundation, 2020). Due to the fact that FMLA does not require paid leave, taking time away from work (without pay) is not possible for many families.

Access to health care is essential for the well-being of all families. As emphasized earlier in this chapter and throughout the book, health and education are interdependent. All family members need to have access to health care. Especially important for early childhood are services such as primary care; well-child assessments; dental, hearing, and vision screening; medication management; and assistance to families in accessing health and social services. Healthy parents are more likely to promote health among their children—and healthy children are more likely to thrive at home, in school, and in the community and enjoy success in learning and all other areas of development.

A loving, supportive, learning-oriented early childhood provides the foundation for lifelong health and well-being. The recommendations presented in this chapter require coordinated, broad-based education and advocacy efforts. Any social movement with a focus on access to quality education and health must address early childhood within its sphere of influence. Educators, physicians, public health professionals, and other stakeholders must be informed initiators, leaders, and engaged participants in moving the early childhood agenda forward.

CHAPTER 4

High School Graduation

Attending, Connecting, Succeeding

Graduating from high school is associated with a range of positive life outcomes, from better employment and income prospects to better health and life expectancy.... The benefits of graduating from high school do not stop with the individual; society also benefits in significant ways.... High school graduates are less likely to be uninsured or engage in criminal activity.   KIDSDATA (n.d.)

I NDIVIDUALS with higher levels of education are more likely to have better health outcomes as adults. Those who graduate with a high school degree have a higher quality of life and live longer than individuals who do not graduate, with the difference growing among those who have graduated from college and increasing even more with those who have advanced degrees. The education-health linkage represents a graded relationship—the greater the difference between education levels (regardless of the comparison levels), the greater the difference between likely health outcomes. Beyond health outcomes, youth who have dropped out of high school have a higher likelihood of being unemployed, having a lower annual income and living in poverty, and being involved in criminal activity (Orpinas et al., 2018). Thus, providing all students with an equal opportunity to graduate from high school is not only an education priority but also a public health priority.

Fortunately, the high school graduation rate in the United States is increasing, but further improvement is needed (Atwell et al., 2020).

Students are more likely to be academically successful and eventually graduate if they are comfortable while in school, minimize being absent, receive adult support, and experience a meaningful program of study with quality teaching. The purpose of this chapter is to analyze two important factors that have an impact on high school graduation: students' connection to school and absenteeism. Other factors that can have an impact on graduation are addressed in other chapters, including social injustices; students' health; early childhood support and education; parental, family, and community support; and the quality of schools. This chapter ends with specific recommendations that are intended to provide direction to minimize barriers and provide direction and support to increase the proportion of students who successfully graduate from high school.

High School Graduation in the United States

Dropping out of school before high school graduation is the result of a mix of factors. It is a process rather than an event. Communities and schools must develop an understanding of the multitude of factors that affect graduation in their local communities and implement strategies to provide all students with equal access to academic success and, ultimately, graduation.   BIRCH (n.d.)

Data from the National Center for Education Statistics indicate that the overall high school graduation rate in the United States for the class of 2019 reached an all-time high, with 86% of students graduating from high school within four years with a regular high school diploma. Eight states reached a 90% or higher graduation rate in 2019, with 40 states reaching an 80%–89% rate. Two states, Arizona and New Mexico, and the District of Columbia were below 80%. Though this overall steady increase is promising, important issues are present. Inequalities exist by race and ethnicity among students regarding 2019 graduation rates. While Asian / Pacific Islander students (93%) and white students (89%) scored above the national average, Hispanic students (82%), Black students (80%), and American Indian / Alaska Native students (74%) were all below the national average (National Center for Education Statistics, 2021). Data from 2018 indicate other groups of students with graduation rates below the national average: low-income students (79.5%), English language learners (68.3%), students with disabilities (67.1%), and homeless students (64%). In 2018, low-income students made up 68.5% of students who did not graduate from high school on time. A total of 2,357 high schools had graduation rates of 67% or less. The overall graduation rate for these schools was 41.8%. Disproportionate numbers of low-income, Black, and Hispanic students attended these high schools (Atwell et al., 2020). Thus, while achieving the highest graduation rate ever in the United States represents important overall improvement, it still translates to many students not graduating and facing increased chances of the personal, social, financial, and health consequences that may accompany not completing high school. Because of the adult health consequences related to education attainment, increasing graduation rates among students of color can serve as a strategy for addressing health disparities.

Few experiences in the life of school-age children do not affect their school experience, academic success, and likelihood of graduating. As already presented, students who have a positive connection to school and are not chronically absent are more likely to succeed academically and are less likely to drop out. In order for schools to initiate interventions to promote students' graduation, educators must be aware of specific factors that are associated with dropping out or staying in school. These factors are interdependent and occur over time. Hammond et al. (2007) emphasized that not graduating is not an event but a process in which factors build and compound over time.

Feldman et al. (2017), in a unique study based on oral histories from 53 students in the state of Washington, examined factors connected to students who did not graduate. Through this research three themes were identified: (1) complex intertwined factors—these included academic challenges such as lack of confidence related to school work, lack of understanding of how to study, disciplinary actions related to behavioral issues, and negative interactions with school staff and peers; (2) relationships and a sense of belonging—many students experienced trauma in transitioning from a comfortable elementary school environment to a larger, less connected middle school environment, creating a sense of not belonging; and (3) less engaging classroom teaching that appeared to be unrelated to their own lives and did not promote interest and motivation related to instruction.

Diplomas Now, an organization focused on evidence-based school improvement, has identified three research-based early warning indicators in middle and high school that are linked to nongraduation. The indicators are poor attendance, disruptive behavior, and course failure in math or English. Research has shown that students who attended the same high-poverty middle school and demonstrated one or more of the three indicators had graduation rates of 20%–30%, while those who did not demonstrate any of the indicators had graduation rates of 70% or higher (Diplomas Now, 2017).

An important factor related to graduation is support from teachers and other school staff. Fisher and Frey (2019) illuminate the importance of support: "The collective interactions we have with students convey to them their importance to us, and to the world. By investing in relationships in an intentional, invitational way, we ensure that each student understands that he or she is able and valuable" (p. 83). A systematic review of 46 research studies found an association between strong student-teacher relationships and important school outcomes such as higher levels of student academic engagement, better attendance, fewer disruptive behaviors and suspensions, and higher school graduation rates (Quin, 2017). Stanley and Plucker (2008) suggest that students should have a strong relationship with at least one adult in the school. Farrington (2017) describes those students who were unable to establish this type of relationship as "young people who were floundering around in plain view, looking for a lifeline, but who didn't seem to have anybody there to effectively reach out and grab onto them" (p. vii).

Research has identified multiple factors that affect the likelihood of students graduating from high school. A comprehensive approach is needed for schools to address these complex, often interdependent factors. Addressing school connectedness and absenteeism can provide a framework for such an approach.

School Connectedness: Feeling Good about School, Being Successful in School

Students who are confident they belong and are valued by their teachers and peers are able to engage more fully in learning. They have fewer behavioral problems, are more open to critical feedback, take advantage of learning opportunities, build important relationships and generally have more positive attitudes about their classwork and teachers. In turn, they are more likely to persevere in the face of difficulty and do better in school.   ROMERO (2018)

Few would disagree that schools should strive to maximize students' level of comfort while in school, minimize student absenteeism, promote students' sense of purpose, demonstrate quality teaching, and provide meaningful support. These actions are all elements of "school connectedness." The concept of school connectedness has received considerable attention in regard to academic success, high school graduation, and the maintenance and development of healthy behaviors. The Centers for Disease Control and Prevention (CDC), National Center for HIV/AIDS, Viral Hepatitis, STD, and TB Prevention, defines school connectedness as "the belief held by students that the adults in their school care about their learning as well as about them as individuals" (CDC, 2009a). Blum (2005) describes students who feel connected as those who feel that they belong in school, believe that teachers care about them and their learning, believe that education matters, have friends at school, believe that the discipline is fair, and have the opportunity to engage in extracurricular activities. A CDC review of various school connectedness studies found four factors that contribute the most to school connectedness: (1) adult support, (2) belonging to a positive peer group, (3) commitment to education, and (4) the school environment (CDC, 2009b).

School connectedness has received attention from both the education and public health sectors. The interdisciplinary nature of the concept was highlighted by a June 2003 conference held with support from the CDC's Division of Adolescent and School Health and the Johnson Foundation. The conference, held at the Wingspread Conference Center in Racine, Wisconsin, engaged a diverse group of education and public health leaders in a review of relevant research and in-depth discussions.

The participants included school principals and superintendents, re-searchers, representatives from national education policy organizations, and representatives from the US Departments of Defense, Education, and Health and Human Services; the White House; the CDC; and various foundations (Blum & Libbey, 2004).

A key outcome of the conference was a statement known as the Wing-spread Declaration on School Connections. The statement included six core elements intended to provide guidance to schools:

1. Student success can be improved through strengthened bonds with school.
2. In order to feel connected, students must experience high expec-tations for academic success, feel supported by staff, and feel safe in their school.
3. Critical accountability measures can be impacted by school con-nectedness such as academic performance, fighting, truancy, and dropout rates.
4. Increased school connectedness is related to educational motiva-tion, classroom engagement, and better attendance. These are then linked to higher academic achievement.
5. School connectedness is also related to lower rates of disruptive behavior, substance and tobacco use, emotional distress, and early age of first sex.
6. School connectedness can be built through fair and consistent discipline, trust among all members of the school community, high expectations from the parents and school staff, effective curriculum and teaching strategies, and students feeling con-nected to at least one member of the school staff (Blum & Libbey, 2004).

Multiple research studies support the importance of connectedness to students' health and school success. Students who report feeling con-nected to school demonstrate better attendance, higher levels of aca-demic achievement, and higher rates of high school graduation (Blum, 2005; CDC, 2018). Research also indicates that higher levels of school connectedness are linked to increased graduation rates among African

American and Latina/o students (McWhirter et al., 2018; Tomek et al., 2017). Relative to health, research has shown associations between connectedness and a lesser likelihood of emotional stress; suicide thoughts and behavior; involvement in physical violence; bullying; vandalism; alcohol, tobacco, and illicit drug use; early sexual activity; and gang activity (CDC, 2018; McCabe et al., 2022).

School connectedness has also been associated with later adult health outcomes. Based on an analysis of data from the National Longitudinal Study of Adolescent and Adult Health, Steiner et al. (2019) found associations between school connectedness during adolescence and positive adult health outcomes such as reduced emotional distress and a decreased likelihood of suicidal ideation, physical violence, victimization and perpetration, multiple sex partners, sexually transmitted infections, prescription drug misuse, and other illicit drug use. Kathleen Ethier, director of the CDC's Division of Adolescent and School Health, stated, "What happens in middle and high school doesn't stay in middle and high school. What we experience as adolescents can set us up for success—including avoiding serious health risks like drug use and STDs. Given the significance and long-lasting protective effects connectedness can have, it is important to take steps to increase this feeling of belonging at home and at school among youth" (CDC, 2020).

Students should feel good about their school experience. Obviously, school connectedness is an important factor for students to move successfully through the various levels of their education. Schools must clearly demonstrate to students that high value is placed on the elements of connectedness.

Attendance

Reducing absenteeism is a compelling indicator for education and an important ingredient for improving population health and health equity and positioning students for lifelong success.   MARTINEZ (2016)

Unfortunately, a high percentage of students in the United States are chronically absent from school on a regular basis. Frequent absenteeism not only jeopardizes a student's opportunity for academic success but also decreases the likelihood of high school graduation and well-being in adulthood. The most common definition for chronic absenteeism is missing 10% or more of the days in the school year (Patnode et al., 2018).

In addition to being less likely to graduate, students who frequently miss school are more likely to have lower standardized test scores, more likely to have lower grade point averages (GPAs), and less likely to enroll in college (Guryan et al., 2021). Based on an analysis of chronic absenteeism in New York City (NYC) public schools, students who demonstrated regular attendance were twice as likely to reach proficiency on standardized examinations as those students who missed a month or more of school (Balfanz & Byrnes, 2013). Research also indicates that students who are chronically absent are more likely to engage in risk-taking behaviors (Grinshteyn & Tony Yang, 2017) and have more limited future employment opportunities and increased mental and emotional health issues in adulthood (Askeland et al., 2015). Chronic absenteeism is more common among students of color, English language learners, and students from low-income families (Malika et al., 2021).

While absenteeism increases at the middle and high school levels, problems from chronic absenteeism can begin at the earliest elementary years. Children who are chronically absent in early elementary grades are especially vulnerable to falling behind in reading skills. This gap often increases as students move through each elementary grade. Students who are reading below grade level at the end of third grade are four times more likely to not graduate from high school than students reading at grade level (American University, 2021). A study of California students found that 61% of students with good attendance in kindergarten and first grade had proficient scores on the third grade English language arts test, compared to 41% of students who were chronically absent during one of those two school years. Only 17% of students who were chronically absent during both school years demonstrated proficiency on the test (Chang & Romero, 2008). A longitudinal study of 340,322 students in Wisconsin found that students who were chronically absent in the first grade had scores on the third grade state reading exams that were approximately 3.5% lower than the average scores for all students. The math scores on the state exam for these students were approximately

5% lower than the average scores for all students. Students of color who were chronically absent in first grade had lower average scores than other chronically absent students. Black students who were chronically absent in the first grade had average third grade reading scores that were approximately 8% lower and math scores that were approximately 11% lower than the average scores of all students. Hispanic students who were chronically absent in first grade also had scores lower than the average scores for all students (4.5% lower for reading and 7% lower for math). Scores were also lower for Native American students who were chronically absent in first grade (4.5% lower for reading and 6% lower for math) (Coelho et al., 2015). The Baltimore City School District, in an analysis of early warning indicators for nongraduation for their students, found that chronic absenteeism was the most common sixth grade indicator for students not graduating. The analysis revealed that the probability for graduation among sixth graders who missed 10 or fewer days of school was 70%, while the graduation rate for those who were chronically absent was 28.6% (Baltimore Education Research Consortium, 2011).

Many US schools experience chronic absenteeism among students. Collecting and analyzing data for absenteeism since 2020 is somewhat complicated because of the varied online instructional methods used by schools as a result of COVID-19. Even defining attendance for various online instructional formats is challenging. In 2021, Attendance Works & Everyone Graduates Center, based on an analysis of US Department of Education data from the 2017–18 school year, reported that one in six students (16%) were chronically absent during the 2017–18 school year. Chronic absence was defined as missing 10% or more of the days in the school year. Chronic absenteeism occurs for at least 20% of the student population in 27% of US schools. Among the schools in this category, 17% are elementary schools and 22% are middle schools. Further, 31% of high schools have at least 30% of students who are chronically absent. A large majority of these high schools are schools with a large percentage of low-income students. More than half of these schools have student bodies that are predominately students of color (Attendance Works & Everyone Graduates Center, 2021).

Many life factors, including social injustices, have an impact on parents and family members, young children, and their school attendance. The 2021 Attendance Works & Everyone Graduates Center report describes chronic absence as "not the result of a once-in-a-century event, but largely the continual grind of poverty and inequitable access to learning opportunities, especially for nonwhite students and students who are differently abled" (p. 4). Because of the early and ongoing impact of chronic absenteeism, schools need to have processes in place beginning at the kindergarten level to identify children at risk for or already demonstrating chronic absenteeism. It is important that the identification and intervention strategies intended for students who are chronically absent address all students, whether they are missing school for excused or unexcused absences. Either type of absence can be potentially harmful to students' success.

At all grade levels, there are numerous factors that contribute to students' frequent absenteeism. Health conditions are a frequent cause. Asthma is one of the leading health-related causes of absenteeism. Other health-related conditions linked to absenteeism include dental pain, depression, diabetes, epilepsy, influenza, and seizures (Grinshteyn & Tony Yang, 2017; Martinez, 2016). Another prominent factor linked with absenteeism is socioeconomic status. Chronic absenteeism is disproportionately present in children living in poverty. In a nationally representative study, chronic absenteeism among low-income students in kindergarten was associated with twice the negative impact on academic performance in comparison to the impact experienced by other chronically absent students (Balfanz & Byrnes, 2013). Student factors at home, including family responsibilities and lack of parent encouragement, can also contribute to missing school (Balfanz & Byrnes, 2012). Fear and embarrassment related to both face-to-face and electronic bullying have been found to be associated with absenteeism (Grinshteyn & Tony Yang, 2017). Fear has also been linked to absenteeism among lesbian, gay, bisexual, transgender, and/or queer (LGBTQ) students (Johns et al., 2019). Safety issues within school or related to travel to and from school have also been connected to fear-related absenteeism (Jordan, 2019). Homelessness and housing instability are also factors linked with chronic absenteeism. Research conducted in Michigan found that students who were homeless had the highest rate of absenteeism of all student demographic groups analyzed in the study (Erb-Downward & Watt, 2018). School refusal is another factor in absenteeism. It is described by Kearney and Bensaheb (2006) as "child-motivated refusal to attend school or difficulty attending classes or remaining in school for an entire day" (p. 3). The behavior may present itself through long periods of absence, partial absences such as skipping classes or missing part of the school day, substantial dread of going to school, and pleading with parents to support staying home from school. Refusal behavior can be linked to legitimate physical, mental, or emotional stressors or nonappropriate reasons such as spending time with friends or sleeping late (Kearney, 2003; Kearney & Bensaheb, 2006). Note that these factors related to absenteeism are not necessarily present in isolation. Multiple influencing factors can be clustered together and present a challenging intersection for children and schools.

The importance of attendance is highlighted by its inclusion in the 2015 Every Student Succeeds Act (ESSA). The law requires states to provide chronic absenteeism rates for schools in their reports to the federal government. Beyond the state reports to the federal government, 36 states and the District of Columbia now require schools to report attendance rates as a measure of school quality (Bartanen, 2020; Martinez, 2016).

Focused efforts in school districts have been shown to be effective in reducing chronic absenteeism. An NYC initiative, under the auspices of the mayor's Interagency Task Force on Chronic Absenteeism and School Attendance, resulted in reductions in chronic absenteeism in schools involved in the study (hereafter referred to as task force schools). These reductions included the following:

- Students in poverty in task force schools were less likely to be absent than those in comparison schools.
- Students from task force schools living in temporary shelter were 31% less likely to be absent than similar students from comparison schools.
- Students working with "Success Mentors" at task force schools

experienced reductions in chronic absenteeism and a higher likelihood of returning to school in the following year.

Important components of the NYC program in this citywide inter-agency effort included the use of data to identify and monitor the progress of chronically absent students, principal-led student success meetings, the connection of local community resources to schools, public accountability, and the promotion of public awareness about chronic absenteeism. Three core findings from the program were identified in the report: (1) students who stop being chronically absent experience academic improvements across the board; (2) cost-efficient, high-impact strategies exist to reduce chronic absenteeism; and (3) the multiagency, public-private partnership that provided direction to the program was able to expand and institutionalize its efforts (Balfanz & Byrnes, 2013).

Other programs experienced promising outcomes. A Philadelphia program sent postcards to families five times throughout the 2014–15 school year informing them of how many days their children had missed school. Research indicated that the communications reduced the number of students who were chronically absent by 10% (Rogers & Feller, 2018). A West Virginia program addressing middle and high schools involved weekly text messages providing information on missed assignments and absences. Among the students whose families received text messages, class attendance increased by 17% (Bergman & Chen, 2019). A program in Pittsburgh that used weekly texts to parents regarding attendance and available resources resulted in a drop in chronic absenteeism from 30% to 13% (Smythe-Leistico & Page, 2018).

Absenteeism has also been reduced through programs focused on health issues. Through the delivery of flu shots, schools in Texas that had the highest vaccination rates had the largest decreases in absences during the peak of flu season. After the opening of a student health center at the Kipp Harmony Academy in Baltimore, the school experienced a 23% drop in chronic absenteeism among students with asthma and a 30% drop among students with attention-deficit/hyperactivity disorder. Another approach to providing school health services has been through telecommunications, including interactive videoconferencing.

Telehealth has resulted in a reduction in asthma attacks in schools in Rochester, New York; a reduction in student absenteeism in schools in Texas and parents' time away from work; and a reduction in absenteeism in Sacramento, California, resulting from the provision of virtual dental care (Jordan, 2019).

Increasing Graduation Rates: Recommendations for the Path Forward

High school graduation for all students must be an important goal for school districts. Promoting school connectedness and reducing chronic absenteeism are essential actions in reaching this goal. The following recommendations are presented for consideration for school leaders and stakeholders. As will be presented in the recommendations, it is important that administrators, teachers, school staff, parents, and all other stakeholders understand the life consequences often faced by students who do not complete high school. It is also important to recognize the complex mix of factors that affect students' likelihood of academic success and graduation. These factors often surface early in a child's life and must be considered and addressed by schools when students begin their education experience. Leading and supporting all students toward graduation must begin as soon as students begin their formal school experience, whether it starts in early childhood education (ECE) or in kindergarten. Fostering movement toward graduation for all students is an important responsibility of schools that can be enhanced by community support and involvement. The following recommendations are important considerations in providing a supportive pathway toward high school graduation.

Engage Parents and Family Members as Active Partners

Parents and family caregivers should be recognized and involved as essential partners in teaching and learning and school decision-making in order to support their child's academic success. While parents will be appropriate partners for many children, for others it might be grandparents, older siblings, or other responsible adults. To maximize this partnership, the schools' relationship with parents and families must be inviting and intentional. It should be evident to all parents that schools want and support their involvement. Parents should be aware of the importance of graduation and the potential implications for children of not graduating. These include limitations on employment opportunities, the likelihood of lower income than that of high school graduates, and potential negative adult health outcomes. It is also crucial that parents clearly understand the importance of attendance as it pertains to graduation. School should make clear to parents that attendance is important at all grade levels, beginning in ECE programs or kindergarten and continuing through elementary, middle, and high school. Communication with parents must start when the child begins school and continue through all years of schooling.

Parents and family members can be involved in promoting graduation in different ways. One essential action on the part of schools is getting the parents' perspectives on their role in the partnership. Through various data-gathering methods, including group meetings, surveys, focus groups, and informal discussions, schools can gain an understanding of how regular student attendance can be supported and how the school can assist in addressing barriers to attendance. Parents and family members' perspectives can be further considered in schools through their involvement as members in school decision-making bodies such as curriculum, policy development, and hiring committees. Schools can support parents as partners by providing updates on current school news and events and parenting information through educational sessions, brochures, online sources, and traditional and social media. It is important to recognize that not all parents have equal access to participation in school activities. An important factor to consider is that, for a variety of reasons, parents may not be comfortable or feel competent in working with teachers and school administrators. Language differences can also be a barrier. It is important that schools communicate with families using translators for programs and educational sessions and present online and print information in multiple languages. Note also that time availability and transportation can be a barrier for the involvement of family members. Missing work to attend an event during regular school hours may not be feasible. A lack of accessible transportation can also be a barrier to engagement. To address these barriers, programs for parent and family engagement should be offered at varying days and times and, if needed, at an alternative location such as a neighborhood site rather than a school. The provision of transportation should be considered. Further information on parent and family engagement is presented in chapter 6.

Engage Community Stakeholders

A strong rationale has been presented for engaging community stakeholders in addressing absenteeism and school connectedness. In regard to the multifactorial challenge of school attendance, Balfanz and Byrnes (2013) stated that "the causes of chronic absenteeism are so complex and varied that no school district can tackle it alone; they include homelessness, asthma, housing mobility, familial responsibilities, fear of gangs, bullying, and parents or students who do not understand the importance of attendance or school" (p. 1). The importance of engaging community stakeholders is captured in the Attendance Works campaign, which includes "A Call to Superintendents." As part of the campaign, school superintendents are urged to mobilize the community to make attendance a widely shared civic priority (Attendance Works, n.d.). Potential stakeholders can include community residents, neighborhood leaders, elected public officials, and representatives from the business community, the faith community, public health and social service agencies, community libraries, museums, parks and recreation agencies, law enforcement, and colleges/universities, among others.

Schools and education advocates need to promote an understanding among stakeholders of the importance of school success and high school graduation; factors that support or present barriers; the economic, health, and social implications for nongraduates and the impact on communities; and the role community stakeholders can play in promoting academic success. Stakeholders can be involved in a variety of ways in supporting academic success and graduation. Similar to parent and family engagement, individuals can be involved in decision-making roles as members of curriculum, policy development, and hiring committees. Organizations and agencies, depending on their areas of expertise, can provide student mentoring, tutoring, individual and group counseling, health and social services, and sites for student out-of-school experiences and internships. Stakeholders can serve as advocates and messengers to promote a community culture that promotes equity in regard to quality education and the supports necessary for all students to be academically successful.

Research supports the engagement of community stakeholders in addressing graduation rates and chronic absenteeism. The American Public Health Association's Center for School, Health and Education's Program to Improve Graduation is designed to advance educational equity to prevent absenteeism and improve graduation rates in schools in urban communities. One of the key lessons learned from evaluation of this multischool program is the importance of multisector partnerships. All participating schools indicated that their relationship with external partners was important to their efforts (American Public Health Association, 2019). A Georgetown University / Attendance Works report on multiple school programs designed to reduce chronic absenteeism cites a team approach as an effective strategy. Based on program evaluation, the most effective models included school counselors, school nurses, parent advocates, and community partners, with principals providing coordination for the team (Jordan, 2019). The mayor's chronic absenteeism project in NYC included a diverse range of agencies, including Child Welfare Homeless Services, the Police Department, the Housing Authority, the Department of Health, and the district attorney. As previously described, the program resulted in reduced absenteeism and other academic benefits (Balfanz & Byrnes, 2013).

Use Attendance Data at All Grade Levels

Numerous programs implemented to address chronic absenteeism have cited the systematic use of data as an important component of their efforts. Precise data analysis can identify students at risk for chronic absenteeism and those who are already experiencing that status. These analyses can provide important direction for the development and implementation of interventions at all grade levels. Balfanz and Byrnes (2013), in their report on the NYC mayor's Interagency Task Force on Truancy, Chronic Absenteeism and School Engagement, emphasized the importance of data: "It cannot be overstated how important this data-sharing component of the NYC effort was to its success" (p. 10). The NYC effort used data to identify students who were chronically absent and those at potential risk for chronic absenteeism to develop preventive strategies and to evaluate strategies in real time. In addition, data were used to obtain support from nonprofit and community-based organizations to address attendance issues (Balfanz & Byrnes, 2013). A report from Attendance Works, a national organization devoted to addressing the problem of chronic absenteeism, identifies the use of data as a key strategy for successful school and district approaches to the chronic absenteeism issue (Jordan, 2019). In the report, best practice is described as checking "weekly or biweekly for students who are missing 10 percent of the school year, or about two days per month for any reason: excused or unexcused or as a result of disciplinary actions" (p. 2).

Using data to identify students who are absent early in the school year can also aid in addressing chronic absenteeism. Attendance Works has presented a three-tiered approach as a framework for school programs. The focus of Tier I is on promoting regular attendance for all students. Tier II interventions focus on students who are close to or have already missed 10% of the school year. Tier II interventions are provided to students and families with emphasis on understanding the importance of regular attendance and the development of a plan to address the attendance barriers faced by the student. Tier III is intended for students with severe attendance problems (20% or more of school days missed). Interventions in this tier usually engage agencies outside of the school such as health, housing, and social services. In addition, Tier III usually includes individual case management that addresses the students' individual attendance challenges (Jordan, 2019).

Another example of the use of data analysis occurred in the Baltimore City School District. Through analysis, the district found that the majority of students in grades K–12 (77%) missed fewer than two days of school in September. Accompanying this finding was the discovery that 8% of the students missed four or more days of school in September. An examination of attendance from October through May found that students who missed two to four days in September were five times as likely to be chronically absent as those who missed less than two days in September, while those students who missed more than four days in September were 16 times as likely (Olson, 2014). The National Association of Chronic Disease Directors (NACDD), in their 2016 report on student attendance and chronic health conditions, presented examples of schools using data to identify health-related reasons for absenteeism that provided the basis for the development of focused interventions for students. One example presented in the report is a program involving multiple school districts in Central Texas that, based on data, implemented programs to address asthma and influenza. Since the program's inception in 2011, schools in the program have experienced increased attendance. One important recommendation from the NACDD report is to include disaggregated data to examine chronic absenteeism among racial, ethnic, socioeconomic, and other groups of students (Martinez, 2016).

It is important that schools, families, and stakeholders consider all absences, both excused and nonexcused (truancy), as potentially harmful to academic success. Students missing school for understandable reasons are still vulnerable to challenges related to frequent or chronic absenteeism. Another important consideration relates to the distinction between the daily percentage of students in attendance and individual student attendance. While the daily percentage of students in attendance presents important data for schools and school districts, individual student data (number of days missed and percentage of total days missed per student) are most important in the identification of students with absenteeism issues. Schools can have high rates of overall attendance but still have individual students with chronic absenteeism.

Address Social Injustices That Affect Students' Connection to School and Attendance

If school is not a comfortable and safe setting, students are less likely to feel a sense of connectedness and more likely to be absent. Subtle or overt discrimination (racism, sexism, homophobia, transphobia, xenophobia, etc.), discriminatory school policies, bullying, fear from danger traveling to and from school and during time in school, homelessness, and poverty are among many challenges that students can face. Administrators, teachers, and other school staff members have a responsibility to connect with all students and prevent the marginalization of any students. Educational, cultural, environmental, and policy-related strategies for addressing the root causes of these challenges must be identified and implemented. The development of these strategies must involve students, school faculty and staff, parents and family members, and representatives from all segments of the community. An excellent resource from the Southern Poverty Law Center, *Critical Practices for Anti-bias Education*, identifies actions that can lead to an affirming, safe environment, including support for teachers and classrooms. These actions place an emphasis on diversity, equity, and justice; support the identity of all students; ensure safety for students to be themselves; and address anti-bias themes in education (Teaching Tolerance, 2016). Bias and discrimination, whether faced during school hours or outside of school in the community, can affect students' education. Teachers, school administrators, staff members, parents, and community partners all play a role in creating a safe, healthy, inclusive environment at the community and school levels.

Promote Student Engagement

School should be meaningful to students. Students are more likely to value their school experience and feel connected if they can link instructional content to their lives. This is more likely if instruction actively involves students in relevant learning opportunities and if their learning is assessed in a manner that allows them to demonstrate it through authentic, real-world application. Active engagement by students in learning is essential. Schools should not only be able to provide a relevant answer if students pose the question "What does this have to do with me?" but also implement teaching and learning that minimizes students' need to ask the question. Fullan et al. (2019) propose an emphasis on "deep teaching" that helps students make connections to the world, think critically, work collaboratively, and empathize. Mehta and Fine (2019), based on an in-depth study of schools, concluded that the richest learning takes place when students have opportunities to develop knowledge and skills, are vitally connected to what they are learning, and are able to demonstrate what is learned through something new and unique.

Instruction should promote meaningful dialogue between the teacher and students, as well as between individual students and groups of students. These approaches to learning are designed to both prepare students for their transition to postsecondary education and careers and provide a foundation for informed, active citizenship as current members of the school community and as current and future members of local communities, their country, and the world.

The assessment of students' learning is also important. The application of knowledge, the demonstration of skills, and the use of critical thinking and analysis, rather than knowledge acquisition, should be the focus of assessment. This approach to assessment can be based on the application of course content to actual or simulated real-world scenarios and meaningful projects rather than forced-choice exams (multiple-choice, true-false) that require extensive memorization rather than actual application.

Positive teacher-student relationships also contribute to students' connection to teaching and learning. Fisher and Frey (2019), in highlighting the importance of teacher/student relationships, present several considerations: (1) relatedness—demonstrating interest in the students' lives; (2) structure—being fair and consistent in regard to classroom policies; (3) autonomy—providing opportunities to make choices; (4) optimism—expressing the belief that all students are capable of learning; and (5) emotional support—acknowledging students' feelings and providing related support. Feldman et al. (2017) emphasize the importance of teachers gaining an understanding about the underlying factors that lead to students' problematic behaviors or academic issues. Other suggestions presented for improving the student-teacher relationship include checking in with students who are struggling, holding periodic individual meetings with all students, and implementing advisory periods or meetings with small groups of students (Feldman et al., 2017). James Ford, 2015 North Carolina Teacher of the Year, emphasized the importance of intentional caring relationships: "Our first job as teachers is to make sure that we learn our student, that we connect with them on a real level, showing respect for their culture and affirming their worthiness to receive the best education possible" (Sparks, 2019, p.8).

Student engagement in learning can also take place outside of the classroom. Various programs either outside of school or beyond the regular school day can enhance a student's learning, community engagement, and overall school experience. These programs include activities such as special-interest clubs, afterschool programs, field trips, service learning, community projects, summer programs, and other activities that promote socialization, positive interaction between students and adults, and community commitment and contribute to the development of life skills. It is essential that these activities are equally accessible to all students. Barriers related to cost, transportation, the need to work, and other issues can make it difficult for some students to participate. When planning these programs, careful consideration should be given to these potential barriers. All students or a group representative of all students should be involved in the planning process. These activities can also present opportunities for parent and community volunteers to connect with students. Volunteers should be provided with preparation to familiarize them with the goals and guidelines for the activities.

Another important avenue for student engagement is their involvement in school decision-making. Milner (2019) emphasized that students should feel that the school values their identity, aspirations, and involvement. Horace Hall (2019), a youth mentor in the Chicago Public Schools, addressed the importance of youth input in the school community, stating that it is important for educators to realize that "in order to reach students academically, they must first know where they 'live' socially, culturally, and emotionally" (p. 53). An example of this type of involvement was implemented at Theodore Roosevelt High School in Des Moines, Iowa. Students were given the opportunity to provide input on the school's mission and vision statement, its disciplinary policy, and the identification of extracurricular activities that reflect students' interests (Superville, 2019). In Canada, the Upper Canada District School Board annually conducted school culture surveys to gather the students' perspectives on various topics, including school engagement. A team including a school administrator, a teacher, and five or six student representatives met to review the data and discuss the school culture (Hardie, 2019). Another possible opportunity for student involvement is the local school board. Some school districts have included a student member on the school board in either a voting or nonvoting capacity. While certainly better than not having a student member, nonvoting status gives students a voice but does not give them full agency and lessens their role as a member. Further information on student engagement in learning is presented in chapter 5.

Provide Health and Social Services to Students

As emphasized throughout this book, education and health are interdependent. Children who are physically ill, faced with stress or trauma, or dealing with mental or emotional health issues are less likely to be able to focus on learning and more likely to miss school. Over time, this can lead to not being connected to school, chronic absence, and a higher likelihood of not graduating. For many reasons, some students may not have access to primary care to address their medical needs. The previously mentioned health issues may then not be addressed and possibly exacerbate the school problems caused by the health condition. Because of the potential impact on learning, the health issue also becomes an academic issue.

One efficient method of addressing these education and health issues is through the provision of health services. In many schools these services are provided through a school nurse. The services can include acute and emergency care, chronic and communicable disease management, family engagement, and care coordination (CDC, 2019). The National Association of School Nurses recommends that every school have one full-time school nurse present during the entire school day. In addition, the American Academy of Pediatrics Council on School Health (2013) recommends that every school district have a school physician.

In order to expand on the school health services model, an increasing number of schools are using the school-based health center (SBHC) model. SBHCs are defined as clinics that provide health services to students from pre-K through grade 12. Services may include immunizations, physical examinations, hearing and vision screening, chronic disease management, reproductive health services, behavior health screening and services, social services, oral health, and health education and counseling (Arenson et al., 2019; Beem et al., 2019). SBHC services may be offered in the school (i.e., school-based centers) or offsite (i.e., school-linked centers). Further information on school health services and SBHCs is presented in chapter 6.

Recognize Students with Regular and Improved Attendance

Providing incentives for attendance and recognition for students who either maintain or improve attendance has been presented as a possible strategy for schools. Jordan (2019) indicates that while research regarding incentives is somewhat mixed, anecdotal evidence indicates that, when done correctly, these strategies can be a motivation for reducing chronic absence. Balu and Ehrlich (2018) recommend several important considerations in regard to incentives, including not focusing on perfect attendance (could disincentivize students who miss one or two days), providing monthly or weekly rewards rather than annual rewards, and accounting for age and grade level when identifying the type of incentive. Attendance Works recommends that incentives be part of a comprehensive attendance plan. Other considerations presented by Attendance Works include offering incentives to all students, considering arrival at school on time as part of credit for attendance (students can't just show up at any time during the day and get credit for attendance), and offering recognition to parents or families for their child's attendance award. Inexpensive awards that are possible incentives include certificates; students' names on an attendance wall; special assemblies; school supplies; special lunches with teachers, school administrators, or local celebrities; and free tickets to school sporting events. In regard to the selection of incentives, opportunities should be provided for student input (Attendance Works, 2015).

Health affects education (healthy kids learn better), and education affects health (adults who attain higher levels of education have better health outcomes). School connectedness and attendance, because of their influence on academic success and high school graduation, are both education and public health issues. Advocacy or social movement efforts to ensure access to quality education for all children must include a focus on these factors that underlie academic success.

CHAPTER 5

Quality Schools

Equity, Social Justice, and Meaningful Teaching and Learning

We should fight to the last ditch to keep open the right to learn, the right to have examined in our schools not only what we believe, but what we do not believe; not only what our leaders say, what the leaders of other groups and nations, and the leaders of other centuries have said. We must insist upon this to give our children the fairness of a start which will equip them with such an array of facts and such an attitude toward truth that they can have a real chance to judge what the world is and what its greater minds have thought it might be.

W. E. B. DUBOIS, quoted in Darling-Hammond (2010)

ALL COMMUNITIES, all parents, and all students deserve quality schools. However, many individuals often look at different factors when considering the quality of schools. Their vision of a school might be affected by their view of the purpose of education, their past experiences with schools, current social issues, personal values, and their understanding of what is important in teaching and learning. The values and perceptions of individual stakeholders can influence the decisions and actions of school decision-makers such as school board members, school administrators, and teachers.

Like all complex systems, the ultimate educational outcomes of schools depend on a variety of interactions among students, parents, administrators, teachers, community members, and local, state, and national governing units. The system will more efficiently meet the needs of the students if there is general agreement on answers to questions such as the following: What does it mean for students to be educated? What is a health-promoting school? What content should be taught within the overall school curriculum? What instructional methods should be used? What are the structures, policies, people, processes, and actions that, if in place, will support teaching, learning, and the health of students and the entire school community? What should students be able to do as a result of their school experiences?

The purpose of chapters 5 and 6 is to provide informed responses to these questions. Chapter 5 presents considerations for structures, policies, people, processes, and actions that lead to quality teaching and meaningful student learning. In chapter 6, the Whole School, Whole Community, Whole Child (WSCC) model is presented as a framework and context for schools to address the interdependence of education and health and prepare students for a fulfilling life. The model includes 10 components that support students' health and learning (Birch et al., 2015). Quality schools should nurture both education and health. Health supports and promotes education, and education supports and promotes health.

Note that additional factors that affect school quality are examined in other chapters in this book. Chapter 2 focuses on equity and social justice issues that affect both education and health. Early childhood education and development and parental support are addressed in chapter 3. All schools should also prioritize promoting school connectedness, reducing absenteeism, and providing support for graduation. Suggestions for school-wide actions to address these issues are presented in chapter 4.

To begin this chapter, important considerations are presented that relate to the identification of a mission and core values that provide direction to the school's curriculum, teaching and learning approaches, school policies, the overall school environment, and the intended outcomes for students. The next section presents the dilemma of standardized testing and its potential impact on a school's mission and values and, more importantly, on curriculum content and instruction. Unfortunately, in the past 20–30 years in the United States, some have viewed students' scores on standardized tests as the only indicator for student learning and school quality, rather than it being one indicator in a mix of outcomes that demonstrate students' progress in learning and their readiness for their post–high school lives. Following the examination of standardized testing, the next section in the chapter is devoted to factors related to teaching excellence. The importance of the schools' commitment to equity and social justice is then examined in regard to its relevance to the overall school community. Directly related to social justice, the next section addresses school discipline with a focus on a restorative justice–oriented approach. Important considerations related to the school response to student trauma are then examined. The chapter ends with an overview of leadership necessary for school excellence and a detailed unpacking of school finances.

A Clear Mission: What Should Students Get Out of School?

You can mandate that people do the same thing, but you've developed a collective purpose only if there is a shared desire to move toward a common destination.

MEHTA ET AL. (2022)

In very simple terms, schools should be able to clearly articulate how students will benefit from their educational experience. In addition, all stakeholders should have a clear understanding of what students should attain from attending school in their community. Schools need to have a clear purpose for their work with students, a clear picture of how to attain their purpose, and core values that form the basis for their work. The purpose or mission should drive the content of the curriculum, the teaching methods, student assessment, and policies related to teaching, learning, health, and safety. In many schools and school districts this is presented through a mission statement, while in other schools it might be expressed in a statement of purpose. Some schools may also have a vision statement, or in some cases a vision statement without a mission statement or statement of purpose. As presented in this book, a mission statement or statement of purpose presents what a school currently values and what it is intending to accomplish at the present time. A vision statement presents a goal for the future. A school's core values can be either incorporated into a mission statement or identified as a separate listing. In whatever format the mission and core values are presented, or however they are named, it is important that these elements clearly express what is important to the school in regard to teaching and learning.

A school's purpose or mission and core values are more meaningful and durable if it is the result of a defined, inclusive process. School district and individual school leaders, parents/family members, students, community members, and other stakeholders should engage in a process to identify what knowledge, skills, and dispositions students should acquire or develop as a result of their school experiences. The knowledge, skills, and dispositions should form the basis for a clear mission statement that is supported by core values. Examples of possible core values include a commitment to equity and social justice, diversity, and inclusion; active student engagement in learning; deeper learning focused on analysis, critical thinking, problem-solving, and skill development; meaningful or authentic assessment of students' learning; and active student engagement as a member of the school community.

General agreement exists that students should master traditional academic content in subjects such as math, reading, science, and the use of technology. However, other outcomes have been identified. Ravitch (2014) suggests that students need to be able to read critically, listen carefully, weigh evidence, and make thoughtful judgments. Schneider (2017) suggests that students should leave school being able to identify personal and professional life aspirations and gain the knowledge and skills to live in and contribute to diverse communities with an understanding of the historical challenges, accomplishments, and current status of various cultures in the United States. Ayers (2004) and Sleeter (2007) believe that students' school experiences should provide them with knowledge, skills, and dispositions that will lead them to become active citizens dedicated to addressing inequity and social injustices. As presented in chapter 1, schools should consider the inclusion of "21st century skills" such as civic literacy, creativity, critical thinking, cultural competency, decision-making, and problem-solving. Based on the consideration of what content, values, and student outcomes are viewed as important, schools should craft a mission statement that indicates the commitment to preparing students for their transition from high school to postsecondary education and careers, their health and well-being, and preparing them for their role as active, informed citizens of their community, their country, and the world.

Once a mission statement is carefully developed, it must be visible to have maximal impact. A meaningful mission statement not only provides direction for how the school functions but also can be an important source of information about the schools for parents and community members. It can be prominently displayed in a common area of the school for administrators, teachers, staff, and students to see; appear on the school's social media venues; and be displayed on the school website, social media communications, and print materials. It can inform students, parents, and community members as to what is important in the education provided by the school and help them understand the expected outcomes of the school experience. In addition, it will provide direction for teaching and learning and serve as an ongoing reminder to administrators, teachers, and school staff members of the important purpose of their work.

Standardized Testing: A Limited View of Students and Their Abilities

However, over two decades of an ed-reform apparatus that has emphasized the production of math and ELA test scores over civics and learning for learning's sake has helped produce an electorate that is ignorant of constitutional democracy and thus is more vulnerable to demagoguery.   GABOR (2018)

Measurement, after all, is merely a means to an end. The deeper purpose of education is the pursuit of goodness, beauty, and justice. However we try to get there, we must not forget where we are trying to go.   SCHNEIDER (2017)

Over the past 30 years, standardized testing of students has grown in prominence in US public schools. Unfortunately, these tests have been perceived by some individuals, both within and outside of education, as a gold standard for assessing student learning and also, unfortunately, as the only factor in judging the quality of schools. It should be recognized that many education leaders and stakeholders do not place the same value on standardized testing as a way to improve student learning (Schneider, 2017).

Several key events have elevated testing within the culture of education in the United States. In the late 1970s and 1980s, questions began to surface about the rigor and quality of US schools and their standing in comparison to schools in other countries. This concern was reflected in the 1983 report *A Nation at Risk*, developed by the National Committee on Excellence in Education. The committee was convened by then US commissioner of education Terrell H. Bell. The report described US education as declining in quality and falling behind other countries. In response to this concern (which was not received with universal agreement), many states developed learning standards in various disciplines, along with statewide tests linked to the standards (Ravitch, 2014).

In 2001, the first legislation passed by the administration of President George W. Bush was No Child Left Behind (NCLB). This law was an update of the 1965 Elementary and Secondary Education Act. NCLB created a more focused emphasis regarding schools' curriculum content through its requirement that all states implement standards-based testing in math and English for all students in grades 3–8 and one year in high school. States were required to develop their own criteria for student proficiency on the tests and have 100% of students meet proficiency in all tests within 12 years of the passage of the law. This outcome turned out to be unattainable. After 12 years, no states had succeeded in having all students meet their levels of proficiency. Many individuals, including some original supporters, judged NCLB to be a failure (Schneider, 2017). The emphasis on national testing received continued support from the administration of President Barrack Obama through its education initiative Race to the Top (Ravitch, 2015).

Unfortunately, there have been negative by-products of the increased emphasis placed on testing. In some school districts, because of the narrow focus of the tests, there was increased attention paid to math and English and a decrease in attention to other subjects (Schneider, 2017). Another consequence was instruction that focused on test-taking skills, including memorization and simple math operations. This focus often eliminated or took time away from deeper learning that engaged students in important life skills such as creativity, critical thinking, writing, decision-making, and problem-solving (Darling-Hammond, 2010). Beyond this negative impact on instruction, as mentioned earlier, for many people the exam results became the sole indicator of school quality.

An additional major concern related to standardized tests is the impact of students' background and out-of-school factors on test results. Family income and parental education are two strong predictors of students' test scores. Students who throughout their school years have access to educational support and resources at home and in the community have an advantage related to performance on standardized testing (Gorski, 2018). Lower scores on tests related to college admission such as the ACT and SAT exams can affect students' opportunities for post-secondary education and possibly decrease their chances for improving their socioeconomic situation.

There has been a small step at the national level in moving toward a more diverse picture in regard to assessing teaching and learning and school quality. In 2015, a new version of the Elementary and Secondary Education Act, the Every Student Succeeds Act (ESSA), was passed by the US Congress. ESSA still required the same grade level and subject testing requirements as NCLB. However, one important difference was in the evaluation of schools. While NCLB and "Race to the Top" used only the testing results to evaluate schools, ESSA uses the test scores but also English language proficiency test scores, high school graduation rates, and one state-selected academic measure for elementary and middle schools. In addition, states select one other factor that has an impact on school quality from options such as kindergarten readiness, access to and completion of advanced coursework, college readiness, school climate and safety, and chronic absenteeism. One other important requirement for ESSA that was not present in NCLB and "Race to the Top" is parent and family involvement. ESSA requires parents or family members to be involved in the development of the state and local plans and the school district reports (Every Student Succeeds Act, 20 U.S.C. § 6301 [2015]). Thus, ESSA, while still including a focus on standardized testing, has expanded to a more holistic view of the impact of the school experience and consideration of the social factors that have an impact on teaching and learning. Hopefully these changes are leading to richer school experiences for students.

It is important to consider that students learn at different rates and best demonstrate what they learn in different ways. Standardized tests assess students at one point in time. The tests are limited in what they contribute to an overall picture of teaching and learning. As noted, factors outside of the school experience can affect test performance. The tests do not assess important skills related to deeper learning such as civic literacy, creativity, critical thinking, cultural competency, decision-making, and problem-solving. These important skills can provide the basis for more meaningful, rich student assessments such as reflective writing, individual and group projects, presentations, application exams, skill demonstrations, and portfolios. Demonstrated achievement through authentic or real-world assessments will provide a much more important and relevant measure of the quality of a school than the use of standardized test results as the primary or sole indicator.

Because of these limitations, standardized test results should not be the primary driver behind the determination of curriculum content, how students' learning is assessed, and how schools are evaluated. Schneider (2017) captures the caution that should be applied toward standardized tests: "We are well down a path that has narrowed our view of education and reduced our understanding of what it means to be a good school, and we must not follow it any further" (p. 57).

Excellence in Teaching

Excellence in teaching is multi-faceted. It is characterized by passion, empathy, professional preparation, pedagogical skill, a commitment to equity and social justice, anti-racism, a positive vision for all students, a commitment to career-long professional development, and an understanding of how schools and teaching exists within the context of the local, state, national and international milieu.   BIRCH (n.d.)

Good schools make a strong commitment to excellence in teaching. Research clearly indicates that teachers' academic background, preparation for teaching, certification status, and experience have an impact on students' achievement (Berliner & Glass, 2014; Darling-Hammond, 2010; Ravitch, 2014). Excellence is further characterized by teachers who are passionate about their job, passionate about the subject matter, and committed to playing a role in helping their students "become all that they can be" both in their present lives and in their future as post-secondary learners, community members, and professionals. While academic background, professional preparation, and certification seem to be logical requirements and are often assumed to be present in all schools, this is not always the case. In some schools, teachers are some-times assigned a limited number of classes outside of their certified sub-ject area. Though teacher certification requirements exist in all states, schools have the ability in certain situations to waive certification. Unfor-tunately, uncertified teachers are more common in financially challenged schools than those with more resources (Black, 2016).

While teachers' primary role is in the classroom, teaching and learning are affected by a variety of factors within the school community and out-side of the school. Teaching and learning should not take place in a vacuum. The following teacher roles and actions are important in the implemen-tation of quality instruction, the promotion of equity, and the provision of equal access to high-quality teaching and learning for all students.

Promoting Active Student Engagement in Learning

An important characteristic of excellence in teaching is the active engagement of students in learning. This approach is based on the prem-ise that high-level, meaningful learning is not focused on the memori-zation of facts presented through class lectures and reading assignments but instead based on skills related to the application of knowledge and deeper learning through processes such as analysis, synthesis, critical thinking, creativity, reflection, and problem-solving. Engagement should occur in an inclusive environment in which the teacher demonstrates a clear expectation that all students are capable of learning. Students should see their teachers as passionate about teaching, passionate about the subject, and committed to their well-being and academic success.

Active engagement is embedded in lessons that engage students in a variety of learning activities based on curriculum objectives that connect instruction to the lives of students and the larger world outside of the classroom. Instruction not only establishes the connection of instructional content to students' lives but also enables active engagement in current school, local community, state, national, and international events and issues. The failure to cover current events related to race, ethnicity, sexual orientation and identity, and poverty can send a message to students directly affected by these issues that school does not address issues that connect to their lives. Not covering these issues can also lead students (especially those not directly affected) to minimize the role of discrimination in US society (Brady et al., 2021). Addressing these issues can occur in classes featuring small group and whole class activities characterized by deeper learning. These activities can include students' reviews and discussion of social justice–oriented videos, articles, and books; analysis or development of various art forms that express social justice themes; and photovoice projects (Birch, 2021).

Other opportunities exist for student engagement. Griggs (2020) recommends that students be given the opportunity to be involved in advocacy activities in their school or community that have the potential to create change and set the stage for this type of involvement throughout their lives. Student engagement in advocacy can occur through the authorship of op-eds, position papers, social media messages, and analyses of political candidates' positions on specific issues (Birch, 2021). Students should also have a voice related to their thoughts on teaching and learning. On a regular basis, students should be given the opportunity to provide anonymous written feedback to teachers regarding their thoughts on their learning experience. This opportunity can be provided weekly, monthly, or at the end of each specific topic or learning unit. An important part of this feedback is that teachers, after receiving the students' input, provide a summary of the feedback to students, along with their reflective thoughts on the input, including possible adjustments in future teaching. This is an important step in validating students and their teacher as partners in teaching and learning.

Engagement is also evident in how students are evaluated. Students' progress in learning can be continually assessed throughout instruction using formative assessment techniques (assessing students' progress while they are learning). Meaningful feedback from teacher to student is provided throughout the teaching and learning process as part of the formative assessment process. Summative assessment (assessing students at the end of a teaching unit or course) is based on individual and group projects; reflective writing; the authorship of op-eds, position papers, and social media messages; expression through traditional media, social media, or the arts; skill demonstrations; and application exams rather than memory-based, forced-choice exams. Whenever possible, students should be given options for how they will demonstrate their learning. Assessments should reflect authentic (as close to real life as possible) application of the instructional content.

Social Justice–Oriented Teaching

Social justice–oriented teaching is focused not only on students' development of subject knowledge and skills but also on students' development of personal agency to address the social injustices that affect their lives and the lives of others. This approach to teaching promotes students' understanding of the societal role of power and privilege, knowledge of the historical background of social injustices, and an awareness of the personal and community assets and challenges that students bring to the classroom. Love (2019) supports this type of instruction: "Pedagogies must call out and teach students how racism, sexism, homophobia transphobia, Islamophobia, and inequality are structural, not just people behaving badly" (p. 55). Love further emphasizes that such instruction must analyze how power remains a constant though laws exist related to equality, thus enabling students to examine the systems that perpetuate injustice.

A social justice–oriented teaching and learning approach should establish the connection of content to students' lives and enable active engagement in current local, state, national, and international issues, including those that relate to inequity and social justice. Recent events in the United States have brought attention to the importance of informed citizens and the dangers of those who are not informed. These events have included the presence of elected officials and US citizens who appear to not understand and value justice and demonstrate a lack of commitment to the well-being of communities and individual members. This lack of understanding and commitment has contributed to a continuation and exacerbation of racism and other types of systemic discrimination and other social injustices. These injustices have played out in the form of police violence, election misinformation and support for policies that inhibit access to voting, lack of an empathetic immigration policy, opposition to equal access to medical care for all, the perpetuation of income and wealth gaps, inaction on environmental issues, and the nonimplementation of meaningful public health and social justice policies and practices. Specific to education, uninformed and biased elected officials have led and contributed to restrictions on social justice–oriented teaching and learning and the banning of books and instructional resources.

Several teaching models or theories have emerged that emanate from a social justice–oriented foundation and employ social justice–oriented teaching and learning experiences. Examples of these models or theories include critical race theory (CRT), culturally responsive teaching, and anti-racist teaching. All three of these models can be adapted for use in a variety of subject areas, including civics, social studies, history, health education, art, music, math, and literature. The models are not specific courses, nor do they prescribe specific instructional activities; rather, they present foundational underpinnings that provide direction for content selection and approaches to pedagogy. The three models or theories for teaching and learning are not mutually exclusive in aspects of their foundational underpinnings, instructional focus, and desired student outcomes. Teachers should view these models or theories as complimentary rather than "either-or" choices for classroom implementation.

Over the past few years, CRT has received considerable attention among elected public officials, school administrators, teachers, and the general public. Unfortunately, a considerable amount of that attention has been influenced by misinformation regarding CRT. It has been mistakenly described as an instructional method that is intended to indoctrinate students, place responsibility for the US history of systemic racism on white students, and, as a result, create discomfort among these students. In some local communities and some states, laws have been passed or policies have been implemented that restrict instruction related to the history and analysis of the past and current state of systemic racism in the United States (Sawchuk, 2021b). The NAACP Legal Defense Fund describes opposition efforts to CRT as attempts to silence discussions of systemic racism and ban the truthful teaching of American history (NAACP Legal Defense Fund, n.d.). CRT is based on the premise that racism not only is a product of individual bias and prejudice but also results from systemic racism embedded in laws, policies, and institutions (NAACP Legal Defense Fund, n.d.). CRT is intended to examine the history and impact of systemic racism in the United States and its effect on individuals and communities. It has been described by George (2021) as "not a substantive course or workshop; it is a practice. It is an approach or lens through which an educator can help students examine the role of race and racism in American society" (p. 24). Rather than a separate course, CRT is an interdisciplinary approach to teaching and learning and can be integrated into a variety of subject areas. For students of color, addressing issues related to racism, rather than ignoring them, validates their lived experiences and connects learning to an important aspect of their being (Howard, 2010).

While the majority of students in US public schools are students of color, schools, through their environment, policies, and approaches to teaching and learning, often reflect only a white American perspective. The customs, values, language, beliefs, culture, and life experiences of students of color are not reflected in this perspective and can create a disconnect from their experiences in their homes and communities (Will & Najarro, 2022). Culturally responsive teaching attempts to address this disconnect. Gay (2000) suggests that culturally responsive teaching incorporates "the cultural knowledge, prior experiences, frames of reference, and performance styles of ethnically diverse students to make learning more relevant to them. It teaches to and through the strengths of these students. It is culturally validating and affirming" (p. 29). Milner (2018) posits that instruction should relate to students' life experiences from a point of view of the students, their families, and their community. Culturally responsive teaching involves the use of teaching resources that illustrate characters and images that represent a variety of ages, genders, ethnicities, and other types of diversity. Discussions about historical and current issues and events provide students with an opportunity for critical thinking and analysis through the consideration of multiple perspectives (Will & Najarro, 2022).

Pertaining to actual teaching and learning activities, Howard (2010) recommends that culturally responsive pedagogy include "dynamic teaching practices, multicultural content, multiple means of assessment, and a philosophical view of teaching that is dedicated to nurturing student academic, social, emotional, cultural, psychological, and physiological well-being" (pp. 67–68). This approach is based on teachers and students valuing different viewpoints on topics. It provides students with opportunities to question, deconstruct, and reconstruct knowledge and offer their insights on various topics and issues (Howard, 2010). Regarding content, it is important that students are exposed to issues and topics that are both familiar to them and outside of their own worldview, cultural experiences, and belief systems (Milner, 2018).

Anti-racist teaching addresses the undoing and dismantling of systems of discrimination and oppression and promotes a commitment to social justice (Pitts, 2020). Similar to CRT and culturally responsive teaching, anti-racist teaching provides students with the opportunity to develop an understanding of the history and effects of systemic racism and other forms of discrimination and consider their potential roles as disrupters rather than perpetuators of social injustices (Alvarez, 2021). It is a philosophical and pedagogical commitment of moving students from being racist, described by Kendi (2019) as "one who is supporting a racist policy through their actions or inaction or expressing a racist idea," to a more engaged anti-racist stance, described by Kendi as "one who is supporting an antiracist policy through their actions or expressing an antiracist idea" (p. 13). Bettina Love, in her book *We Want to Do*

More Than Survive: Abolitionist Teaching and the Pursuit of Educational Freedom, presents the essence of anti-racist teaching through Bernice Johnson Reagon's compelling statement, "Anti-racist teaching is not just acknowledging that racism exists but about consciously committing to the struggle of fighting for racial justice, and it is fundamental to abolitionist teaching" (Love, 2019, p. 54). Christina Torres (2019), citing the importance of anti-racist education, suggests that anti-racist teaching can support a cultural shift that promotes the dismantling of racist beliefs and moves toward a society that no longer nurtures hate but actively challenges hateful beliefs.

Social justice–oriented teachers must know their students and their communities and understand the assets and challenges that each student brings to the classroom. Teachers should have an understanding of factors related to inequality and social injustices such as systemic racism and other forms of systemic discrimination; be committed to informing students of the accurate, honest history of oppression and privilege; and possess a repertoire of authentic instructional activities that engage students in meaningful learning. An important factor in connecting teaching to students' personal lives and social justice issues is the teacher's comfort level. The teacher's comfort and an emotionally and socially safe classroom environment will contribute to the personal comfort level among students in addressing sensitive issues related to prejudice or other social justice topics.

The ultimate goal of social justice–oriented teaching is for students to successfully apply what has been learned in the classroom to real-life situations in the present and future. Social justice–oriented teaching should prepare students to understand the past and present implications of equity, privilege, power, and systemic discrimination; analyze anti-racism and other anti-discriminatory behaviors; be informed voters; contribute to the well-being of individuals and communities; and advocate for education, health, and social justice in order to contribute to the quality of their lives and the lives of others. Lowenberg Ball captures the important potential of social justice–oriented teaching: "Teachers educate the next generation who can fight for human rights, build institutions, make laws, create knowledge and art, and imagine and make possible a just world . . . teachers can challenge power and privilege and consistently open the histories of our past so that we can achieve our shared ideals of justice and freedom . . . they can intervene on patterns of marginalization, changing our society by helping the young people whose lives they touch to thrive" (Turn and Talk, 2018, p. 10).

Teacher Advocacy for Equity and Social Justice

While a teacher's primary role is in the classroom, they can play a key role in advocacy for social justice–oriented education. Recently very visible, organized, and vocal opposition has surfaced among parents, stakeholders, and public officials regarding social justice–oriented teaching. Examples of these concerns include opposition to teaching that incorporates CRT, opposition to instruction that presents accurate portrayals of the long US history of systemic racism, and book banning. While in some cases this opposition appears to flow from personal and systemic racism and other forms of discrimination, it also emanates from a lack of understanding of the goals, content, and teaching methods related to social justice–oriented instruction. This organized opposition has led to efforts to persuade local school decision-makers and state legislatures to prohibit social justice–oriented teaching (Pendharkar, 2021; Sawchuk, 2021b; Schwartz, 2021).

Teachers can be important community advocates and educators. Teachers' commitment to their students, while focused on their work in the classroom, should not be limited to social justice issues related to teaching and learning. Beyond the classroom, teachers should be informed, committed, and in some cases collectively organized to advocate for education, health, and equitable, social justice–oriented laws, policies, and practices within their school and their community. This does not mean that teachers should devote endless hours beyond their professional responsibilities. However, teachers can present an informed voice in regard to issues related to education, health, and social justice issues that influence access to quality education for all students. Addressing systemic racism and other forms of discrimination and social injustice may have a greater collective impact on the current and future well-being of students than the highest quality of instruction.

The opportunities for teachers to present their voice outside of the classroom can take place in a variety of venues. Within the school, these advocacy opportunities might take place during faculty meetings, grade- or subject-level teacher meetings, committee meetings, individual meetings with administrators, meetings with parents, and incidental discussions with colleagues. These efforts might focus on curriculum content; teaching methods; student assessment; school policies; allocation of school resources; equal access to all school courses, programs, and activities for all students; parent and community engagement; issues related to the school environment; or social justice within and outside of the school.

Social justice issues that affect students extend beyond the school setting. An important aspect of teachers' caring for students is providing advocacy and support for addressing challenges and social injustices in the community that affect students and their school experience. At the community level, teachers can organize to educate the public about issues affecting the school and students and mobilize to influence elected and nonelected officials at the local, state, and national levels. Love (2019), in emphasizing the importance of teachers' involvement in social change, stated, "Pedagogy, regardless of its name, is useless without teachers dedicated to challenging systemic oppression with intersectional social justice" (p. 19). This approach could be reflected in work to address inequity and discrimination in the community related to race, sexual orientation, gender identity and expression, language, immigration status, poverty, ability/disability, and other identities. Teachers can also be advocates regarding community issues such as safety, living-wage jobs, housing, food security, environmental dangers, and police brutality. These issues affect students and their family members, and they ultimately affect students' school performance. Going beyond advocacy efforts, teachers, as citizens, should be well-informed voters and make efforts to gain an understanding of all candidates' positions related to education, health, and social justice.

Supporting Excellence in Teaching

Teaching and learning is evolutionary. What is known about how students learn, how schools thrive and adapt in a changing world, and the impact of social issues and change present the need for ongoing support and professional development for teachers. Schools must demonstrate how they value teachers and students by providing meaningful, ongoing professional development and supporting and rewarding excellence in teaching.   BIRCH (n.d.)

Schools and school districts should clearly demonstrate their support for teachers, as well as excellence in teaching and learning. One very clear indicator of this support is teacher salary. Teacher pay needs to be commensurate with their educational level, experience, and salaries in the best-paying school districts. All children should have teachers who are fairly and equitably compensated. Competitive salaries that reflect the importance of the work of teachers will enhance recruitment of new teachers, promote retention of current teachers, and provide teachers with the evidence that there work is valued.

Including teachers in school decision-making is a clear indicator that schools support and value the presence and voice of these professionals. Because of their ongoing observation of and interaction with students, teachers are important sources for identifying the collective and individual needs of students. Teacher leadership connects school decision-making at all levels, local, state, and national, to the everyday experiences of students. Teachers' expertise and voice are essential in school decision-making in areas such as school policies, the school curriculum, approaches to teaching and learning, student discipline, and the overall school environment (Bondono et al., 2021).

Teachers must be lifelong learners. Placing value on professional development for teachers is an essential component of a school district's support for excellence in teaching. Bryk et al. (2010), in their work with Chicago Public Schools, identified principals' support of professional development as an important element for school improvement and the enhancement of teachers' professional capabilities. It is important that these ongoing education efforts are planned with teacher input; are included as part of a coordinated effort rather than disconnected one-shot efforts; relate directly to the school's teaching and learning methods and environment; consider community and students' assets, needs, and challenges; and be designed to lead to quality, culturally responsive teaching and students' school success. Important considerations related to the quality of this support from the school or school district are the processes used for the identification and development of topics, the time allocation for teachers to engage in professional development, and teachers' perception of the value of their professional development (Darling-Hammond, 2010; Khalifa, 2018; Schneider, 2017). Khalifa (2018) presents a unique and worthwhile consideration for professional development in which teachers are allocated a certain amount of time in the community to interact with parents and community members and learn more about their students' home communities.

One example of support for professional development is time allocated for teachers to work together. Research supports teacher collaboration to analyze students' work and to review areas in which teaching and learning appear to be successful and those areas that need improvement. Through this type of professional community activity, teachers collaboratively assess students' learning and instructional needs and identify and develop effective teaching methods. Studies indicate that these opportunities promote a collective responsibility for student learning and can increase teachers' knowledge and skills and improve instruction (Darling-Hammond, 2010).

A key aspect of providing support to teachers and maintaining and improving quality instruction is the evaluation system used for teachers. It is essential that this process be viewed as a method to improve teaching and learning. The evaluation process should be comprehensive and not be based only on a few disconnected classroom observations during the school year. Hall (2019) suggests that teacher evaluation include a clear description of high-level performance, frequent and meaningful feedback, a clear account of any concerns, and consistent support and resources. Exhibits used for teacher evaluations can include multiple artifacts such as teaching units, samples of students' work, and observations and videotapes of classroom instruction accompanied by the teacher's reflection related to the instruction. The evaluation should promote insight into teaching and learning and, if needed, form the basis for a plan for improvement, including pertinent professional development.

Schools should also support the well-being of teachers and all staff members. School employee wellness is an important component of the WSCC model and is presented in detail in chapter 6.

Equity and Social Justice: The Total School Context

The cumulative effects (of institutionalized and socialized racism) are exacerbated when we do not structure schools to address the inequitable distribution of advantages and opportunities experienced by students and generations of their families outside of school. We cannot expect students to engage in learning in a system that mirrors the racial and ethnic bias that they experience on a daily basis.   SHEETZ & SENGE (2016)

The importance of social justice–oriented teaching has been emphasized. This approach to teaching will have more impact when it takes place within the context of a social justice–oriented school. Schools with a focus on equity and social justice demonstrate this commitment daily in their actions related to teaching and learning; a safe and inviting school environment; interactions with students, staff, parents, and family members; and connections with the community. The commitment can be evident to stakeholders through the school mission statement, school policies, curriculum content, teaching and learning approaches, the school discipline policy, the allocation of resources, and a parent and family engagement policy. All components of a school's operation should be developed, implemented, and evaluated with careful consideration of the impact on equity and social justice. These school components are interdependent. Examples of this interdependence include a mission statement supporting social justice–oriented teaching and learning, culturally respectful policies influencing the school environment and practices, culturally sensitive communication enhancing parent and family engagement, and the equity-based allocation of resources supporting teaching and learning, student success, and school operations. The commitment to equity and social justice must be evident to all stakeholders—students, parents and family members, teachers, staff members, and the community. The school commitment should be not only evident to all stakeholders but also institutionalized as an essential part of the school culture. It should be an ongoing component of the school's professional development plan for teachers, a consideration in the development of all policies, and an ongoing focus in the review of school data.

Many schools or school districts present their commitment in their school mission statement, vision statement, statement of core values or beliefs, or other documents. The Northshore School District in Bothell, Washington, provides an example of a strong commitment through the district's "Our Mission and Work" statement:

> WE ARE COMMITTED to supporting and sustaining an educational community that is inclusive, diverse, and equitable. The values of diversity, inclusion and equity are inextricably linked to our mission of excellence, and we embrace these values as being critical to development, learning, and success. To fully realize our mission it is imperative we recognize the institutional barriers, including racism and bias, that contribute to the pervasive, disparate educational outcomes within our school system.
>
> WE WILL TAKE ACTION to eliminate barriers as we strive for educational equity for all student groups. We expect nothing less than an accessible, multicultural community in which civility and respect are fostered, and discrimination and harassment are not tolerated. We recognize that our work to respect diversity and to include all in our community has roots in a history that has privileged certain groups while excluding and oppressing others. In our work with our schools and community, we work to address the detrimental effects of this history through our teaching, practice, training, and service.
>
> MOREOVER, WE ARE VIGILANT to advance the voices and needs of our marginalized populations, given the existing power differentials within our community and in the larger society. (Northshore School District, n.d.)

The Northshore statement not only informs stakeholders but also, just as importantly, presents direction to the school administration, teachers, and staff members. Once developed, this type of statement should be consistently and widely disseminated via school documents, websites, traditional and social media, and messages to families, as well as displayed in prominent locations within and outside of school buildings.

Equity and cultural responsiveness in teaching is a critical school responsibility. Rimmer (2016) suggests inquiry via multiple data sources as an important activity for principals, teachers, and other instructional leaders to assess factors that influence teaching and learning. Rimmer (2016) suggests some specific questions: "What are the patterns of achievement among our students? Which students are doing well? Why? How will this initiative help the low-performing students? Who is taking honors courses? Who is in special education? Who is caught in-between systems and supports? Why? Are we hearing student voices about their learning experience in our school? What are the methods we're using to hear and be in dialogue with students? Are they deep enough or authentic? How does behavior impact learning? Who is being suspended? For what reasons? What teachers are being successful with which students, within which disciplines? Why?" (p. 104).

The school curriculum must demonstrate deep learning through a multicultural lens rather than a more limited Eurocentric focus. Literature that students read should be representative of authors from diverse racial and ethnic backgrounds and present a range of viewpoints on selected topics. History should be taught in a student-engaged manner that connects the topic to the lives of all students through instruction that presents both the positive and negative aspects of US history, addressing topics such as power, privilege, oppression, and other forms of discrimination. In civics instruction, students should engage in deep learning activities that engage students in critical thinking that focuses on past and current events at the local, state, national, and global levels. All instruction should use multiple instructional methods and various student assessment strategies to provide students with the opportunity to learn through different methods and demonstrate what they have learned in different ways.

Schools must also have a process in place for monitoring the school environment regarding incidents and situations that demonstrate discrimination. The process should include methods for addressing discrimination-related transgressions. The Southern Poverty Law Center's Teaching Tolerance project developed an excellent resource for schools titled *Responding to Hate and Bias at School*. The document includes five suggestions for monitoring the school environment and responding to troubling situations:

1. "Listen, Watch and Learn." Be attentive for possible threats, slurs, tension between groups, certain students marginalized from a majority of other students, and situations that could become dangerous. Emphasis should be clear that this monitoring is the responsibility of all within the school. To support monitoring, the school should develop a reporting system that can be used by all with responsibility—students, teachers, administrators, staff, bus drivers, cafeteria staff, and so on. Areas for observation include hallways, cafeteria, playgrounds, buses, and other central areas.

2. "Stay Current, Stay Connected." Monitor appropriately all student communication, including social media. Because of privacy concerns, a policy should be in place related to monitoring student communication. The school's legal representative should be involved in the development of this policy.

3. "Set High Expectations." No hate, no disrespect, and no intimidation should be an expectation of all in the school community—this expectation should be made clear to all.

4. "Make the Most of Teachable Moments." When a discrimination, injustice, or hate-related incident occurs at school or at another school in the local community or receives public coverage, discussions should be facilitated among staff and in classrooms with students—social justice–oriented incidents should always be on the table for discussion.

5. "Speak Up." Always respond to verbal or nonverbal incidents—appropriate responses such as "we don't use that word at this

school" or "stop—that is totally wrong—we don't accept that here" can be used in response to a slur, joke, or even some type of nonverbal taunt. All members of the school community should be aware of the importance of safe responses to incidents (Willoughby, 2012).

Schools should also have a policy in place in case a bias-related incident or hate crime has occurred in the school, on school grounds, on school buses, or in some other venue connected to the school. Teaching Tolerance recommends nine considerations for this type of policy: (1) put safety first, (2) denounce the act, (3) investigate, (4) involve others, (5) work with the media, (6) provide accurate information and dispel misinformation, (7) support targeted students, (8) seek justice and avoid blame, and (9) promote healing (Willoughby, 2012).

Another key aspect of equitable and culturally responsive schools is the expectation on the part of administrators, teachers, and staff members that all students, not just advantaged students, are capable of learning. This is an underlying foundation of schools that practice an asset-based approach to education rather than a deficit approach. Fundamental to an asset-based approach is an understanding among school personnel of the institutional and structural discrimination that disadvantaged students and their families face and a recognition of the assets that these students and families can bring to their school situation, including knowledge, skills, and curiosity that are important to learning; caring for their community and an interest in addressing factors that negatively affect their lives; parental aspirations for school success; and personal goals for academic achievement and adulthood. Social justice–oriented schools recognize these assets and build on them to steer students toward school success and overall well-being.

Unfortunately, not all schools operate on an asset-based foundation. Schools using a deficit approach view disadvantaged students as facing family and community challenges and lacking the necessary knowledge, skills, and motivation to learn at the highest level. This often plays out in these students receiving lower-level instruction that emphasizes passive learning rather than active engagement and focuses primarily on basic knowledge acquisition, worksheet activities and other individual seatwork, and single-focused assessment dependent on forced-choice exams based on memorization rather than teaching, learning, and evaluation that addresses higher-level thinking and multiple methods of engaged student assessment. A deficit mindset can also lead to increased assignment of students to special education, placement in lower academic tracks, lesser access to higher-level courses, emphasis on teaching that focuses on passing tests, and decreased opportunity for student awards and recognition (Gorski, 2018). Haberman (2000), addressing this issue through the lens of students living in poverty, observed that children living in poverty often do not experience instruction that prepares them to think through complex problems, use their own creativity, and develop their consciousness to address inequity in their own lives. Burch (2001) reinforced this observation, positing that students in well-resourced school districts (overwhelmingly white) are educated to govern, while students from resource-challenged districts are educated to be governed.

Keeping Students in School: A Restorative Justice–Based Discipline Approach

Unlike punitive models for regulating schools, restorative justice practice provides school communities with the flexibility to address, confront, and resolve conflicts. . . . While there is no single answer to school discipline, studies of school based restorative justice programs unequivocally demonstrate the positive impacts of restorative justice within school communities.

GONZÁLEZ (2012)

School discipline policies and practices can negatively affect students' connectedness to school, attendance, academic performance, likelihood of high school graduation, and postsecondary opportunities. Attention has been given to the association between punitive school discipline, such as in-school and out-of-school suspension, and students' future life issues, such as dropping out of school and experiencing a higher likelihood of unemployment and incarceration (Okonofua et al., 2016). The pathway from school discipline to incarceration has been referred to as the "school-to-prison pipeline" (Collins, 2021). Bacher-Hicks et al. (2021) describe the school-to-prison pipeline as "the connection between exclusionary school punishments like suspensions and expulsions and involvement in the criminal justice system" (p. 52).

Students of color, those living in poverty, and those with disabilities are disproportionality suspended from school, overrepresented in other school disciplinary actions, and, thus, more vulnerable to the school-to-prison pipeline. Often the reason for these more frequent suspensions and disciplinary actions affecting Black students are nebulous offenses such as disrespect, defiance, disruption, excessive noise, threat, and loitering (Welsh, 2021). Keels (2020) suggests that educators often view a behavior as more defiant when acted out by a student of color than when the same behavior is demonstrated by a white student. Khalifa (2018) identifies tone and manner of speech, clothing, modes of play and competition, and perceptions of aggressiveness as specific examples of the behaviors for which students of color are more likely to be suspended than white students. In addition to being subject to more suspensions, Black students often receive longer terms of punishment than white students who have committed the same misconduct. Morris and Perry (2016), based on a review of data from Kentucky schools, concluded that suspensions were responsible for one-fifth of the racial achievement gap. Relevant to the racial disparities among students, note that the rates of suspensions and expulsions are lower among Black students when they have a Black teacher (Welsh, 2021).

The implementation of zero tolerance policies by schools has been suggested as one underlying cause of the school-to-prison pipeline. Zero tolerance policies were originally developed and initiated in the 1990s to address drug issues in schools (Skiba & Rausch, 2006). In many cases, the policies were expanded beyond drug issues to address other school discipline issues (American Psychological Association Zero Tolerance Task Force, 2008). Zero tolerance policies are based on mandatory consequences for violations of school rules without consideration of the seriousness of the behavior, mitigating circumstances, or situational context. Students who violate rules subject to zero tolerance are suspended, expelled, or, in some situations, referred to the juvenile justice system (Heitzeg, 2009).

The increased presence of police officers or school resource officers (SROs) has also been called out as a contributing factor to the school-to-prison pipeline. SROs first appeared in schools in limited numbers in the 1950s. However, in the 1990s, SROs became more common in the United States. Sawchuk (2021a) cites three factors as responsible for this increase: a rise in juvenile crime, federal funding for Community Oriented Policing Services, and the 1999 Columbine (CO) High School shooting. Further increases occurred following the Sandy Hook (CT) Elementary School shooting in 2012 and the 2018 mass shooting at Marjory Stoneman Douglas High School in Parkland, Florida (Sawchuk et al., 2021). During the 2017–18 school year, approximately 45% of schools in the United States had an SRO for at least one day per week. However, because of a distrust of policing following recent police violence, including the George Floyd murder, at least 33 school districts have eliminated police officers (Sawchuk et al., 2021).

SROs serve in a variety of roles in schools, including law enforcement, mentoring, counseling, and teaching (Sawchuk, 2021a). In some situations, SROs have engaged with students in noncriminal behaviors that were previously discipline issues dealt with by school administrators. This type of engagement with SROs increased the likelihood of students being arrested and subsequently entering the juvenile justice system (Counts et al., 2018; González, 2012). To minimize inappropriate SRO actions, the following recommendations have been presented (Counts et al., 2018; Crosse et al., 2021; Justice Policy Institute, 2011; Pigott et al., 2018):

- Determine whether SROs are necessary for the school.
- If SROs are necessary, develop a policy that clearly defines the SRO roles and responsibilities regarding engagement with students.
- Provide school-specific training for SROs.
- If available, require state SRO certification.

- Conduct ongoing evaluation related to the presence, actions, and impact on students of SROs.

Suspensions are associated with negative student outcomes, including lower student achievement (Skiba et al., 2014), higher levels of involvement with the juvenile and criminal justice systems (Fabelo et al., 2011; González, 2012), and students dropping out of school (Flannery, 2015; Noltemeyer et al., 2015). Sparks (2021), based on a review of an American Institutes for Research study that analyzed over a decade of academic and discipline data from the New York City (NYC) public schools, identified several key findings: suspensions do not improve school behavior, suspensions negatively affect students' academic success, excluding students who exhibited discipline problems does not improve learning for the rest of the students in the class, and suspensions disproportionately affect students of color, especially Black students. Beyond the actual impact during the school day, student suspensions also create a national financial consequence because of the higher likelihood of suspended students not graduating from high school. Numerous researchers have estimated substantial financial costs to government and taxpayers resulting from exclusionary discipline such as suspension and expulsion and subsequent nongraduation from high school. Based on an analysis of national data from the 2002 Education Longitudinal Study, Rumberger and Losen (2016) estimated that school suspensions among students in tenth grade alone increased the number of dropouts in the United States by more than 67,000, costing taxpayers more than $11 billion.

The attention given to the school-to-prison pipeline has generated interest in and led to an increasing presence in schools of the restorative justice approach to school discipline. Awareness is increasing among education stakeholders that punitive discipline systems do not change students' behaviors or result in students learning positive replacement behaviors (Fisher & Frey, 2019). Restorative justice has been described as "a growing social movement to institutionalize nonpunitive, relationship-centered approaches for avoiding and addressing harm, responding to violations of legal and human rights, and collaboratively solving problems" (Fronius et al., 2019, p. 1). The restorative justice approach is a whole school effort intended to bring together stakeholders, including family members, to resolve discipline issues and build, nurture, and repair relationships rather than control student misbehavior through punitive exclusionary approaches such as in-school and out-of-school suspension and expulsion (Augustine et al., 2018; González, 2012; Hopkins, 2003). It focuses on inclusionary consequences rather than exclusion, and it emphasizes communication, accountability, conflict resolution, restitution, and restoration of the school community (Augustine et al., 2018; González, 2012). Fisher and Frey (2019) posit that restorative justice helps offending students gain an awareness of harm caused by their actions and provides opportunities for them to make amends.

The restorative justice approach uses various strategies such as mediations and family and group conferences to address disciplinary situations. The conferences include both family members and members of the school community directly involved in the problem situation in an attempt to repair relationships among these individuals. Another strategy, circle conferencing, is similar to family and group conferences but goes beyond engaging only those directly involved and includes members or representatives of the broader school community who were indirectly affected or harmed by the incident (González, 2012). Participants in these processes attempt to determine a reasonable restorative sanction for the offender rather than exclusionary punitive actions. Possible restorative sanctions can include community service, restitution, apologies, or specific behavioral change agreements (Stinchcomb et al., 2006). Another important aspect of restorative justice is that it gives students a voice within the school and can serve as a real-life lesson in community justice. It is also suggested that by giving students a voice in the school disciplinary process, students will perceive it to be legitimate and fair (Morrison & Vaandering, 2012; Tyler, 2006). Others have posited that giving students agency in the process could lead to more self-regulation and greater compliance (Tyler, 2006; Zehr, 2002).

Important evaluation findings regarding the implementation of a restorative justice initiative in an urban school district emanated from a randomized control study conducted by the RAND Corporation during two academic years (2015–16 and 2016–17) in schools at all levels in the Pittsburgh (PA) Public School system. The implementation of the restorative justice initiative was led by the International Institute for Restorative Practices. Findings from the evaluation indicated that almost all staff in the intervention schools developed at least some understanding of restorative practices and used the restorative practices over the two-year implementation period, with an increase in use from the first year to the second year. Teachers in the intervention schools also reported that the intervention improved the overall school climate, including higher ratings than the control schools pertaining to conduct management, teacher leadership, school leadership, relationships with students, and overall teaching and learning conditions. Suspension rates were lower overall in the intervention schools compared to the control schools. This difference was primarily due to reductions in suspensions at the elementary grade level. The students in the restorative justice schools were less likely to be suspended and less likely to be suspended multiple times. Regarding race and socioeconomic status, fewer African American and low-income students were suspended in the intervention schools than in control schools. Though many positive findings were identified through the evaluations, academic outcomes were not improved among students in the intervention schools (Augustine et al., 2018).

In addition to the Pittsburgh evaluation, studies of Tulsa (Oklahoma) Public Schools, Denver (Colorado) Public Schools, and two public high schools in Worcester, Massachusetts, have identified reductions in suspensions after the implementation of restorative justice programs (Lewontin, 2017). Fried (2019) presents several research-based considerations for restorative justice programs. These include considering no form of suspension for addressing nonviolent misbehavior but, in some cases of violent behavior, considering time away from school as a consequence; not eliminating consequences but instead connecting the consequences to the student's processing of their misbehavior; and working with community agencies to help schools and students in addressing misbehavior and planning how to move forward.

Restorative justice approaches promote a positive school environment, give students a voice in school discipline, and keep students in school rather than suspending or expelling them from the school community. Schools should consider restorative disciplinary policies as a method to provide support for students who have engaged in inappropriate behavior and for students, teachers, and staff members directly and indirectly affected by the behavior. Rather than punitive or exclusionary in nature, disciplinary outcomes should focus on nonpunitive, relationship-centered approaches that use communication and collaboration to mediate conflict; promote a supportive, safe school environment; and result in accountability, restitution, and the restoration of the school community. The individual and school community benefits that result from a restorative justice approach to disciplining students clearly outweigh the immediate and long-term impact of students being expelled or suspended from school.

Trauma Informed and Trauma Responsive

Students can't learn unless they feel safe. When it comes to student trauma, there is much that is beyond educators' power, but there is also a great deal they can do to build a supportive and sensitive environment where students feel safe, comfortable, take risks, learn, and even heal.   MINAHAN (2019)

Unfortunately, trauma is experienced by many school-age children and adolescents. The events children face that are linked to trauma may be episodic or constant. The National Dropout Prevention Center suspects that every school has students affected by trauma, with many schools having hundreds of trauma-impacted students (Gailer et al., 2018). Childhood trauma has been described by Temkin et al. (2020) as an "actual or threatened harmful event that leads to emotional pain and overwhelms the child's ability to cope" (p. 940). Tomlinson (2020) has described trauma as "not a single thing but a constellation of symptoms and challenges of varying duration and intensity, stemming from an array of experiences" (p. 29). Children may experience trauma such as physical, sexual, and emotional abuse; emotional and physical neglect; having a mother who experienced violence; living with someone mentally ill or who abused alcohol or drugs; the incarceration of a member of their household; and the divorce or separation of parents. Chapter 3 includes an examination of a specific type of trauma, adverse childhood experiences. While examples of trauma occur within the household, experiences can also take place in a child's social environment. These can include poverty, homelessness, neighborhood violence, natural disasters and pandemics, and racism and other types of discrimination (Temkin et al., 2020). Schools can also be a site for childhood trauma. Bullying, microaggressions, biased disciplinary actions and policies, and other discrimination-based sources of trauma can occur in schools. Other experiences can also cause childhood trauma, including serious injuries or illnesses, medical procedures, and the death of a loved one. While some children may experience one traumatic event, other children may experience multiple events (Gailer et al., 2018).

Exposure to trauma can lead to issues and behaviors that affect school success and have a negative effect on overall well-being. These issues include anxiety; depression; trouble eating and sleeping; relationship problems; lack of engagement in learning; difficulty with memory, recall, and response to instruction; withdrawal and lack of connection to other students and school; frequent school absenteeism; disruptive school behavior issues; and dropping out of school (Hoover, 2019; Rumsey & Milsom, 2017).

While trauma screening in schools can identify students, it comes with challenges. These challenges can include inadequate capacity to screen all students, missing some students who have experienced trauma, and creating a situation where the screening itself can be traumatic (Gailer et al., 2018; Nadeem et al., 2021; Temkin et al., 2020). This does not imply that screening should be abandoned, but it should be conducted carefully with consideration of the noted challenges.

As with any education or public health issue, it is important to consider the social injustices such as individual and structural discrimination and poverty that underlie childhood trauma. Children of color and children living in poverty are at increased risk for experiencing trauma as a result of inequitable distribution of resources and systemic racism and oppression (Ellis, 2020; Simmons, 2020). Childhood trauma will not be dealt with in a comprehensive manner if social injustices faced by students and their families are not addressed. Earlier in this chapter, the importance of teachers implementing culturally responsive teaching and advocating for equity and social justice was emphasized. Racism and other forms of discrimination and social injustices must be addressed not only inside the classroom and school building but also in communities where students and families live. Simmons (2020) captures the importance of dealing with racism: "To ensure that all children especially Black youth have the privilege to live full lives, educators must confront racism and the resulting trauma from it. If we don't, we are not really trauma-informed or trauma-sensitive. We are just saying we are. We are just maintaining the status quo and making ourselves feel better" (p. 81).

It is also important for schools to recognize that some types of trauma may be unique to students of color and other minoritized students. Henderson et al. (2019) describe race-related trauma as occurring at both the individual and institutional levels and leading to the same physical, psychological, and social harm as other forms of trauma. Race-related trauma may include events or situations such as students being exposed to teaching and learning from a Eurocentric orientation, microaggressions, a lack of equity regarding resources, and policies and practices that disproportionately affect students of color and other minoritized students in a negative manner, including discriminatory discipline policies. It is also important that recognition be given to sources of trauma that students may face through their observation or awareness of current events such as police violence and racism among elected leaders (Simmons, 2020). Simmons (2020) emphasizes that confronting white privilege with all students is a necessary aspect of addressing race-based trauma because of its underlying role in racism.

Schools should go beyond being trauma informed and be trauma responsive. Schools that are trauma informed include administrators, teachers, and staff members who recognize that all schools can include students who are dealing with trauma, that many factors can lead to trauma, and the impact of trauma on student's overall well-being and school performance. Trauma-responsive represents systemic action including the implementation of policies and strategies that address trauma from a comprehensive school-wide approach and act to avoid re-traumatization. These actions can include providing teachers and school staff members with ongoing professional development; understanding the underlying factors related to students' trauma; being empathetic; maintaining student dignity; recognizing the assets within children, their family, and their community; building and nurturing relationships with all students; demonstrating consistency; encouraging students' engagement, voice, and agency; and collective action among school administrators, teachers, and staff members to identify and address policies, actions, and environmental factors within the school that contribute to trauma.

The National Child Traumatic Stress Network (NCTSN) recommends a multitiered system of supports and services (MTSS) in schools. Implementation of MTTS involves engagement between the schools and communities, along with partnerships with students and families. It addresses social and environmental factors and policies and social norms that affect mental health. The MTSS includes services and supports for all students, with specific attention to supporting trauma-affected students and staff members. While the number of tiers varies, a common approach is based on three tiers:

1. Universal services and supports: this tier is represented by activities that support the social, emotional, and mental health of all students whether or not they are at risk for mental health issues.
2. Selective services and supports: the focus of this tier are students identified through needs assessments and school teaming processes as being at risk for a given concern or problem.
3. Indicated services and supports: this tier is based on interventions to address the needs of student who are displaying mental health concerns, problematic behaviors, or significant functional impairment (Hoover, 2019).

Within the various tiers, NCTSN has identified the following actions for schools to implement to address trauma:

- Identifying and assessing traumatic stress
- Addressing and treating traumatic stress

- Trauma education and awareness
- Partnerships with students and families
- Creating a trauma-informed learning environment
- Cultural responsiveness
- Emergency management / crisis response
- Staff self-care and secondary traumatic stress
- School discipline policies and practices
- Cross-system collaboration and community partnerships

Outside of the school, trauma responsiveness also includes administrator, teacher, and staff commitment to addressing the social injustices in communities, states, the nation, and the world that underlie the events and situations that lead to trauma. Because trauma is often rooted in inequitable conditions, Ellis (2020) emphasizes the importance of collective action that reaches the entire community. Gorski (2020) suggests that the best approaches to addressing trauma include a commitment to helping students cope with the impact of traumatic events and confronting racism, other forms of discrimination, and oppression in the school and the community. These efforts can include schools supporting and collaborating with community organizations that address societal issues such as systemic racism and other forms of systemic discrimination, police violence, the lack of living-wage jobs, inadequate public transportation, community safety, and environmental injustices.

Leadership

Based on research since 2000, the impact of an effective principal has likely been understated, with impacts being both greater and broader than previously believed: greater in the impact on student achievement and broader in affecting other important outcomes, including teacher satisfaction and retention (especially among high-performing teachers), student attendance, and reductions in exclusionary discipline. — GRISSOM ET AL. (2021)

Earlier in the chapter, emphasis was placed on the importance of schools having a clear mission or purpose that describes what students will gain from their school experience. Additionally, the importance of excellent teaching has been presented, which is highlighted by social justice–oriented instruction, the active involvement of students in learning, and authentic student assessment. These characteristics are demonstrated within the context of a school that values social justice, is trauma responsive, and practices restorative justice–based discipline. Beyond these characteristics, there is another essential factor that must be present—outstanding school leadership. In this section, an overview is presented of several important characteristics of leadership excellence.

The Role of the Principal

Outstanding leadership in schools has a presence. People "feel" it. This presence is evident to students, teachers, staff members, parents, and community members. It shows up in the classroom, in hallways, in the cafeteria, at school events, on the playground, in meetings, and in all other locations within the school community.

A key person in this leadership climate is the principal. Based on an analysis of more than 22,000 principals in four states and two urban districts, Grissom et al. (2021) identified four principal leadership behaviors improving school outcomes: engaging in instructionally focused interactions with teachers, building a productive climate, facilitating collaboration and professional learning communities, and managing personnel and resources strategically. The research team also identified three important principal skills: (1) people skills actions that promote human development and enhance relationships such as demonstrating caring, communication, and trust; (2) instructional skills that support teachers' classroom instruction; and (3) organizational or management skills that transcend schools, such as data use, strategic thinking, and resource allocation.

The principal's passion and commitment to student success must be evident to all stakeholders. The principal's leadership can have an impact on every student and teacher in the school, as well as the overall community. Principals demonstrate important leadership in roles such as the development of a school mission statement and the identification of core values, engaging teachers and staff in shared leadership, securing the commitment of the school community to the mission and values, promoting commitment and action related to equity and social justice, recognizing the linkage between students' health and academic success, maintaining a safe and supportive environment, monitoring curriculum development and implementation, expecting and supporting excellence in teaching, leading necessary change, and actively engaging parents and community members in all aspects of the school's activities and culture. Important to a principal's leadership success are personal and interpersonal characteristics such as the ability to develop trusting relationships, strong communication skills, being able to adapt to change, practicing personal and professional reflection, a level of comfort in difficult discussions and situations, a commitment to equity and social justice, placing value on leadership development for colleagues, and practicing self-care (including nutrition, physical activity, rest, and stress management).

Building and Maintaining the School Community

An essential aspect of the leadership of the principal, teachers, and other staff members is the formation and ongoing nurturance of the school community. The school community is focused on the daily life of students, teachers, administrators, and staff in the school building but also extends to interactions and events with parents and family members, community members, and outside organizations.

A thriving school community is based on all members feeling valued by others in the community. Reciprocal respect is a requirement. It is important that schools view communities from an asset-based approach rather than a deficit approach. Similar to using an asset-based approach with students, schools look for the assets that family and community members and organizations can bring to a school rather than assuming that certain segments of a school community might not have knowledge, resources, and aspirations that would be useful to schools.

Schools must be invitational to promote accessibility and engagement. In order to maximize the benefits of family and community engagement, it is important that all members are continually informed and aware of the school's mission, how various policies and actions relate to the mission, and their role in supporting the mission. Members of the school community can be engaged in school decision-making through their role in committees and other groups and through the provision of feedback via public meetings and document and facility reviews. Another form of engagement is the open invitation and encouragement to attend events in the school. These could be classroom activities, student demonstrations of schoolwork, concerts, plays, and other activities. School leaders, staff, and teachers should also have a presence in the community. Principals and other leaders can allocate time in their schedules for meetings in locations outside of the school with community leaders and parents. It is also important to consider times that work best for participants. Work, transportation issues, and other life issues can often make attending meetings at school during the workday a challenge.

Another important feature of an engaged school community is shared leadership. Principals play a key role in facilitating shared leadership and engaging members of various segments of the school community with the opportunity to assume leadership roles. Examples of shared leadership include two teachers co-coordinating a curriculum development committee, a student or students being a member or members of a committee reviewing the school environment, and a parent serving as co-coordinator of a committee developing a school safety policy. In an engaged school community, leadership should be viewed not as a position but rather as a way of being. In this approach, the principal assumes the role of being a "leader among leaders." Further information on family and community engagement is presented in chapter 6.

Commitment to Equity and Social Justice

Social justice–oriented school leaders have an important role in working with members of the school community to institutionalize a commitment to address social injustices that affect the school environment, teaching and learning, students, teachers, parents, families, and other school community members. Principals should ensure that teachers and staff members demonstrate a recognition of the underlying impact of privilege and structural discrimination on the challenges and advantages experienced by students and members of the school community. This recognition should be evident in curriculum content and the presence of social justice–oriented teaching, the school environment, school policies and practices, and interactions with all school community members, as well as through the provision of equity and social justice–focused professional development. Teaching and learning should also reflect this type of awareness and commitment to cultural inclusivity. The Austin (TX) Public Schools, under the leadership of chief equity officer Stephanie Hawley, developed a three-question equity-focused framework for consideration before district and school decisions are finalized: (1) Are diverse voices, with actual power, represented in the process? (2) Will the solutions proposed work for marginalized populations? (3) Are there built-in accountability measures so that school leaders can see the true impact of their decisions (Samuels, 2020)?

When considering important characteristics of principals, race and ethnicity should be viewed as an important factor. The racial and ethnic diversity of principals and teachers in US schools does not reflect the diversity of students. Research conducted by Bartanen and Grissom (2019) suggests that the presence of a Black principal in a school is associated with an increased number of Black faculty members. Beyond the diversification of school faculty members, Bartanen and Grissom (2019) found that in schools with Black principals, Black students increased their math test scores at a higher rate and were less likely to experience in-school suspension. These findings were reinforced in a systematic synthesis of two decades of research on principals' impact on schools and students. The research synthesis suggests that the presence of a principal of color leads to an increase in the hiring and retention of teachers of color. In addition, students of color in schools with principals of color demonstrated a higher likelihood of placement into gifted programs (Grissom et al., 2021).

Characteristics of social justice–oriented schools were presented earlier in this chapter. Principals and other school leaders are responsible for promoting and maintaining a commitment to equity and social justice.

Data Informed

Data-informed school decision-making can provide direction to schools regarding the operationalization of best practices in many areas. Bernhardt (2015), in suggesting that data can have a positive impact on both teachers and students, stated that "schools must gather and analyze data that will help them understand where they are now as a system, why they're getting the results they're getting, and, if they're not happy with current results, how to get better results for everyone" (p. 56). One important example relates to curriculum development and teaching and learning. Relevant data can provide direction regarding curriculum content and the selection of specific teaching techniques and student assessments. These data should go beyond standardized test scores. Both quantitative and qualitative data generated from assessments of students' learning can be a source for informing this level of decision-making. These data can be used to evaluate students' success and challenges in learning and assess students' perceptions of the quality and meaning-fulness of instruction. Possible indicators of students' progress in learning can include measures related to skill development, artistic expression, social-emotional learning, "21st century skills," and postgraduation readiness for community life, higher education, and professional training. Disaggregated data can be used to examine whether differences related to teaching and learning exist among subgroups of the student population in regard to race, ethnicity, socioeconomic status, and so on. Gina Davenport, a high school principal in Maryland, in analyzing student differences, reviewed disaggregated school data pertaining to standardized test scores, graduate rates, participation in advanced courses, and disciplinary actions with teachers and staff members. The data were disaggregated by race, economic status, and language acquisition (Davenport, 2022). Data can also be used to identify problems that individual students may be experiencing with attendance. More information is presented in chapter 4 regarding the use of attendance data.

Student data can also be generated regarding the school environment and culture. Various qualitative and quantitative techniques can be used to evaluate aspects of school culture issues such as the physical and social-emotional environment, the use of school health and social services, the school schedule, the food services program, and extracurricular activities.

Beyond the use of data to inform school decision-making, data can be used to inform stakeholders. Data can provide a focal point for meetings and discussions with teachers and staff, students, parents, and community members. These meetings provide excellent forums for engaging various members of the school community and contribute to school and school district transparency. In addition, hard copies of reports and online reports based on various data can be made available for parents and community members.

Equitable School Funding: Meeting the Needs of All Students

It is astounding to observers from other countries that we spend more on the education of affluent children than poor children.   COOKSON (2013)

Funding for schools in the United States is based on federal, state, and local revenue sources. During the 2017–18 school year, the average funding allocation for public school districts was 8% from the federal government, 47% from the state, and 45% from local sources. The range of allocations among states was 4%–16% from federal sources, 31%–90% from the states, and 2%–63% from local funding (National Center for Education Statistics, 2022).

The two largest sources of federal funding for public schools are the Title I program and Individuals with Disabilities Education Act (IDEA). Title I funding provides educational support for students who are economically disadvantaged, while IDEA funding is used to support educational programs for students with disabilities. A variety of other sources of federal funds are provided to public schools to support English language learners, professional development, teacher quality, reading programs, student support, and career and technical education (Edgenuity, n.d.).

While federal funding is a necessity, the largest portions of public school funding come from state and local sources. States use different criteria for determining the amount of their budget that will fund education and employ different methods for the allocation of funds to local school districts. Typically, state funding is based on factors such as the number of students in a school district, special education needs, programs for English language learners, support of at-risk and gifted and talented students, and the unique needs of districts such as small size or higher regional costs (Education Commission of the States, 2019). In many states, equity is not a consideration in providing funding to local school districts. Only 25 states provide higher levels of funding to high-poverty school districts than to low-poverty school districts.

Most school districts in the United States receive a considerable portion of their local funding from community property taxes. For the 2017–18 school year, an average of 81% of local public-school funding came from property taxes. Other local revenue sources include investments, student fees, food services revenues, and contributions (National Center for Education Statistics, 2022). Thus, those districts that have higher property tax bases and wealthier residents bring in more local money for school spending than less affluent districts.

Differences in the amounts of private funding can present disparities among school districts. In 2014 the Kohler School District in Wisconsin generated $863 per pupil in private contributions, while in the neighboring Sheboygan Falls district private contributions accounted for $27 per pupil (Lloyd & Harwin, 2019). Parent-teacher associations (PTAs) can serve as a source of disparities in private funding for public schools. In NYC, the Public School 87 PTA, located on the Upper West Side in Manhattan, generated over $1.5 million in revenue. This is considerably higher than the PTA funds generated in other NYC public schools (Goldstein, 2017). Several school districts, including those in Seattle, Washington, Portland, Oregon, and Evanston, Illinois, have attempted to reduce PTA funding disparities among district schools. Using different formulas and funding allocation, these districts have implemented models in which a percentage of funds raised in well-resourced schools is shared with schools that receive lesser PTA funding (Cope, 2019).

The amount of funding that schools receive and allocate toward students makes a difference. Baker (2016) stated that rigorous evidence shows that "substantive and sustained state school finance reforms" are important for improving both the level and distribution of short-term and long-term student outcomes (p. 6). Multiple studies demonstrate specific results that indicate that increases in school funding are associated with higher graduation rates, increased college enrollment, improved education outcomes for children from low-income families, higher adult wages, and less adult poverty. Common uses of the increased funding included increases in teacher salaries, with accompanying increases in teacher retention, and the hiring of additional teachers, in order to lower student-teacher ratios (Barnum, 2019; Jackson et al., 2016).

While some federal and state funding streams have attempted to eliminate gaps between districts, often these funds are only sufficient to reduce gaps rather than eliminate them (Cascio & Reber, 2013). Disparities in the funding received by school districts continue to exist at the local level and continue to play a role in perpetuating inequality. A 2018 Education Trust report shows that students educated in high-poverty districts receive approximately $1,000 less per pupil than students in districts with less poverty. School districts serving large populations of Black, Latino, and American Indian students average about $1,800 less per student than students in districts serving fewer students of color (Morgan & Amerikaner, 2018). This inequity often results in lower-paid and less experienced teachers, a higher proportion of uncertified teachers, larger class size, less connection between individual students and teachers, and lesser and lower-quality instructional resources (Darling-Hammond, 2010; Gorski, 2018). It also contributes to a continuation of discrimination and racism in education and a perpetuation of intergenerational poverty.

Various leaders in education have acknowledged that while equitable funding is essential, how money is used is also of great importance (Lesley, 2018). Additional funding is especially important when it is used to decrease student-to-teacher ratios and increase teacher salaries (Jackson et al., 2016).

All students deserve an equal opportunity to receive the optimal benefit from their school experience. Equitable federal, state, and local funding is an important consideration in providing equal opportunity.

Some school districts, schools, and students will need more financial support than others.

To address the current funding inequity and provide all students in the United States with an equal opportunity for quality education, the following recommendations are posed for advocates, policy makers, education leaders, parents, and community members:

- All stakeholders should gain an understanding of how schools are funded in the United States and in their local school district and consider the relationship between equity in funding and equality in opportunity.
- Additional federal and state funding should be provided to address the past and current inequity in per-pupil spending at the local funding level. Education support and quality should be based on equity and school and student needs rather than where students live.
- Funding within local school districts, including most or all private funding, should be allocated through an equity lens with amounts based on school and students' needs.
- The allocation of discretionary funding at the local level should, whenever possible, be evidence based or reflect best practices determined through input from thought leaders in education, administrators, teachers, and other stakeholders, including students, parents, families, and community members.

Equity in resources and equality in opportunity should be the bottom-line consideration in school funding decisions. Diane Ravitch (2010), a thought leader in education, addressed the issue of inequality: "We should work toward a national consensus that prioritizes equitable resources for schools. At present, many of our states base funding on property taxes and affluent districts have far more per-pupil allocations than urban districts, where students are far needier. We are one of the few nations in the world that spends more on affluent students than poor students. That is wrong" (p. 250).

All students deserve equal access to quality schools that engage them in meaningful teaching and learning and extracurricular experiences.

Schools should prepare students to attain their post–high school aspirations and to be engaged citizens who are active contributors to healthy, socially just communities. Advocates from the education–medical–public health sectors must have an awareness of the characteristics of schools that can accomplish these outcomes.

CHAPTER 6

The Whole School, Whole Community, Whole Child Model

A Commitment to Health and Learning

Health and education are related. They are interrelated. They are symbiotic. There is a connection between the two sectors. When one fails, so does the other. When one succeeds, that success feeds the other. We do not just have an isolated duty to want the child to be healthy and educated—we have a moral imperative.

GENE CARTER, former executive director and CEO of ASCD,
quoted in ASCD (2014)

A CONSISTENT MESSAGE throughout this book has been the importance of recognition of the reciprocal relationship between education and health. Healthy students are more likely to be academically successful, graduate from high school, and attend college or engage in some type of post–high school education or training (Allensworth, 2015). Research clearly indicates that as adults achieve higher levels of education, they are more likely to have better adult health outcomes (Institute of Medicine, 2015).

Because of this reciprocal relationship, schools should view health and learning as inseparable. Students are more likely to achieve academic success if health issues are recognized and addressed by schools. Chapter 5 emphasized the importance of a relevant mission, excellence in teaching, equity and a social justice focus, trauma responsiveness, restorative justice–based discipline, leadership, and equitable funding as important considerations for school success. The health of students is linked to all of these considerations.

The focus of this chapter is on the Whole School, Whole Community, Whole Child (WSCC) model. This model enables schools to place emphasis on health and education as essential interdependent priorities. The development of the WSCC model was initiated in 2013 by ASCD and the Centers for Disease Control and Prevention (CDC). Leaders in education, public health, and school health were identified by the two organizations to engage in the developmental process for the new model. Upon finalization, the new WSCC model was introduced at the 2014 ASCD national conference and the 2014 Society for Public Health Education (SOPHE) national conference. The WSCC model evolved from a combination and expansion of two existing models: the Coordinated School Health (CSH) model promoted by the CDC and first presented by health education leaders Diane Allensworth and Lloyd Kolbe in the late 1980s, and the ASCD Whole Child approach first presented in 2007 (Birch & Videto, 2015).

The Origin of WSCC: Coordinated School Health and the Whole Child Approach

The CSH model was presented in a special issue of the *Journal of School Health* in December 1987 (the original term "Comprehensive" was later replaced by "Coordinated" when referring to CSH). In the introductory article of the journal, Allensworth and Kolbe (1987) presented an overview of the new approach to school health. The model included eight components:

1. School health services
2. School health education
3. School health environment
4. Integrated school and community health promotion efforts
5. School physical education
6. School food service
7. School counseling
8. School site health promotion programs for faculty and staff

The journal also included articles written by invited national leaders that addressed each of the eight components. Two important principles were presented in the overview article: the need for collaboration by professionals representing the various components of CSH in the planning and implementation of health programs for students, and the linkage between positive health behaviors and students' academic achievement (Birch & Videto, 2015). Though CSH received national attention in the late 1980s, and the CDC's Division of Adolescent and School Health funding was provided to selected state departments of education, state departments of health, and nongovernmental organizations, implementation in local school districts was less than optimal. A possible contributing factor for this limited implementation on the local level was that school administrators and leaders viewed CSH as focusing only on health outcomes, rather than being a program that also supported academic outcomes (Allensworth, 2015). To emphasize the inclusive and coordinated nature of the model, Allensworth (1994) identified the following strategies:

- Coordinating the efforts of all faculty, staff, and administration by focusing on priority behaviors interfering with learning and well-being within a school or school district.
- Coordinating programming with interdisciplinary and interagency work teams, and using the program planning process in a cycle of continuous improvement.
- Enhancing health instruction through a health promotion model using strategies such as policy, environmental change, role modeling, social support, and media.
- Addressing structural and environmental changes, as well as lifestyle changes.
- Providing staff development to enhance professional skills.
- Ensuring that all students have access to needed services.
- Viewing students as resources by soliciting their involvement in health promotion initiatives.

The Whole Child Initiative: An Overview

ASCD, in 2006, convened the Commission on the Whole Child (ASCD, 2007). Members of the commission included thought leaders, researchers, and practitioners from a variety of disciplines. The commission's charge was to change the definition of a successful learner from being based entirely on academic test scores to one that reflects more holistic or well-rounded outcomes. Based on the work of the commission, the ASCD Whole Child Initiative was introduced in 2007 (Slade, 2015a). The initiative called on communities, educators, and key decision-makers to work together to develop and implement policies that would result in students who are knowledgeable, emotionally and physically healthy, civically active, artistically engaged, prepared for economic self-sufficiency, and ready for adulthood (Allensworth, 2015). A key element of the ASCD Whole Child approach were five tenets identified as necessary for health and learning:

1. Healthy—each student enters school healthy and learns about and practices a heathy lifestyle.
2. Safe—each student learns in an environment that is physically and emotionally safe for students and adults.
3. Engaged—each student is actively engaged in learning and is connected to the school and broader community.
4. Supported—each student has access to personalized learning and to qualified and caring adults.
5. Challenged—each student is challenged academically and prepared for success in college or further study and for employment and participation in a global environment (Slade, 2015b).

To initiate or enhance the implementation of the Whole Child concept, 10 indicators were developed for each tenet. The indicators were developed to provide direction for schools to assess needs, analyze assets, and plan for improved health and education alignment (Slade, 2015a). The 10 indicators are presented later in this chapter.

The WSCC Framework

> The more that education can see its role as expanding beyond mere academic achievement to social emotional, mental, and physical development and the more that health can see how it plays a critical role in aiding the functions of education, the greater the benefit will be for the development and growth of our youth. Each sector along with the critical roles of individual community members and organizations serves the same youth in the same location.   SLADE (2015b)

As previously stated, in 2013 ASCD and the CDC initiated the development of a new model designed to promote students' health and academic success in schools. A consultation group developed drafts of the model and related documents. These products were continually reviewed for feedback by a second group of individuals, the review group. Both groups consisted of leaders in both education and health (Birch & Videto, 2015). The result of this collaboration was the WSCC model.

The WSCC model combines and builds on the components of CSH and the tenets of the ASCD Whole Child model. WSCC is designed to engage the whole school in the promotion of health and learning through policies, processes, and practices. The child is at the center of the model, and the model itself is placed within the entire community. It includes 10 components, indicating an expansion of the original eight-component CSH model. Its placement within the community demonstrates that education and health in schools should be supported and influenced by the entire community (Slade, 2015b). In presenting an overview of WSCC, ASCD (2014) describes the new framework as an "ecological approach directed at the whole school; the school draws its resources and influences from the whole community and serves to address the needs of the whole child" (p. 6). A diagrammatic representation of the WSCC framework is presented in figure 6.1.

The Child at the Center

As represented in figure 6.1, the center of the model features a depiction of a child engaged in movement. The child represents something obvious but also something that is not given an adequate level of

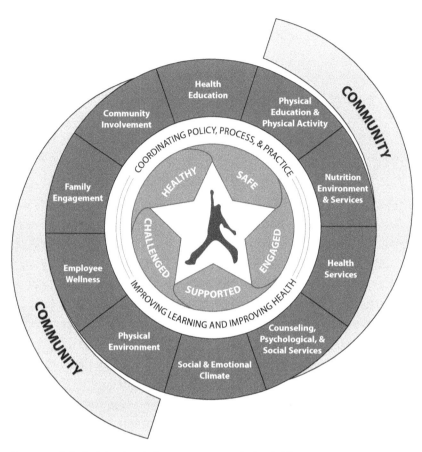

Figure 6.1. Whole School, Whole Community, Whole Child (WSCC) Model.
SOURCE: Centers for Disease Control and Prevention. (2021). *Whole School, Whole Community, Whole Child.* US Department of Health and Human Services. https://www.cdc.gov/healthyschools/wscc/index.htm

attention—the well-being of children and youth should be the primary focus for all school decisions regarding policies, processes, curricula, teaching and learning, the school environment, and the allocation of resources.

Having students at the center of the model that is focused on developing the whole child also validates the importance of promoting students' agency in school and community decision-making. Examples of opportunities for students to be engaged in these activities include service on school committees, the school board, and community committees. Classroom instruction in all subjects can inform students and engage them in the analysis of local, state, national, and global issues. This instruction can address current issues through student-centered activities such as the review of relevant social and traditional media; the analysis or development of various issue-related art forms; the authorship of op-eds, position papers, and social media messages; photovoice projects; engagement in advocacy; and the analysis of the positions of elected officials and candidates for elected office (Birch, 2021).

The Five Tenets

The five tenets—healthy, safe, engaged, supported, and challenged—can serve as a focal point for school or curriculum decision-making, as strategic goals and outcomes, as a framework for policies and processes, or as the definition of key components of a whole child approach to education. Ten indicators have been identified for each tenet:

Tenet 1: Healthy
1. Our school culture supports and reinforces the health and well-being of each student.
2. Our school health education curriculum and instruction support and reinforce the health and well-being of each student by addressing the physical, mental, emotional, and social dimensions of health.
3. Our school physical education schedule, curriculum, and instruction support and reinforce the health and well-being of each student by addressing lifetime fitness knowledge, attitudes, behaviors, and skills.
4. Our school facility and environment support and reinforce the health and well-being of each student and staff member.
5. Our school addresses the health and well-being of each staff member.
6. Our school collaborates with parents and the local community to promote the health and well-being of each student.
7. Our school integrates health and well-being into the school's ongoing activities, professional development, curriculum, and assessment practices.

8. Our school sets realistic goals for student and staff health that are built on accurate data and sound science.

9. Our school facilitates student and staff access to health, mental health, and dental services.

10. Our school supports, promotes, and reinforces healthy eating patterns and food safety in routine food services and special programming and events for students and staff (ASCD, n.d.-c).

Tenet 2: Safe

1. Our school building, grounds, playground equipment, and vehicles are secure and meet all established safety and environmental standards.

2. Our school physical plant is attractive; is structurally sound; has good internal (hallways) and external (pedestrian, bicycle, and motor vehicle) traffic flow, including for those with special needs; and is free of defects.

3. Our physical, emotional, academic, and social school climate is safe, friendly, and student centered.

4. Our students feel valued, respected, and cared for and are motivated to learn.

5. Our school staff, students, and family members establish and maintain school and classroom behavioral expectations, rules, and routines that teach students how to manage their behavior and help students improve problem behavior.

6. Our school provides our students, staff, and family members with regular opportunities for learning and support in teaching students how to manage their own behavior and reinforcing expectations, rules, and routines.

7. Our school teaches, models, and provides opportunities to practice social-emotional skills, including effective listening, conflict resolution, problem-solving, personal reflection and responsibility, and ethical decision-making.

8. Our school upholds social justice and equity concepts and practices mutual respect for individual differences at all levels

of school interactions—student to student, adult to student, and adult to adult.

9. Our school climate, curriculum, and instruction reflect both high expectations and an understanding of child and adolescent growth and development.

10. Our teachers and staff develop and implement academic and behavioral interventions based on an understanding of child and adolescent development and learning theories (ASCD, n.d.-d).

Tenet 3: Engaged

1. Our teachers use active learning strategies, such as cooperative learning and project-based learning.

2. Our school offers a range of opportunities for students to contribute to and learn within the community at large, including service learning, internships, apprenticeships, and volunteer projects.

3. Our school policies and climate reinforce citizenship and civic behaviors by students, family members, and staff and include meaningful participation in decision-making.

4. Our school uses curriculum-related experiences such as field trips and outreach projects to complement and extend our curriculum and instruction.

5. Each student in our school has access to a range of options and choices for a wide array of extracurricular and cocurricular activities that reflect student interests, goals, and learning profiles.

6. Our curriculum and instruction promote students' understanding of the real-world, global relevance and application of learned content.

7. Our teachers use a range of inquiry-based, experiential learning tasks and activities to help all students deepen their understanding of what they are learning and why they are learning it.

8. Our staff works closely with students to help them monitor and direct their own progress.

9. Our school expects and prepares students to assume age-appropriate responsibility for learning through effective decision-making, goal setting, and time management.
10. Our school supports, promotes, and reinforces responsible environmental habits through recycling, trash management, sustainable energy, and other efforts (ASCD, n.d.-b).

Tenet 4: Supported
1. Our school personalizes learning, including the flexible use of time and scheduling to meet academic and social goals for each student.
2. Our teachers use a range of diagnostic, formative, and summative assessment tasks to monitor student progress, provide timely feedback, and adjust teaching and learning activities to maximize student progress.
3. Our school ensures that adult-student relationships support and encourage each student's academic and personal growth.
4. Each student has access to school counselors and other structured academic, social, and emotional support systems.
5. Our school staff understands and makes curricular, instructional, and school improvement decisions based on child and adolescent development and student performance information.
6. Our school personnel welcome and include all families as partners in their children's education and significant members of the school community.
7. Our school uses a variety of methods across languages and cultures to communicate with all families and community members about the school's vision, mission, goals, activities, and opportunities for students.
8. Our school helps families understand available services, advocate for their children's needs, and support their children's learning.
9. Every member of our school staff is well qualified and properly credentialed.
10. All adults who interact with students both within the school

and through extracurricular, cocurricular, and community-based experiences teach and model prosocial behavior (ASCD, n.d.-e).

Tenet 5: Challenged

1. Each student in our school has access to challenging, comprehensive curriculum in all content areas.
2. Our curriculum and instruction provide opportunities for students to develop critical thinking and reasoning skills, problem-solving competencies, and technology proficiency.
3. Our school collects and uses qualitative and quantitative data to support student academic and personal growth.
4. Our curriculum, instruction, and assessment demonstrate high expectations for each student.
5. Our school works with families to help all students understand the connection between education and lifelong success.
6. Our curriculum and instruction include evidence-based strategies to prepare students for further education, career, and citizenship.
7. Our extracurricular, cocurricular, and community-based programs provide students with experiences relevant to higher education, career, and citizenship.
8. Our curriculum and instruction develop students' global awareness and competencies, including understanding of language and culture.
9. Our school monitors and assesses extracurricular, cocurricular, and community-based experiences to ensure students' academic and personal growth.
10. Our school provides cross-curricular opportunities for learning with and through technology (ASCD, n.d.-a).

Coordinating Policy, Process, and Practice: Improving Learning and Improving Health

Encircling the tenets and the child in the diagrammatic depiction of the model is the phrase "Coordinating Policy, Process, and Practice—

Improving Learning and Improving Health." The WSCC model in practice includes numerous education and health policies, processes, and programs within and across the model's 10 components that engage a range of individuals, units, organizations, and stakeholders. For WSCC to maximize its potential and sustain its presence, carefully planned coordination is essential. WSCC leaders recommend that coordination emanate from two bodies, a school health council and school health teams. School health councils provide leadership at the school district level, while school health teams do the same at the individual school level. While the school health council will identify policies, processes, and practices for district-wide WSCC implementation, school health teams will translate district-wide direction for implementation at the local school level, taking into account the school's grade levels, resources, facilities, individual school mission and values, and local community characteristics (Allensworth, 2015).

Each of these groups should have a designated coordinator. The coordinator is responsible for planning and facilitating council or team meetings, maintaining the group's vision and commitment, providing leadership related to the group's work, and providing coordination among the diverse interests and activities. Members of the school health council should include the coordinator of the school health team from each of the district's schools and district representatives from each of the 10 WSCC components. Additional members for both the school health council and school health team can include school administrators, parents and family members, students, community representatives, and other stakeholders such as representatives from health and youth-focused community organizations, law enforcement, and the business and faith communities. The members of both bodies should reflect the diversity of the community and include individuals who understand its cultural, political, geographic, demographic, and economic structure (Murray et al., 2015). Communication between the district body and local school group is essential.

Both groups, whether at the district level or school level, engage in WSCC planning activities such as gaining administrative support, eliciting input from stakeholders within the school and community, gathering relevant qualitative and quantitative data at the district or school level, and assessing WSCC-related policies, processes, and programs (Hodges & Videto, 2015). WSCC action steps that evolve from the planning process include developing an implementation plan with specific goals and objectives, putting the plan into action, providing support for all individuals and groups engaged in or affected by WSCC, conducting formative and process evaluation throughout implementation, and maintaining forward movement by the school health council or team and all parties responsible for various aspects of the WSCC plan (Valois, 2015; Videto & Birch, 2015).

The 10 Components

The WSCC model is intended to permeate all school programs, policies, processes, and practices. The model's 10 components provide a framework for the infusion and coordination of the essence of WSCC. In this section of the chapter, a description including characteristics of quality structure and implementation is provided for each of the 10 components.

Health Education

School health education is characterized by planned, sequential learning experiences taught by teachers who are qualified and professionally prepared. The health education curriculum should be based on relevant health behavior theories; focus on the emotional, intellectual, physical, and social dimensions of health; provide students with exposure to diverse instructional techniques; and evaluate student achievement through a variety of assessment strategies (Joint Committee on National Health Education Standards, 2007). The learning experiences embedded within the curriculum should be designed to promote students' learning through

- the acquisition of functional health information;
- the identification of personal values that support healthy behaviors;

- the development of health-related skills;
- the analysis of the influence of family, peers, media, technology, and social injustices on personal and community health; and
- the development of advocacy skills for health, social justice, and equal opportunity to well-being for all members of society (Birch, 2021; CDC, 2019d; Joint Committee on National Health Education Standards, 2007).

The potential of quality school health education has been recognized as an important strategy for maintaining and improving public health. Examples of this recognition are reflected through multiple CDC resources, including *Characteristics of an Effective Health Education Curriculum* (CDC, 2019a) and *Health Education Curriculum Analysis Tool* (CDC, 2019b). The inclusion of health education as 1 of the 10 components of the ASCD/CDC-supported WSCC model also provides validation of its importance (Mann & Lohrmann, 2019).

Unfortunately, even with this recognition of the importance of school health education for all students, few school districts provide quality school health education from the elementary grades through high school. Numerous factors have been identified for this problem, including an increased emphasis placed by schools on standardized testing that does not assess student learning in health education, emphasis on a small number of selected topics (e.g., physical activity, nutrition, drug education) rather than a coordinated comprehensive approach that is skill based and addresses a wider range topics, a lack of academically prepared health education teachers, and—because few adults have observed or experienced quality programs—a lack of understanding of what quality health education is on the part of stakeholders (teachers, school administrators, parents) (Videto & Dake, 2019). One issue related to teacher preparation is a lack of understanding of the distinction between health education teachers and physical education teachers. While the subjects are related, teaching and learning in the two disciplines takes place in different venues, is based on separate instructional standards, involves different teaching methods and student assessments, and requires distinct professional preparation (Birch et al., 2019). It is not unusual for schools to assign health education instruction to a physical education teacher who, while well qualified to teach physical education, is often not qualified and, in some cases, is not excited about teaching health education. This distinction was affirmed by the SOPHE Accreditation Working Group statement: "School health education and physical education are separate and unique disciplines and require distinct quality assurance standards and processes. All those assigned to teach health education in schools should be professionally prepared in health education" (Taub et al., 2014, p. 355).

While issues exist in the quality of school health education, direction has been provided on how to move forward for improvement. SOPHE's National Committee on the Future of School Health Education published four articles in the November 2019 issue of the SOPHE journal *Health Promotion Practice*. These articles presented 12 challenges and related recommendations for each of the challenges. The challenges identified in the articles address needs such as an improved understanding of the meaning and characteristics of quality school health education, collaborative coordination of and advocacy for school health education, enhanced capacity for the delivery of quality school programs and related research and evaluation, increased rigor for teacher certification in health education in some states, and improved professional preparation for prospective health education teachers and improved professional development for current teachers (Birch & Auld, 2019; Birch et al., 2019; Mann & Lohrmann, 2019; Videto & Dake, 2019).

Direction at the school level is provided through the third edition of the National Health Education Standards: Model Guidance for Curriculum and Instruction. The standards were developed by the National Consensus for School Health Education, a group consisting of six nongovernmental health organizations: the American School Health Association, Eta Sigma Gamma, the Foundation for the Advancement of Health Education, the National Commission for Health Education Credentialing, the Society for Public Health Education, and the Society of State Leaders of Health and Physical Education. The development process for the standards included a national review and subsequent input from over 500 school health education stakeholders. The standards are

TABLE 6.1. National Health Education Standards (Third Edition)

Standard 1	Students comprehend functional health knowledge to enhance health.
Standard 2	Students analyze the influence of family, peers, culture, social media, technology, and other determinants on health behaviors.
Standard 3	Students demonstrate health literacy by accessing valid and reliable health information, products, and services to enhance health.
Standard 4	Students demonstrate effective interpersonal communication skills to enhance health.
Standard 5	Students demonstrate effective decision-making skills to enhance health.
Standard 6	Students demonstrate effective goal-setting skills to enhance health.
Standard 7	Students demonstrate observable health and safety practices.
Standard 8	Students advocate for behaviors that support personal, family, peer, school, and community health.

SOURCE: National Consensus for School Health Education. (2022). *National health education standards: Model guidance for curriculum and instruction* (3rd ed.). www.schoolhealtheducation.org

not a prescriptive curriculum but provide guidance to school districts related to curriculum development and content, instructional methods, and student assessment. The standards are intended to be applicable for instruction in all health education topic areas. A description, teaching suggestions, and performance expectations for grades 2, 5, 8, and 12 are provided for each of the eight standards (National Consensus for School Health Education, 2022). The standards are presented in table 6.1.

Further direction for school districts and individual schools has been given through the identification of characteristics for consideration for quality health education programs. The following listing is an adaptation and expansion of CDC recommendations for school health education (Birch et al., 2015; CDC, 2019a):

- Involves stakeholders in the planning/curriculum development process.
- Focuses on clear health goals and related behavioral outcomes.
- Is research based and theory driven.
- Incorporates issues related to health equity and health-related social justice issues.

- Based on National Health Education Standards.
- Taught by teachers professionally prepared and passionate about teaching health education.
- Addresses individual values, attitudes, and beliefs.
- Addresses individual and group norms that support health-enhancing behaviors.
- Focuses on reinforcing protective factors and increasing perceptions of personal risk and harmfulness of engaging in specific unhealthy practices and behaviors.
- Addresses social pressures and influences.
- Addresses the influence of social injustices, including systemic racism and other systemic discrimination, on health disparities and overall well-being.
- Builds personal competence, social competence, and self-efficacy through skill development.
- Provides functional health knowledge that is basic, accurate, and directly contributes to health-promoting decisions and behaviors.
- Uses strategies designed to personalize information and engage students.
- Addresses content sequentially from elementary school through middle school and high school.
- Provides age-appropriate and developmentally appropriate information, learning strategies, teaching methods, and materials.
- Incorporates learning strategies, teaching methods, and materials that actively engage students in learning and are culturally inclusive.
- Provides adequate time for instruction and learning.
- Provides opportunities to reinforce skills and positive health behaviors.
- Provides opportunities to make positive connections with influential others.
- Evaluates learning through authentic assessment techniques.
- Includes teacher information and plans for professional develop-

ment and training that enhance effectiveness of instruction and student learning.

- Is a component of an active WSCC model.

Physical Education and Physical Activity

Physical activity is recognized as an important research-based healthy behavior for individuals of all ages from early childhood through adulthood. Numerous benefits, including weight management, cardiovascular health, metabolic health, and musculoskeletal health, as well as a decreased risk of certain types of cancer, falls during older adulthood, and premature death, are linked to regular engagement in physical activity (CDC, 2022). The Aspen Institute's Sports and Society Program reports that children and youth engaged in physical activity are less likely to be obese; are more likely to have lower levels of depression, smoking, drug use, pregnancy, and engagement in risky sex; have higher levels of self-esteem and higher test scores; and are more likely to go to college (Project Play, n.d.). Schools can play an important role in providing opportunities for regular physical activity for students through the attainment of knowledge and skills, which can lead to engagement in lifelong physical activity. These opportunities can be provided through quality physical education programs and other physical activities within and beyond the school day.

Unfortunately, many adults and some school-age children have not experienced the type of broad-based physical education described by prominent national organizations. The Society of Health and Physical Educators (SHAPE), a leading professional organization for physical educators, defines physical education as "an academic subject that provides a planned, sequential, K–12 standards-based program of curricula and instruction designed to develop motor skills, knowledge, and behaviors for healthy, active living, physical fitness, sportsmanship, self-efficacy and emotional intelligence" (SHAPE America—Society of Health and Physical Educators, 2015). The CDC has described physical education as an academic subject characterized by a planned, sequential K–12 curriculum (course of study) that is based on the national standards for physical education and provides cognitive content and instruction designed to develop motor skills, knowledge, and behaviors for physical activity and physical fitness (CDC, 2020).

As a subject or course, physical education has a long history of inclusion in the public school curriculum. At times it has received increased attention. One example of this was during and after World War I, when a large number of men were not eligible for the military draft because of medical reasons. A similar situation occurred during both World War II and the Korean War, which generated an increased emphasis on physical fitness in many physical education programs (Goodwin, 1993). Historically, physical education has not received the same attention from educators, parents, and the general public as other subjects such as math, science, history, and reading (Birch et al., 2015). Over the past 20 years, two social forces have created opposing impacts on physical education. One of these forces, an increased public emphasis on standardized test scores, has, in some situations, resulted in a reduction or elimination of physical education to allow schools to allocate more time to subjects addressed on standardized tests (Kohl & Cook, 2013). In contrast, in some schools a surge of interest has emerged in physical education in response to the increase in obesity among both children and adults (Birch et al., 2015). The US government plan to promote and strengthen the nation's health, Healthy People 2030, includes an objective directly related to physical education: "Increase the proportion of adolescents who participate in daily school physical education" (Office of Disease Prevention and Health Promotion, n.d.). In 2013 the Institute of Medicine recommended that the federal government designate physical education as a core subject because "it has commensurate values that are foundational for learning and therefore essential" (Kohl & Cook, 2013, p. 3). In addition, the American Academy of Pediatrics (AAP), the American Heart Association, SHAPE America, the US Department of Education, the US Department of Health and Human Services, and the President's Council on Physical Fitness and Sport all support the need for high-quality physical education and physical activity (SHAPE America et al., 2016).

Physical education has developed national standards to provide direction to school districts and schools. Each of the standards relates to the knowledge, skills, and attitudes of a "physically literate individual." The five standards are defined as follows:

1. The physically literate individual demonstrates competency in a variety of motor skills and movement patterns.
2. The physically literate individual applies knowledge of concepts, principles, strategies, and tactics related to movement and performance.
3. The physically literate individual demonstrates the knowledge and skills to achieve and maintain a health-enhancing level of physical activity and fitness.
4. The physically literate individual exhibits responsible personal and social behavior that respects self and others.
5. The physically literate individual recognizes the value of physical activity for health (SHAPE America—Society of Health and Physical Educators, 2015).

Further direction for schools was provided by the SHAPE America Opportunity to Learn Guidelines (SHAPE America—Society of Health and Physical Educators, 2010). These guidelines are intended to describe essential physical education program elements that provide effective learning foundations for elementary, middle, and high school students. The following list is derived from these guidelines:

- Highly qualified physical education teachers
- A comprehensive, sequential, standards-based curriculum
- A healthy and safe learning environment for physical education
- Appropriate class size
- Quality facilities to promote learning, student participation, and safety
- Safe materials and equipment that maximize learning
- Appropriate time allocation for instruction
- Up-to-date instructional technology and related teacher training

- Formative and authentic summative assessment of student learning
- Annual program evaluation

While quality physical education should be an essential component of the school curriculum and can provide a pathway to lifelong physical activity, by itself it is not able to provide the recommended 60 minutes per day of physical activity for school-age children and youth (Kohl & Cook, 2013). The CDC (2018) defined physical activity as any bodily movement that is produced by the contraction of skeletal muscle and that substantially increases energy. A 2013 Institute of Medicine report titled *Educating the Student Body: Taking Physical Activity and Physical Education to School* (Kohl & Cook, 2013) includes several recommendations, beyond physical education, that relate to the schools' role in increasing physical activity. These suggestions include increasing the amount of time that youth spend in physical activity through brief classroom breaks, incorporating physical activity directly into academic sessions, providing active recess breaks throughout the school day, offering intramural sports and physical activity clubs, and providing access to school facilities during nonschool hours.

Interest in the use of classroom-based physical activity among students has increased in recent years. These activities may take place within the context of classroom instruction or occur during breaks from instruction. These opportunities for increasing physical activity during the school day require minimal planning and no equipment (Kohl & Cook, 2013). The CDC reports that classroom-based physical activities are more likely to be required and implemented at the elementary and middle school levels than in high schools (CDC, 2018). Additional research suggests that classroom-based physical activity can improve on-task classroom behaviors, reduce negative off-task behaviors, and have a positive impact on academic outcomes (Watson et al., 2017).

For many years, recess has presented an opportunity for physical activity during the school day for children. Recess is more common in elementary schools and is rare in secondary schools. It not only provides students with an opportunity for physical activity but also supplies a venue for the development of life skills related to communication, conflict resolution, cooperation, creativity, decision-making, problem-solving, taking turns, and sharing (Kohl & Cook, 2013). Evidence also suggests that recess has physical benefits for children and promotes positive emotional health, social development, school behavior, and cognitive performance (Massey et al., 2021). A Robert Wood Johnson Foundation study of elementary school principals done in collaboration with the National Elementary Principals Association surveyed a balanced sample of principals from urban, suburban, and rural schools with varied income levels. The principals' responses overwhelmingly indicated that recess has a positive impact not only on the development of students' social skills but also on achievement and learning in the classroom (Kohl & Cook, 2013).

Strong advocates are present in support of recess. An AAP policy statement supporting recess describes it as a "fundamental component of a child's normal growth and development." The policy statement also includes a recommendation that recess should not be withheld for punitive or academic reasons (Murray et al., 2013, p. 186). Recess also has support from education organizations. The National Association of Early Childhood Specialists in State Departments of Education (2001) posits that "recess is an essential component of education and that preschool and elementary school children must have the opportunity to participate in regular periods of active play with peers" (p. 1). In addition, the National Association of Elementary Principals, the National Association for the Education of Young Children, the National Association for Sport and Physical Education, and the National Parent Teacher Association have all presented statements supporting recess as an important component of students' overall school experience (Kohl & Cook, 2013). A practical tool, the Great Recess Framework Observational Tool, provides direction for schools to assess the quality of their recess offerings through the examination of safety and structure, adult supervision and engagement, student behaviors (communication, interpersonal interactions, conflict resolutions), and transitions to and from the recess environment (Massey et al., 2018).

School sports, both interscholastic and intramural, also provide students with opportunities for physical activity. Intramural sports take place within one school, while interscholastic sports involve competition between schools or between individual students in different schools. Since both intramural and interscholastic sports take place beyond the school day, students face different levels of accessibility regarding participation. Factors that can affect accessibility include the socioeconomic status of the student's family, the student's need to have a job outside of school, home responsibilities, and a lack of transportation or other travel issues. Money matters—the financial resources of school districts and individual schools can have an impact on the number of sports or programs offered, the quality of equipment and facilities, the number of coaches and their qualifications, and access to medical care and athletic trainers (Mohl & Patel, 2015; Wallace et al., 2017). All of these factors can affect not only the number of students engaged in these activities but also the quality of that engagement. Merkel (2013) presented a glaring example of an athletics funding disparity in 2009–10 between two school districts in New Jersey. In that school year, the Newark School System (an urban district) spent approximately $1,000,000 on athletics for approximately 40,000 students, including approximately 10,000 high school students. In comparison, the Millburn Public Schools (a suburban district), located close to Newark, spent approximately the same amount for about 5,000 students, including 1,500 high school students.

While research on the impact of intramural sports participation involving high school students is limited, there is a considerable body of research focused on interscholastic sports. Research related to interscholastic sports participation suggests that participation in interscholastic sports is associated with increased levels of college enrollment and educational attainment (Shifrer et al., 2015).

While research suggests academic benefits from participation in high school sports, most students are nonparticipants. Data from the Aspen Institute indicate that only 39% of high school students are engaged in school sports, and engagement is even lower in urban (32%) and high-poverty (27%) schools (Farrey, 2020). To expand participation in both interscholastic and intramural programs, schools need policies and practices in place that support the involvement of students. The following recommendations, unless noted, relate to both interscholastic and intramural sports:

- Equal access for all students to sports regardless of ability—while some limitations might be necessary for interscholastic sports, intramural opportunities should be available for all students.
- Equal emphasis should be placed on boys' and girls' sports—this should be reflected in attention, budget, facilities, and so on.
- Safety and injury prevention should be top priority. This includes not only the prevention of physical injuries but also emotional and social well-being. Participants should have access to an on-site certified athletic trainer during athletic participation.
- Students who are interested in participation in multiple sports should be encouraged to follow their interests. Specialization in one sport at the high school level should not be a priority for students, coaches, or others.
- Parents and students should be engaged in decision-making related to school sports and have representation on advisory boards, committees, and other groups.
- Ongoing professional development should be provided to coaches and all individuals with responsibility related to both intramural and interscholastic sports.

Active transport—walking, biking, skateboarding, or some other type of physically active travel to and from school—presents another opportunity for increasing students' daily physical activity. It might involve walking the entire distance to and from school, or it might mean being transported by car, school bus, or public transportation to a certain point and then walking the remainder of the way (Kohl & Cook, 2013). Active transport not only can increase physical activity for students but also can enhance students' social interaction and community and school connectedness (Victoria State Government, 2022). Factors that may affect the feasibility of active transport can include the location of schools; existence of sidewalks, walking and bike paths, pedestrian crossings, and traffic lights; neighborhood safety; weather conditions; and the possible need for adult supervision.

One structured method of active transport for students is the "walking school bus" (WSB). WSBs involve a group of children walking together to and from school with adult supervision. Each group of children and the adult supervisor(s) walk along a predetermined route and may pick up other children at designated stops along the way. On the way to school, the adult supervision starts at the beginning point of the route; after school, the adult(s) meets the children at the school and reverses the route to lead all children home (County Health Rankings and Roadmaps, 2019). An adaptation of the WSB model is the "bicycle train." In this model, the group of children and adult leaders ride together on bikes to and from school (National Center for Safe Routes to School, n.d.-b).

Obviously the WSB approach presents an opportunity for contributing to students' overall level of physical activity. However, other benefits may also be present, including an increase in social interaction among students and with adults, increased parent and community member engagement with schools, reduced traffic to and from schools, enhanced sense of community among student walkers and adult supervisors, and increased traffic safety knowledge and skills among students (Blue Zones, n.d.; National Center for Safe Routes to School, n.d.-a).

WSBs can also present an opportunity for extracurricular health education. In a pilot program, Kong et al. (2010) provided messages to students during the walks about nutrition and physical activity.

Important considerations have been identified for the initiation and maintenance of WSB programs. Smith et al. (2015) presented the importance of a paid program coordinator. The coordinator can reach out and secure parents and other adult volunteers, provide ongoing support to the volunteers, maintain community and school support, and work with the community to promote safe walking routes. An excellent resource guide titled *Step by Step: How to Start a Walking School Bus at Your School* (Moening et al., 2016), a collaborative project of the California Department of Public Health and Safe Routes to School National Partnership, presents detailed direction for the development, maintenance, and evaluation of WSB programs, along with a listing of additional resources.

Afterschool programs show promise as a vehicle for providing students with an opportunity for physical activity. The programs engage children and youth of all ages through interventions such as academic support and tutoring, mentoring, youth development, arts, health, and sports and recreation. These efforts may be addressed through formal instruction, individual and group advising, community service projects, field trips, organized physical activity, and health education (Youth .gov, n.d.).

Similar to all programs, adequate funding is important to afterschool program success. Federal funding is available from the 21st Century Community Learning Center. This funding provides support to community learning centers that offer students a broad array of academic enrichment services, including tutoring, homework help, and community service, as well as music, arts, sports, and cultural activities. This funding is awarded to state education agencies, which then manage statewide competitions to grant funds to eligible organizations (Youth .gov, n.d.).

Nutrition Environment and Services

Schools are an important factor in the diet of children and youth. For some students, school meals may be the primary or only daily source of nutritious foods. The school nutrition environment includes the school lunch and breakfast programs, foods sold outside of the school meal programs (vending machines, school stores, school fundraisers, concession stands), and food provided at classroom or school parties or celebrations. Food may also be provided to students in school-based afterschool programs (CDC, 2019d).

In fiscal year 2018, the federal National School Lunch Program (NSLP) operated in approximately 100,000 public and nonprofit private schools (grades pre-K–12) and residential childcare institutions. All students in participating schools can purchase an NSLP lunch. Eligible students in these schools can receive free or reduced-price lunches. Students in households at or below 130% of the poverty level are eligible for free lunch, while those between 130% and 185% are eligible for reduced-price lunch (Economic Research Center, 2020).

The Food Research and Action Center has identified a range of research-based benefits from school food service programs. As might be expected, research findings indicate that free and reduced-price lunch programs decrease food insecurity among participating children. In addition, children consuming school meals are more likely to eat fruit, vegetables, and milk at breakfast and lunch and less likely to have nutrient inadequacies. Research also indicates that school lunches have less calories, fat, saturated fat, and sugar and more protein, fiber, vitamin A, and calcium than packed lunches from home. Researchers have also concluded that participation in school meals can be influential in reducing obesity among students (Hartline-Grafton, 2016).

Additional research findings reported by the Food Research and Action Center provide support for the role of school meals in reducing hunger and improving school behavior and learning. Children experiencing hunger are more likely to have behavioral, emotional, and mental health issues; experience hyperactivity; have attention problems; be tardy and absent; repeat a grade; and receive mental health counseling or special education services. Teens who have experienced hunger are more likely to have been suspended from school and to have had issues related to getting along with other students (Hartline-Grafton, 2016). The Healthy, Hunger-Free Kids Act of 2010 (HHFKA) required the US Department of Agriculture (USDA) to update school nutrition standards. The new regulations went into effect in 2012. These regulations require cafeterias to offer more fruit, vegetables, and whole grains and limit sodium, calories, and unhealthy fat in every meal offered by participating schools. Since 2012, the USDA has made adjustments to the whole grain, sodium, and milk mandates. The 2020 standards require larger portions of fruits and vegetables with every lunch, as well as weekly vegetable offerings that include legumes and dark-green and red/orange vegetables. Every school breakfast must offer a full cup of fruits or vegetables. Students are required to take at least one half-cup serving of fruits or vegetables with every school breakfast and lunch. At least half of the grains offered with school meals must be whole grain rich (at least 51% whole grain). Meals must also meet age-appropriate calorie minimums and maximums that have been determined by the USDA. Regarding dietary fats, meals cannot contain added trans fat, and no more than 10% of calories can come from saturated fat. All school meals must also offer one cup of fat-free or 1% milk. In addition, free drinking water must be available in the cafeteria during lunch and breakfast (School Nutrition Association, n.d.-a).

As of July 1, 2014, HHFKA put into effect the "Smart Snacks in School" standards. These standards apply to foods and beverages sold in competition with reimbursable meals. These "competitive foods" are sold in vending machines, snack bars, and a la carte lines. Under the standards, competitive foods must be a "whole grain–rich" product or have as the first ingredient a fruit, vegetable, dairy product, protein food, or a combination food that contains at least one-fourth of a cup of fruits or vegetables. In addition, there are requirements that place limitations on the amounts of calories, sodium, dietary fats, and sugars. The standards also place restrictions on the types of liquid drinks that can be available for sale. The standards do not apply to food and beverages brought from home or sold during nonschool hours, on weekends, or at off-campus events such as school sporting events and school plays. Individual states may establish exemptions for local schools for items sold at infrequent fundraisers or bake sales (School Nutrition Association, n.d.-a, n.d.-b).

The USDA has encouraged school districts to use locally produced foods in school meals and to implement farm-to-school activities to spark students' interest in trying new foods. Research indicates that these activities are more common in school districts with enrollment above 5,000 students, urban districts, and districts located in counties with a higher density of farmers' markets. Higher-income districts and districts located in states with more policies supporting farm-to-school programs were also more likely to engage in farm-to-school activities (Economic Research Center, 2020).

The School Nutrition Association (2019) provides an important resource for school nutrition programs titled *Keys to Excellence: Standards of Practice for Nutrition Integrity.* The resource is intended to assist schools in achieving nutrition integrity goals at the administrative, management, and operational levels. It describes 10 "Best Practices" in nutrition and nutrition education as part of a comprehensive school nutrition program. Multiple indicators are presented for each of the practices. In addition to nutrition and nutrition education, "Best Practices" are presented for physical activity, operations, administration, and marketing and communication. The following listing presents the 10 "Best Practices" for nutrition and nutrition education:

1. School meals and snacks are planned and prepared to improve and sustain the health and well-being of all students and to contribute to the development of healthy eating habits.
2. Competitive foods are planned and served to encourage healthy choices and comply with federal guidelines.
3. The school nutrition program addresses competitive food issues to reflect the best interest of student health.
4. The school nutrition program participates in national, state, or local initiatives to encourage students to consume healthy foods.
5. The school nutrition program participates in the Farm to School Program.
6. The school nutrition program encourages and supports nutrition education.
7. The school dining area serves as a dynamic nutrition learning center where students are engaged in healthy eating.
8. The school nutrition program ensures that school nutrition personnel receive training that meets the USDA's Professional Standards for School Nutrition Program Personnel.
9. The school nutrition program provides opportunities for the community to learn how school meals are a model for healthy eating.
10. The school nutrition program is engaged in wellness activities in the schools and community (School Nutrition Association, 2017).

School Health Services

All schools should have a robust health services program that meets the health, medical, and educational needs of students. While many professionals, including pediatricians and other physicians, physician assistants, nurse practitioners, dentists, and allied health personnel professionals, can be engaged in various ways with the health services program, the school nurse should serve in the coordination and leadership role (CDC, 2019c). The National Association of School Nurses (2017) describes school nursing as "a specialized practice of nursing" that protects and promotes student health, facilitates optimal development, and advances academic success. As the coordinator of a school's health services, the school nurse's responsibilities can include leadership in the development of policies, programs, and procedures at the school and district level; the development, implementation, and evaluation of students' individualized health care plans; communication about students' health issues and needs with teachers, administrators, parents, and, in some cases, the community; case management for students' health care in the context of the school, family home, and medical home; the establishment of relationships and referral procedures with medical partners and social agencies; elicitation of program support; and the development of school safety emergency management plans (McClanahan & Weismuller, 2015; National Association of School Nurses, 2016). Beyond the coordination responsibilities, specific school services provided in schools can include primary health care, such as emergency care for illness or injury; referral to specialized medical care; daily care of students with chronic conditions such as asthma and diabetes; preventive care such as flu shots and hearing and vision screening; and health education for students and parents (CDC, 2019c). Note that the health education provided by school nurses is not intended to take the place of classroom health education for students. Because of the impact of social determinants and social justice on students' health and academic achievement, school nurses may also address student issues related to poverty, housing and homelessness, immigration, violence, transportation, and access to health care (Holmes et al., 2016).

The National Association of School Nurses (2020) recommends that every school have one full-time registered professional nurse. The bottom line is that all students should have access to the school nurse all day, every day. In large schools providing access may mean having more than one nurse. As school populations change, school nursing capacity should be assessed on a regular basis. Assessment should consider not only the number of students in a school but also the special health, education, and safety needs of students (National Association of School Nurses, 2020). A review of research related to the influence of school nurses on academic outcomes indicated that the presence of a school nurse is associated with decreased student absenteeism and less missed class time (Yoder, 2020). Additional research indicates that school nursing is a cost-saving investment based on a reduction in emergency room visits and a decrease in parents' time away from work to care for sick children (Wang et al., 2014).

Physicians are important members of the health services team. The AAP's Council on School Health recommends that every school district have a school physician. In the AAP 2013 Policy Statement, *Role of the School Physician*, it is recommended that school physicians should possess expertise in pediatrics or be nationally board-certified pediatricians (Devore et al., 2013). It is also recommended that school physicians possess knowledge related to public health, adolescent health, infectious disease, immunizations, medical-school legal issues, health and learning, social services resources, environmental and occupational health, emergency preparedness, sports medicine, and coordinated school health (similar to the WSCC model) (Devore et al., 2013). School physicians may have part-time status as an independent contractor with a school district or have full-time employee status. School physician assignments and responsibilities are dependent on the social and medical needs or demands of the community, the school district's priorities, and state laws (Devore et al., 2013).

Many schools offer an expanded health services program through school-based health centers (SBHCs). School-based health care offered through centers does not replace the school nurse but complements the nurse's work by providing a readily accessible referral site for students who are without a medical home or in need of more comprehensive services such as primary, mental, oral, or vision health care (School-Based Health Alliance, n.d.). SBHCs are located in the school or, in some cases, outside of the school grounds (referred to as "school-linked centers";

Knopf et al., 2016). SBHCs are located in urban, suburban, and rural school settings at the elementary, middle, and high school levels. Since the first SBHCs were implemented in the 1960s, the numbers have increased steadily, to approximately 2,580 in the 2016–17 school year (Love et al., 2019). The AAP has recommended SBHCs as a health care resource for children who are uninsured, are underinsured, or have limited access to health care (Council on School Health, 2012). The CDC, based on evidence that indicates effectiveness in improving both health and educational outcomes, recommends that SBHCs be implemented and maintained in low-income communities (Community Preventive Services Task Force, 2016).

The overall goal of SBHCs is to promote and support students' health and academic performance through the provision of primary health care, mental health care, social services, dental care, and health education. Services may be available during the school day or, in some SBHCs, outside of school hours. Some centers may offer services to school staff, student family members, and others within the surrounding community. In some schools and school districts, services are also provided from outside of the school system by a qualified hospital, health department, medical practice, or academic institution (Knopf et al., 2016). Some centers may have an advisory board that includes community representatives, parents, youth, and family organizations (Keeton et al., 2012).

In regard to services offered, the School-Based Health Alliance reported that 29.2% of SBHCs provide "primary care only," whereas 33.4% also provide mental health services and 37.4% offer additional services. In addition, a majority of SBHCs report providing comprehensive health assessments; treatment of acute illness; prescriptions; asthma treatment; screening for vision, hearing, and scoliosis; immunizations; counseling for healthful eating / active living / weight management; violence prevention activities; pregnancy testing; oral health education; dental screenings; dropout prevention programs; and substance abuse counseling and treatment (Lofink et al., 2013).

Research indicates that SBHCs can have positive effects on both students' health and their academic outcomes. In a systematic review of 46 studies that evaluated on-site SBHCs serving urban, low-income, and racial or ethnic minority high school students, the findings indicated that SBHCs were associated with improved educational outcomes, including grade point average (GPA), grade promotion, and reduced suspension rates, and improved health-related outcomes, including vaccination and other preventive services, asthma morbidity, contraceptive use among females, prenatal care, birth weight, decreases in emergency department use and hospital admissions, and decreases in illegal substance use and alcohol consumption (Knopf et al., 2016). Soleimanpour and Geierstanger (2014) coauthored a guide documenting links between SBHCs and academic indicators. The guide provided an overview of studies that demonstrated positive effects of SBHCs, including reduced absences and tardiness among high school students in urban settings that included a large population of Hispanic immigrants (Gall et al., 2000); a reduction in hospitalization and an increase in school attendance among elementary students with asthma in the Bronx, New York City (Webber et al., 2003); and a lesser likelihood of being sent home during the school day among students in two urban high schools in western New York (Van Cura, 2010).

In addition, in a comparison of schools with and without SBHCs in a large northeastern city, students in schools with SBHCs were more likely to report a favorable learning environment than students in schools without SBHCs (Strolin-Goltzman et al., 2012). McNall et al. (2010), in a two-year prospective study of middle and high school students in matched schools with and without SBHCs, found in year two that students who used SBHCs reported a higher satisfaction with their health, more involvement in physical activity, and a higher consumption of healthy food than students who did not use SBHCs. Specific to positive educational outcomes, student use of SBHCs has been associated with increased school connectedness, attendance, and GPA and reduced suspension rates (Arenson et al., 2019). Beyond these specific examples, Arenson et al. (2019) present an extensive review of literature focused on SBHC research published between 2000 and 2018. The authors present the findings of the research in four categories: financial, physical health, mental health, and educational outcomes.

Research also indicates economic benefits related to the presence of

SBHCs. Based on a systematic review of papers published from 1985 to 2014 that focused on cost and/or benefits, Ran et al. (2016) concluded that the economic benefits of SBHCs exceeded the intervention cost.

Counseling, Psychological, and Social Services

According to the American School Counselor Association (ASCA), counseling, psychological, and social services are essential in schools to promote and support students' mental, behavioral, and social-emotional health; academic success; career development; and progress toward a productive and fulfilling adulthood. Certified school counselors, school psychologists, and school social workers are key members of the school team relative to the attainment of these student outcomes. The services provided by these professionals include psychological, psychoeducational, and psychosocial assessments; interventions such as individual or group counseling and consultation to address barriers to learning; and, when needed, referrals to school and community support services. School mental health professionals can also provide assessment, prevention, intervention, and programs that address the overall school environment and contribute to the health and learning needs of all students. In addition, these professionals engage in consultation with other school staff and community resources and providers (ASCA, 2020b).

School counselors are an important part of the school team and should have a presence at the elementary, middle, and high school levels (ASCA, 2020c). ASCA recommends that, at a minimum, school counselors have a master's degree in school counseling, meet certification/licensure standards, and uphold ASCA ethical and professional standards. The organization identifies 250:1 as an ideal student-to-counselor caseload. The school counselor's responsibilities include the provision of individual student academic planning and goal setting, school counseling classroom lessons, short-term counseling to students, referrals for long-term support, collaboration with families/teachers/administrators/community for student success, advocacy for students at individual education plan meetings and other student-focused meetings, and data analysis to identify student issues, needs, and challenges.

Research supports the positive impact of school counseling on student outcomes, including increased academic success, better school behavior, more informed career awareness and college preparation, increased college enrollment, and enhanced ethnic and racial identity. Research also supports the importance of an appropriate student-to-counselor ratio in regard to services having a positive impact on students. ASCA has compiled an accessible compendium of research studies related to the value of school counseling programs titled *Empirical Research Studies Supporting the Value of School Counseling*. The studies presented in the report have been identified from national peer-reviewed journals and research reports (ASCA, 2020a).

School psychologists are mental health professionals who play an important role in supporting students' academic success and overall well-being. All schools have access to the services of a school psychologist. However, because psychologists serve two or more schools, some schools may not have on-site access each day. School psychologists work with students, families, educators, and community members to help them understand and resolve students' chronic problems and issues. Specifically, school psychologists' responsibilities focus on improving academic achievement, promoting positive behavior and mental health, supporting diverse learning, creating safe and positive school climates, strengthening family-school partnerships, providing direct support, improving school-wide assessment and accountability, and monitoring individual student progress in academics and behavior. To attain these outcomes, school psychologists engage in interventions with students; consult with teachers, families, and other school-employed mental health professionals (i.e., school counselors, school social workers); work with school administrators to improve school-wide practices and policies; and collaborate with community providers to coordinate needed services. The National Association of School Psychologists (NASP) recommends a ratio of 1 school psychologist per 500–700 students (NASP, n.d., 2020).

School psychologists complete specialized advanced graduate preparation that includes coursework and practical experiences relevant to both psychology and education. In most cases, school psychologists complete a specialist-level degree program (at least 60 graduate semester hours) or a doctoral degree (at least 90 graduate semester hours). Both degrees require a year-long, 1,200-hour supervised internship. Through their graduate study, school psychologists develop knowledge and skills related to topics such as school-wide practices to promote learning, resilience and risk factors, consultation and collaboration, academic learning interventions, mental health interventions, behavioral interventions, instructional support, special education services, and crisis preparedness, response, and recovery. School psychologists must be credentialed by the state in which they work and may also be nationally certified by the National School Psychology Certification Board (NASP, 2020).

Research documents the positive impact of the work of school psychologists. A research summary compiled by the NASP presents multiple studies that have been presented in peer-reviewed articles, books, and research reports. These studies describe the impact of the work of school psychologists on improving instruction and learning, supporting healthy successful students, creating safe and positive school climates strengthening family-school partnerships, and improving assessment and accountability (NASP, 2015).

School social workers represent a specialized area of practice within the social work profession. According to the National Association of Social Workers (NASW), responsibilities include the provision of services and the coordination of efforts with students, families, teachers, administrators, and other school staff to promote students' school and life adjustment and academic achievement. Examples of specific responsibilities include (NASW, 2012) addressing students' mental health concerns and behavioral issues; providing academic and classroom support; consulting with teachers, family members, administrators, and other staff members; providing individual and group counseling therapy; assisting in special education planning; mobilizing family, school, and community resources to support individual students; developing and conducting professional development sessions; and advocating for community services to meet the needs of students and families (MSW@USC, 2019; School Social Work Association of America, n.d.-a, n.d.-b).

According to the *NASW Standards for School Social Work Services*, school social workers must have a graduate degree in social work from a program accredited by the Council on Social Work Education. The recommended entry-level requirement should be a master's in social work degree. Because school social work requires specialized knowledge and understanding of education systems, focus on the school setting should be part of the professional preparation. If not included, it should be addressed through professional development. School social workers are licensed by state boards of social work and, if available at the state level, certified through state departments of education. School social workers should also have knowledge and an understanding of past and current issues in education and be knowledgeable about evidence-informed approaches to teaching and learning that promote positive academic outcomes for all students (NASW, 2012).

As noted, counseling, psychological, and social services are essential in schools to promote and support students' mental, behavioral, and social-emotional health; academic success; career development; and progress toward a productive and fulfilling adulthood. While there is some overlap in the contributions provided by professionals in these areas, each provides unique services to schools. It is important that professionals in these three areas collaborate to delineate specific roles and collaborative opportunities among the three professions within a school or school district.

Social and Emotional Climate / Social-Emotional Learning

While the WSCC framework includes a social and emotional climate component, because of the overlap of purpose, policies, and programming, social-emotional learning (SEL) is presented in this section of the chapter as an additional element of the social-emotional component of the WSCC model. Griffith and Slade (2018) have presented the ASCD Whole Child approach, a foundation of WSCC, as an overarching component to SEL. Osher and Berg (2017) view SEL as co-influential in that a positive school climate creates the conditions for SEL and the social and emotional competence of each member of the school community affects school climate on both an individual and a collective level. Because of this relationship, Osher and Berg view the alignment of the school climate and SEL as creating synergies and reducing fragmentation.

The school social and emotional climate refers to the quality of life within the school for students, teachers, and all stakeholders. The National School Climate Council describes school climate as the quality and character of school life (Center for Social and Emotional Education, n.d.). Characteristics of a positive social and emotional climate include equity and inclusivity; academic challenge and engagement; empowerment; respect; meaningful relationships among teachers, administrators, staff members, parents, and students; physical, social, and psychological safety; norms, values, and expectations; a student-centered disciplinary policy; a safe and supportive learning environment that provides academic opportunities for all students; and opportunities for student involvement in decision-making (Osher & Berg, 2017). Interactions within the social and emotional climate take place in hallways, playgrounds, cafeterias, classrooms, and other sites for teaching and learning.

A positive school social and emotional environment does not just happen. DeWitt and Slade (2014) suggest that focused planning can result in a supportive, protective, and nurturing environment that leads to effective teaching and learning. The National School Climate Council enlisted the involvement of education leaders from across the United States to develop school climate standards (Center for Social and Emotional Education, n.d.). The five standards each include 16 indicators and 30 subindicators. The five standards are presented in table 6.2.

School Health Index: A Self-Assessment and Planning Guide is a guide developed by the CDC to provide schools with a tool to identify strengths and weaknesses of health and safety policies and programs in order to develop an action plan for improving student health. The School Health Index (SHI) uses the 10 WSCC components as a framework for reviewing policies, programs, and services. For the assessment of the Social and Emotional Climate component, the tool addresses the following areas:

- Positive school climate
- Positive student relationships
- Professional development on meeting diverse needs of students
- Collaboration to promote social and emotional learning
- School-wide social and emotional learning

TABLE 6.2. National School Climate Standards

Standard 1	The school community has a shared vision and plan for promoting, enhancing, and sustaining a positive school climate.
Standard 2	The school community sets policies specifically promoting (a) the development and sustainability of social, emotional, ethical, civic, and intellectual skills, knowledge, dispositions, and engagement; and (b) a comprehensive system to address barriers to learning and teaching and to reengage students who have become disengaged.
Standard 3	The school community's practices are identified, prioritized, and supported to (a) promote the learning and positive social, emotional, ethical, and civic development of students; (b) enhance engagement in teaching, learning, and school-wide activities; (c) address barriers to learning and teaching and reengage those who have become disengaged; and (d) develop and sustain an appropriate operational infrastructure and capacity-building mechanisms for meeting this standard.
Standard 4	The school community creates an environment where all members are welcomed, supported, and feel safe in school: socially, emotionally, intellectually, and physically.
Standard 5	The school community develops meaningful and engaging practices, activities, and norms that promote social and civic responsibilities and a commitment to social justice.

SOURCE: National School Climate Center. (n.d.). *National School Climate Standards: Benchmarks to promote effective teaching, learning and comprehensive school improvement.* Center for Social and Emotional Education. http://www.casciac.org/pdfs/school-climate-standards-csee.pdf

- Community partnerships to promote social and emotional learning for students in school
- Prevention of harassment and bullying
- Active supervision
- Engagement of all students
- Prevention of school violence (CDC, 2017)

Research supports the linkage between a positive school climate and improved teaching and learning and improved health and education outcomes for students. Specifically, research findings include increased bonding with teachers and peers, respect for school rules, reduced aggression and violence, better classroom behavior, improved grades, increased satisfaction with school, reduced absenteeism, decreased suspension rates, and a higher level of school connectedness (Daily et al., 2020; Michael et al., 2015).

It is important for school leaders to note that students may have varied perceptions of the school climate or may be affected in different ways. Osher and Berg (2017) report that students of color and students who are economically disadvantaged are more likely to report lower perceptions of school climate than their peers. A positive, inclusive approach to the school climate, including policies and practices, can not only be supportive to marginalized students but also present opportunities for engaging parents and family members of students from marginalized groups (Osher & Berg, 2017). In presenting the perspectives of members of the school community in regard to school climate, Temkin et al. (2019) report that students commented on the importance of having multiple sources of support. One specific suggestion provided by the students was to have more than one guidance counselor in case students did not feel comfortable with a specific counselor and had no one else to connect with in a meaningful way.

SEL, while not a new concept, has received increased emphasis in recent years. SEL is defined as the "process through which children and adults acquire and effectively apply the knowledge, attitudes, and skills necessary to understand and manage emotions, set and achieve positive goals, feel and show empathy for others, establish and maintain positive relationships, and make responsible decisions" (Osher & Berg, 2017, p. 1). Jones et al. (2019) describe SEL as providing students with the opportunity to learn and apply social, emotional, behavioral, and character skills that are important in schooling, work, relationships, and citizenship. SEL is often addressed structurally through two components: classroom-based instruction and an emphasis on a safe and supportive total school environment (Durlak et al., 2011). Five overarching competencies have been identified for classroom-based SEL instruction: self-awareness, social awareness, self-management, relationship skills, and responsible decision-making. Specific capacities, presented in table 6.3, have been linked to each of the five competencies (Collaborative for Academic, Social, and Emotional Learning, 2020). A report from the Harvard Graduate School of Education, focused on elementary-level SEL, presents a

TABLE 6.3. Core Competencies in Social and Emotional Learning

Competency	Description	Examples
Self-awareness	The abilities to understand one's own emotions, thoughts, and values and how they influence behavior across contexts	Integrating personal and social identities Identifying personal, cultural, and linguistic assets Identifying one's emotions Demonstrating honesty and integrity
Self-management	The abilities to manage one's emotions, thoughts, and behaviors effectively in different situations and to achieve goals and aspirations	Managing one's emotions Identifying and using stress-management strategies Exhibiting self-discipline and self-motivation Setting personal and collective goals
Responsible decision-making	The abilities to make caring and constructive choices about personal behavior and social interactions across diverse situations	Demonstrating curiosity and open-mindedness Learning how to make a reasoned judgment after analyzing information, data, and facts Identifying solutions for personal and social problems Anticipating and evaluating the consequences of one's actions
Relationship skills	The abilities to establish and maintain healthy and supportive relationships and to effectively navigate settings with diverse individuals and groups	Communicating effectively Developing positive relationships Demonstrating cultural competency Practicing teamwork and collaborative problem-solving
Social awareness	The abilities to understand the perspectives of and empathize with others, including those from diverse backgrounds, cultures, and contexts	Taking others' perspectives Recognizing strengths in others Demonstrating empathy and compassion Showing concern for the feelings of others

SOURCE: Collaborative for Academic, Social, and Emotional Learning. (2005). *Core SEL competencies*. https://casel.org/Core-Competencies/

framework that includes skills in three domains: cognitive regulation (attention control, inhibitory control, working memory / planning, cognitive flexibility), emotional processes (emotion knowledge/expression, emotion/behavior regulation, empathy/perspective-taking), and social/ interpersonal skills (understanding social cues, conflict resolution, prosocial behavior). These three domains and related skills are intended to lead to both short- and long-term outcomes linked to academic achievement, behavioral adjustment, and emotional health and well-being (Jones et al., 2017).

The placement of SEL may occur as a separate instructional unit with skills presented and taught as applicable to a variety of life situations faced by students or incorporated within instruction in various health education–related content areas such as substance abuse prevention, mental and emotional health, sexual health, nutrition, and physical activity. Simmons (2019) views SEL as a vehicle for initiating important conversations that enable students to confront injustice, hate, and inequity by addressing issues related to racism, poverty, violence, sexism, homophobia, transphobia, and all other forms of marginalization. Through addressing these issues, students can develop an understanding of power and privilege, examine their own personal stances and actions, and explore their role as a community member in issues regarding social justice. Because social and emotional development is influenced by school, family, and community factors, school programs must address SEL through a systems approach across multiple settings using a variety of strategies (Jones et al., 2019).

Though SEL and a safe, supportive social and emotional climate are complimentary, both approaches are sometimes not emphasized in schools. In some school settings, SEL may be addressed only through skill-based classroom instruction without systematically reinforcing and supporting the instruction through the overall school climate and the daily lives of students. In combination with SEL instruction, a safe and supportive school climate not only reinforces what is taught via SEL classroom instruction but also provides students with the opportunity to interact within that environment and supplies a venue for students to apply SEL skills. SEL leaders view a combined approach (instruction and climate) as an essential component of safe, supportive, and academically successful schools (Osher & Berg, 2017). Tomlinson (2018) captures the importance of a combined approach: "SEL is not a program or curriculum but a way to be together" (p. 88).

Two meta-analyses support the implementation of SEL programs. In a 2011 meta-analysis of 213 school-based studies involving approximately 270,000 students in grades K–12, results indicated that, in comparison to control groups, students who received SEL instruction demonstrated significantly better outcomes in six areas: social and emotional skills, attitudes toward self and others, positive social behaviors, conduct problems, emotional distress, and academic performance. These findings were applicable to schools at all grade levels (elementary, middle, and high school) and in urban, suburban, and rural settings (Durlak et al., 2011). Note that programs were most effective when the instruction included (1) sequential activities for teaching skills, (2) active engagement of students in learning skills, (3) focused time on SEL skill development, and (4) explicit targeting of SEL skills (Durlak et al, 2011). A second 2017 meta-analysis based on 82 schools involving approximately 97,400 students revealed significantly positive outcomes for SEL students in the six areas addressed in the 2011 meta-analysis. Some of the studies in the 2017 meta-analysis included long-term follow-up of students. The results from these studies indicated that more of the SEL students had graduated from high school and attended college, and fewer had been arrested (Taylor et al., 2017). Beyond the direct educational benefits to students, SEL programs are cost-effective. A cost analysis of four SEL programs found that calculated benefits of the interventions easily exceeded the cost of implementing the programs (Belfield et al., 2015).

There are a variety of SEL curriculum approaches that have been implemented in schools. National resources that provide direction for SEL include the Aspen National Commission on Social, Emotional, and Academic Development; the Collaborative for Academic, Social, and Emotional Learning; and the Harvard Graduate School of Education's Taxonomy Project (Jones et al., 2019).

Physical Environment

The provision of a healthy and safe learning environment for all students and staff members is an essential responsibility of school leadership. Prior to graduation, students spend over 15,000 hours in a school building, second only to the time spent at home (Eitland et al., 2017). The physical environment of a school is an important influence on students' academic success, their enjoyment of the school experience, and their safety and overall well-being. An accessible, healthy, safe, learning-centered, and physically attractive school environment will not only benefit students but also enhance the instructional environment for teachers and, in general, make the school a better place to work for all school staff members and a more appreciated place for visitors, including family and community members.

Research has provided direction for the identification of important factors within the school physical environment that are linked to students' health and learning. In an extensive report that can serve as a resource for schools, the Healthy Buildings Program, Harvard University, T.H. Chan School of Public Health, under the direction of Dr. Joseph Allen, developed a report titled *Schools for Health: Foundations for Student Success—How School Buildings Influence Student Health, Thinking and Performance*. As the title indicates, the report focuses on the impact of school buildings on the health and productivity of students, teachers, and staff members (Harvard Healthy Buildings Program, n.d.).

Based on 30 years of scientific evidence, the Healthy Buildings team identified nine fundamental building factors that have an impact on students' health and academic performance:

1. Air quality
2. Thermal heat
3. Moisture
4. Dust and pests
5. Safety and security
6. Water quality

7. Noise
8. Lighting and views
9. Ventilation

For each of the nine factors, the report presents extensive research and the evidence-based impact of each factor on student health, student thinking, and student performance. For the purposes of the report, student health is defined as the overall physical and biological health of students; student thinking refers to the short-term effects on cognitive function and mental well-being such as attention, comprehension, and irritability; and student performance is based on long-term academic outcomes (Harvard Healthy Buildings Program, n.d.).

As described earlier in the chapter, *School Health Index: A Self-Assessment and Planning Guide* is a guide developed by the CDC to provide schools with a tool to identify strengths and weaknesses of health and safety policies and programs in order to develop an action plan for improving student health.

The following eight areas and related factors for each provide a framework for the SHI review of the school physical environment:

Safe Physical Environment
1. Flooring surfaces are slip-resistant and stairways have sturdy guardrails.
2. Poisons and chemical hazards are labeled and are stored in locked cabinets.
3. First-aid equipment and notices describing safety procedures are available.
4. First aid / school nurse office is equipped with running water.
5. All areas of the school have sufficient lighting, and secluded areas are sealed off or supervised.
6. Smoke alarms, sprinklers, and fire extinguishers are installed and operational.
7. Pedestrians are offered special protection, including crossing guards, escorts, crosswalks, and safe bus and car loading.
8. A variety of methods are used to keep weapons out of the school environment.

9. School buses do not idle while loading or unloading students, to reduce emission of diesel exhaust and fine particles.
10. Spaces and facilities for physical activity (including playgrounds and sports fields) meet or exceed recommended safety standards.
11. The campus and buildings are pleasant and welcoming (e.g., uncluttered, uncrowded, well lit, graffiti free).

School Environmental Health Program
1. Effective cleaning and maintenance
2. Mold and moisture prevention
3. Chemical and environmental contaminant hazard reduction
4. Ventilation maintenance
5. Pest prevention and pesticide exposure reduction

Effective Management of an Environmental Health and Safety Program
1. Organize key school staff to develop, implement, and monitor the environmental health and safety program, based on an established action plan and tracking system.
2. Communicate the goals of the program to school staff, teachers, students and/or families.
3. Regularly assess the school environment for potential health risks.
4. Train staff on how to use personal protective equipment.
5. Develop plans to address potential environmental health and safety risks.
6. Evaluate the implementation of policies and practices developed as part of the program.

Professional Development for School Environmental Health
1. Provide professional development and training for key staff (e.g., facility manager, maintenance staff, custodian, teachers, etc.) on managing school environmental health and safety.

Student Involvement in Promoting Environmental Health
1. Incorporates environmental health curricula and lesson plans in classroom learning.

2. Encourages students to complete school projects related to environmental health.
3. Engages students in extracurricular activities related to environment or environmental health.
4. Gives students opportunities to contribute to maintaining school environmental health.

Cleaning and Maintenance Practices

1. Schedule routine cleaning when students are not in the building.
2. Use cleaning products as instructed on the product label.
3. Store cleaning products in locations that are not accessible to students.
4. Maintain an up-to-date inventory of all cleaning products used.
5. Regularly clean and remove dust from hard, impermeable surfaces with a water-dampened cloth.
6. Wipe up paint chips with a wet sponge or rag.
7. Vacuum using high-efficiency vacuums and filters (e.g., high-efficiency particulate air filters).
8. Ensure that garbage is stored in appropriate containers and disposed of properly at the end of each day.
9. Use floor mats at building entrances to reduce the amount of dust and soil tracked into school buildings.
10. Thoroughly clean kitchens, cafeterias, and other food-use areas.
11. Monitor the interior of the roof for water damage.
12. Inspect windows and doors for physical damage and improper seals.
13. Ensure that all windows and doors are functioning properly.
14. Cut back overgrown vegetation near exterior walls.
15. Inspect ceilings and duct work for deteriorating tiles and heating, ventilation, and air conditioning (HVAC) lining, as well as loose insulation.

Implement Indoor Air Quality

1. Regularly clean and vacuum when students are not in school (consider using vacuums with high-efficiency particulate air filters or central vacuums where carpeting exists).

2. Respond quickly to signs of moisture, including mold, mildew, and water leaks in the building (e.g., plumbing) and around the building envelope (e.g., doors, windows, roof).
3. Prevent exhaust fumes from entering the school or accumulating in the outdoor areas by prohibiting buses and cars from idling outside of the school building.
4. Maintain adequate ventilation with humidity control throughout the building.
5. Schedule regular maintenance and repair for HVAC system.
6. Select interior building materials, office furniture, and equipment that minimize exposure to indoor air contaminants.
7. Reduce or eliminate exposure to furred and feathered animals.
8. Schedule painting, floor resurfacings, and major building maintenance or renovations during times when school is not in session, and isolate renovation areas so that dust and debris are confined.
9. Install carbon monoxide detectors and test for indoor radon levels.

Implement Integrated Pest Management Practices
1. Monitor potential pest infestations with regular and detailed inspections.
2. Use adequate sanitation practices (e.g., cover trash cans, place dumpsters away from buildings and entryways) and structural modifications (sealing holes and openings, repair screening, door sweeps) to minimize pests.
3. Use proper food handling, preparation, and storage techniques.
4. Use pest removal strategies first before using pesticides, such as sticky traps, pheromone traps, vacuuming, and insect light traps.
5. Use low-risk pesticides (herbicides, fungicides, insecticides) after all other nonpesticide removal strategies have been tried and when no alternative measures are practical.
6. Be sure no students and staff members are in the area during pesticide application.

7. Refrain from calendar-based pesticide applications; use baits when possible.
8. Notify parents, employees, and students of all pesticide applications.

Schools for Health: Foundations for Student Success—How School Buildings Influence Student Health, Thinking and Performance and the CDC's *School Health Index* are resources that provide direction to schools in the development and maintenance of a physical environment that maximizes the health and safety of students and school staff members and contributes to an optimal climate for teaching and learning. However, schools must also be prepared to protect students and staff from episodic threats emanating from events such as natural disasters, disease outbreaks, crime, and violence. To be as prepared as possible, schools must involve community partners, governmental agencies, various public health and safety representatives, and other stakeholders in the development of a school Emergency Operations Plan (EOP) to be able to provide a coordinated response in case of an occurrence of any type of threat to school safety.

The US Department of Education has developed two complementary EOP resources, one for schools, *Guide for Developing High-Quality School Emergency Operations* (US Department of Education et al., 2013), and the other for school districts, *The Role of Districts in Developing High-Quality School Emergency Operations Plans* (US Department of Education & Office of Elementary and Secondary Education, 2019). These two guides are intended to be used together. The district guide provides direction to school districts in the provision of coordination and support to schools, while the school guide provides step-by-step direction in the development of a school EOP.

The school guide indicates five areas that provide a framework for the US government's approach to preparedness (US Department of Education et al., 2013):

1. Prevention: the capabilities necessary to avoid, deter, or stop an imminent crime or threatened or actual mass casualty incident.

Prevention is the action districts and schools take to prevent a threatened or actual incident from occurring.

2. Protection: the capabilities to secure districts and schools against acts of violence and man-made or natural disasters. Protection focuses on ongoing actions that protect students, teachers, staff, visitors, networks, and property from a threat or hazard.

3. Mitigation: the capabilities necessary to eliminate or reduce the loss of life and property damage by lessening the impact of an event or emergency. Mitigation also means reducing the likelihood that threats and hazards will happen.

4. Response: the capabilities necessary to stabilize an emergency once it has already happened or is certain to happen in an unpreventable way, to establish a safe and secure environment, to save lives and property, and to facilitate the transition to recovery.

5. Recovery: the capabilities necessary to assist districts and schools affected by an event or emergency in restoring the learning environment.

Regarding the actual planning of the school EOP, the school guide emphasizes a collaborative process that considers principles for best addressing a wide range of possible threats and hazards that may impact schools. These principles include support from district and school leadership; the consideration of all possible threats and hazards; planning for access and needs of the whole school community, including individuals with disabilities and others with unique needs, those from religiously, racially, and ethnically diverse backgrounds, and individuals with limited English proficiency; and consideration of incidents that may occur during and outside the school day, as well as on and off campus (e.g., sporting events, field trips).

Emergency preparedness actions such as the installation of security cameras, classroom safety locks, safety glass, and secure entries and conducting lockdown drills are essential, but schools should also make efforts to address the underlying causes of threats to safety. The October 2019 issue of *Educational Leadership* focused on "Making School a Safe Place." Actions to address underlying causes of potential danger that are presented in the articles in the journal include but are not limited to addressing school climate problems, helping students feel safe and valued and a sense of connection and responsibility to one another, promoting positive relationships between students and teachers, providing instruction that helps students develop skills in areas such as interpersonal relationships and stress management, distinguishing between transient and substantial safety threats, implementing a specific safety assessment protocol for any student who is considered to be a possible safety threat, using a coordinated approach with students who are deemed to be threatening, providing mental health services for students, and being a trauma-informed school. In other words, a positive social and emotional climate and a positive physical environment are essential in schools that are safe and doing all that is possible to prevent and prepare for emergencies.

One additional and extremely important consideration regarding the school physical environment is equity. Like other factors related to quality education, equity in funding is essential in regard to building new schools and the renovation of the physical characteristics of older buildings. Research has identified disparities in the allocation of funding for the construction and renovation of school facilities. These disparities exist among schools serving students of varying family and community income levels and students of different racial and ethnic backgrounds (Kitzmiller & Rodriguez, 2021). These disparities not only present challenges to teaching and learning but also send messages of "lesser value" to stakeholders in underfunded schools. Equity must be a high-level consideration in the allocation of funding at all levels designated for improving the quality of the physical environment of schools. Based on concern related to funding disparities, Filardo et al. (2006) stated, "It is only fair that we give all students, especially the most disadvantaged, every opportunity they need to succeed. Providing decent, modern school buildings for all students is crucial to their academic achievement and overall well-being. We know that a well-educated population is crucial to our economy and democracy, and modern, safe, and well-functioning school facilities are one way that we can begin to build a better future for ourselves, our children, and generations to come" (p. 32).

Employee Wellness

School employees, like those in other work settings, can benefit from employee health promotion or employee wellness activities. Programs for teachers, administrators, and all school staff members are intended to both promote the health of individual school employees and support the health and academic success of students. The importance of employee wellness for school employees is validated by its inclusion as 1 of the 10 components of the WSCC framework. Note also that schools are one of the largest employers in the United States. Going beyond direct benefits to schools, reaching this large group of employees can make an important contribution to the nation's efforts to improve the health of the US population (Herbert et al., 2017). Employee wellness programs for teachers, administrators, and other staff members should consist of a coordinated set of activities, policies, benefits, and environmental supports implemented to promote the physical, mental, emotional, and social health and safety of school employees (Lewallen et al., 2015).

In comparison to nonschool worksites, schools can take advantage of existing on-site resources for employee wellness activities. These resources can include gyms, walking and running tracks, and other sites for physical activity; equipment for physical activity; health educators, physical educators, school nurses, and other professionals who can serve as content specialists and program instructors; instructional materials; and classroom and conference room space. Program activities can include employee assistance programs; health risk appraisals; health screening (blood pressure, diabetes, serum cholesterol); physical activity programs such as walking, running, resistance activities, aerobics, swimming, and yoga; health education sessions addressing topics such as nutrition, injury prevention, mindfulness, and stress management; ongoing information sources such as a program website, social media communication, a newsletter, and bulletin boards; and healthy social events.

A variety of outcomes have been identified as potential benefits resulting from the implementation of school employee wellness programs such as increased physical activity, improved diet, reductions in hypertension, weight loss, better stress management, and improvements in overall well-being (Kolbe, 2019). Because of these outcomes, wellness programs have been presented as a strategy for reducing school employee health care costs (Lewallen et al., 2015). Aldana et al. (2005) posit that while the impact of reduced health care costs may be limited in the short term, financial benefits may increase over time as the impact of costly chronic diseases is reduced later in life. Research also indicates that programs associated with a decrease in teacher absenteeism result in a reduction of costs through decreased payments for substitute teachers (Herbert et al., 2017; Miller, 2008). A study based on two years of implementation of a school employee wellness program in the Washoe County (NV) School District found a 20% difference in absenteeism between teachers who participated in the program and nonparticipants (Aldana et al., 2005). Evaluation based on one year of implementation of a teacher wellness program in a large metropolitan school district found an average of 1.25 fewer days missed among program participants in comparison to nonparticipants (Blair et al., 1986). In addition to the financial benefit, reduced teacher absenteeism results in less disruption in teaching and learning. Substitute teachers are often not academically qualified for their assignment (Miller, 2008). The importance of decreasing teacher absenteeism is demonstrated by the state of Rhode Island's implementation plan for the federal Every Students Succeeds Act. The plan designates a decrease in chronic teacher absenteeism as a possible indicator of school success (Rhode Island Department of Education, 2017). Teacher absenteeism is also a factor in education disparities. Schools serving students from predominately low-income families have higher rates of teacher absences than schools with students from more affluent families, thus contributing to increased academic challenges for students (Clofelter et al., 2007).

Wellness programs for school employees can improve job satisfaction and teacher morale and have a positive impact on the overall school climate (Lloyd et al., 2019). Frequent work-related stress can have an impact on even the most dedicated teachers. Frequent teacher turnover can be a disruptive factor to school stability and students' academic success. Job satisfaction and a positive school climate can influence teaching and learning through the retention of quality teachers and valuable staff members and enhance a school district's ability to recruit new teachers (Kolbe, 2019).

Teacher involvement in school wellness programs can also have a positive impact on students. Through their engagement in positive health behaviors and their demonstration of a visible commitment to well-being, teachers can serve as health role models for the students (Schultz et al., 2019). In addition to role modeling, teachers involved in wellness programs can become more committed to the promotion of an overall healthy school environment for their students. In a qualitative study of school employees in socioeconomically disadvantaged, racially diverse school districts in a northeastern US state, "investment in student health" was one of three overarching themes identified as a supporting factor for a wellness program. The employees emphasized that supporting teacher and staff wellness could, in turn, facilitate efforts in supporting students' health and academic achievement (Schultz et al., 2019). It is reasonable to suggest that teachers who are involved in employee wellness programs could develop a stronger commitment to health promotion programs for students such as the WSCC model.

School employee wellness programs will best attain school- or school district–level support, implement meaningful activities, experience high levels of participation, and be sustained over time if, from the very beginning, a systematic planning, implementation, and evaluation process is in place. The following steps are recommended for sequential inclusion in this process:

1. Initiate the Idea: Starting a program can begin with one person or a small group of individuals. Those employees with interest in an idea or a vision of a health activity for faculty members or even a vision of a more comprehensive program can connect and initiate movement forward. This idea initiation could involve discussion of individual visions for a program, reviewing literature on school employee wellness, contacting individuals in school districts that have employee wellness programs, and recruiting additional employees who have interest.

2. Gain Support: This next step involves mobilizing the group to develop a proposal or presentation for discussion with the school principal or other appropriate administrator. The presentation or proposal should highlight possible school district, school, employee, and student benefits resulting from a program; a tentative planning process; and examples of programs in other schools or school districts.

3. Form a Wellness Team: Identify members for the wellness team from the school or school district who have an interest in employee wellness. The members should reflect the diversity of the school, with consideration for race, ethnicity and gender, years of experience (both beginning and more experienced employees), teachers from various academic disciplines and grade levels, and representatives from various nonteaching positions. Early in the process of forming a team, one or two individuals should be designated as the coordinator or co-coordinators.

4. Identify Needs, Interests, and Assets: Determine through a survey and, if possible, small group meetings the needs and interests of faculty members in regard to promoting their health. In addition, an assessment can be considered to determine existing school or district assets, including individuals with health knowledge and skills, and existing equipment and facilities. The results of this information gathering can be summarized in a brief report and shared with school administrators. Consideration can also be given to a meeting with interested employees to share results and elicit their thoughts regarding future wellness programming.

5. Identify Administrative Goals and Objectives and Initial Activities: This step, based on the results of step 4, includes the identification of administrative goals for the overall program (number of sessions, number of participants, identification of topics, etc.) and specific program activity objectives that will lead to the attainment of these goals. Initial activities, linked to the goals and objectives, should then be scheduled. The objectives for these activities should contribute to the attainment of overall

program goals. Starting with a small number of activities can be a consideration in getting the program off the ground. As the program moves forward and gains a higher degree of institutionalization, additional activities can be included as part of the program offerings.

6. Get the Word Out—Market the Program Activities: Let all employees know of the activities. Using email, social media, newsletters, bulletin boards, written announcements, and other communication vehicles, recruit employees for the first wave of wellness activities. While these messages should originate from the wellness team, an invitation for involvement from the school administration can also contribute to these efforts.

7. Implement the Program Activities: After marketing the program, actual program activities can begin. In the beginning stages, wellness committee members should be present to welcome participants and ensure that initial implementation is moving forward in a smooth manner. Process evaluation (described in step 8) will serve as an essential method for participant feedback. Ongoing interaction with activity instructors and supervisors will also serve as an important source of feedback.

8. Conduct Program Evaluation: All program activities should be evaluated throughout the program. Process evaluation should be conducted periodically during the implementation of program activities. This level of evaluation is intended to gauge the participants' satisfaction with the process of program implementation and can also assess participants' perceptions related to program accessibility, instruction and instructional resources (for classes), facilities, equipment, and overall satisfaction. Activity instructors and supervisors can also be a source of process evaluation information. This information can serve as a source for immediate "mid-flight" or future program adjustments. Impact evaluation is conducted at the end of the program. This level of evaluation is linked to specific activity objectives to determine the impact of the activity on program participants (for instance, adherence to regular physical activity, changes in diet, use of

stress-management techniques, reduction in employee absentee-ism, etc.). Both process and impact data can be useful in future program decisions.

9. Maintain Interest and Involvement: Wellness programs are not short-term plans. Sustaining a program is essential for maximum impact. One step that is important in maintaining interest and involvement includes sharing evaluation results from recent program activities with school administrators, current participants, and potential participants. These results can include impact evaluation data, testimonials from participants, ongoing program announcements, and current health updates. It is also important to continue gathering input from employees on existing activities and thoughts on possible new activities.

Teachers, administrators, food service staff, school nurses, bus drivers, custodians, and other staff members are all contributors to a safe and supportive school environment, quality teaching and learning, and the academic success and overall well-being of students. In order to maximize their contributions, school employees must be valued and supported in order to maintain and improve their own health. School employee wellness programs can serve as a foundation for this effort.

Family Engagement

Well-planned family engagement programs are intended to support teaching and learning and promote both academic success and the overall well-being of students, families, and all school staff members. Research indicates that teachers and administrators recognize the importance of school partnerships with families and that the majority of parents want to be partners with schools to support their children's education (Epstein et al., 2018). Epstein et al. (2018) posit that school partnerships with families can improve the school climate, strengthen school and classroom programs, provide family service programs, enhance parents' skills, connect families with others in the school and community, and support teachers. All of these outcomes will contribute to students' success in schools. Bryk et al. (2010), based on research in Chicago schools, identified positive school and family relationships as an essential component for sustained school improvement.

Terminology related to family engagement is important and has evolved for important reasons. Students live in a variety of family structures and situations and may not have parents who are able to engage in a partnership with their school. Family engagement may involve other primary caregivers such as grandparents, foster parents, guardians, siblings, and other influential adults. Thus, the term "family" is more appropriate than "parent." The concept of involvement has evolved from opportunities for family members to be involved in activities identified by the school, often referred to as "parent involvement," to activities emanating from true partnerships between the school and family members, or "family engagement." Ferlazzo (2011) has suggested that engagement is "doing with" rather than "doing to" and that communication is two-way rather than one-way. Common parent involvement activities have included school-identified activities such as beginning-of-the-school-year orientations for parents, parent-teacher conferences, attendance at student performances, and parent volunteer opportunities. Parents are often invited through communication from the school to attend these activities. While these activities are still important, family engagement refers to a broader concept in which a partnership between the school and family members is based on a recognition that schools and families are both essential to students' education and overall well-being. In this type of engaged partnership, schools are clearly invitational to family members, and activities are collaboratively identified, planned, and evaluated through active participation among family members, teachers, administrators, and other school staff members. Engagement includes family input into school decision-making through membership on committees and decision-making bodies, the use of focus groups, and family surveys.

An extensive body of research supports family engagement as having a positive impact on students' academic achievement at all grade levels and across a diverse range of students. While "family engagement" is the suggested term, the term "parent involvement" is still commonly used in both research and practice. This terminology is reflected in the following research findings. A plethora of meta-analyses have been conducted at the pre-K–12 levels to systematically review multiple studies that address the relationship between parent involvement and academic achievement for students. Smith et al. (2020; in a meta-analysis of 77 parent involvement studies), Castro et al. (2015; based on 37 studies), Higgins and Katsipataki (2015; based on 13 studies), and Hill and Tyson (2009; based on 50 studies) all found positive associations through their analyses between parent involvement and academic achievement. The 50 studies in the Hill and Tyson (2009) meta-analysis focused on middle school grades, while the other three focused on studies at multiple grade levels, pre-K–12. Jeynes (2012, 2016, 2017) conducted three separate meta-analyses that investigated the relationship between parent involvement and academic achievement among African American students (42 studies), Latino students (28 studies), and urban students (51 studies). All three of Jeynes's meta-analyses reviewed studies that included students from grades pre-K–12. For each of the three analyses, Jeynes concluded that there was a positive association between parent involvement and academic achievement.

Additional research has demonstrated benefits of family engagement regarding students' school behavior. Domina (2005), based on an analysis of a national database, concluded that parent involvement contributed to prevention of school behavior problems. Sheldon (2018), in linking parent involvement to academic achievement, identified several studies of large data sets that demonstrate linkages between parent involvement and students' improvements in school behavior (Beyers et al., 2003; El Nokali et al., 2010; Hill et al., 2004). Sheldon and Epstein (2002) found that an improvement from one year to the next in schools' family and community involvement efforts resulted in a decrease in student referrals to the principal, detention, and in-school suspensions. Research has also linked parent involvement with improved school attendance (Michael et al., 2015; Sheldon, 2018).

Students are at the center of the WSCC model and at the center of family-school partnerships. Epstein et al. (2018) recommend that the partnerships promote both family-like schools and school-like families. Family-like schools welcome and reach out to all families, recognize the uniqueness of students and their families, and clearly demonstrate that all students and their families are valued and included. School-like families reinforce the importance of education to their children, emphasize and promote regular school attendance, and support students' involvement in activities that help them develop academic and life skills and lead them toward success.

Epstein has developed a framework for family engagement that has been heavily cited in the professional literature and widely used by schools over the past 20 years. The framework, supported by research and practical experience in schools, is based on six types of engagement that are intended to provide direction for the development of comprehensive programs for school, family, and community engagement. Comprehensive programs should include activities in each of the following six components:

1. Parenting: providing supportive home environments and helping school personnel gain an awareness and understanding of the students' families.
2. Communicating: implementing and sustaining ongoing two-way communication using a variety of methods, including technology.
3. Volunteering: recruiting family members to provide assistance at school, home, and other locations.
4. Learning at Home: providing opportunities for parents to develop knowledge and skills to support their children's learning and enhance their own knowledge and skills.
5. Decision-making: inviting parents to serve as members and leaders in decision-making situations in the school, including committees and other important roles.
6. Collaborating with the Community: identifying resources and services in the community that support and engage families and provide a venue for student engagement (Epstein et al., 2018).

In order to maximize the benefits of family engagement, several considerations are of high-level importance:

- It should be clear to family members that the school values and invites family engagement. This may be evident through a school family engagement policy; the inclusion of reference to family engagement in the school mission statement, core values, and philosophy; and invitational wording to family members in all forms of school communication.

- Two-way communication is an important aspect of family engagement. Through this communication it should be clear not only that schools want to provide information to families but also that schools place equal value on providing opportunities for communication from families. Two-way communication may include regular updates from the school on events and initiatives, a dedicated phone line at the school for parents' messages and questions, parent columns and comments in school newsletters, and two-way communication via social media. Schools should not only listen to the voices of families but also provide venues for those voices to be heard and initiate dialogue.

- All school administrators, teachers, and staff members must clearly demonstrate cultural responsiveness in their partnership with families. Schools must demonstrate that all families are valued. Culturally responsive family engagement is highlighted by an invitational school environment; an understanding of the various assets, challenges, and needs of the cultures represented by families in the school community; trust between families and the school; a spirit of collaboration; teaching and learning that respects and addresses the presence and needs of all students; and school policies and an environment that reflect a commitment to equity and academic success.

- Language can be a barrier to communication. It is important that schools identify the various languages spoken by parents and key family members. Whenever possible, there should be at least one school staff member who is fluent in languages spoken by students' family members. All written materials, both hard copies and online content, should be printed in English and other appropriate languages. Translation should be provided during individual and group meetings.

- Access to engagement varies among family members. Difficulty in leaving work, the need to provide childcare, and lack of transportation can create barriers to on-site school engagement. Whenever possible, opportunities for on-site engagement should be offered on different days of the week at different times. For some situations, alternative meeting sites outside of the school using convenient locations within the community can be considered, along with evening and weekend events and meetings. In addition, opportunities should be provided that can engage family members at home.

• Transparency is essential. As presented earlier, students' families should be provided the opportunity to understand and provide input to the school's mission, core values, and philosophy. Family members should have opportunities to understand and provide input to operational information such as the school budget, staffing, and the curriculum.

• All school personnel should be provided with professional development related to family engagement. These programs should be designed to enable personnel to understand the value of family engagement, promote cultural humility and responsiveness, gain awareness of specific methods or activities to promote engagement, and address current issues that have an impact on partnering with families.

• Evaluation should be conducted at both the process and impact levels. Process evaluation addresses the question, "Are we engaging in our partnership with parents in the best way possible?" All stakeholders are sources of process evaluation data. Items addressed through process evaluation can include the stakeholders' perception of the quality of program activities, communication, family's accessibility to programs, cultural responsiveness, and sense of engagement. Impact evaluation addresses the question, "What difference did the family engagement efforts make for families, students, school administrators, teachers and other school staff members?" This level of evaluation can address items such as number of families involved; changes in students' attendance, commitment to leaning, and overall academic achievement; changes in the family members' perception of the school; and administrators', teachers', and other staff members' perceptions of the impact of the family engagement programs. Questions addressed in impact evaluation for the most part should emanate from the goals and objectives of the family engagement program. Process evaluation is typically conducted throughout the program, while impact evaluation is conducted after the completion of an activity or school year. Both process and impact evaluation results are used to inform program revisions and determine whether to continue or terminate activities within an overall program.

Parents and family members, school personnel, and community members want students to be successful in school. Research clearly indicates that family engagement promotes students' school success. Schools need to be invitational to families and engage family members in collaboratively planning comprehensive programs for engagement in all aspects of schools' operation and governance. Family engagement can be a powerful strategy in building a supportive community of families, teachers, administrators, and school staff that benefits all stakeholders and, most importantly, supports students throughout their total school experience.

Community Involvement

Community members, businesses, organizations, and facilities present opportunities for partnerships with schools that can provide benefits to students, families, schools, and the community itself. Research supports community partnerships as beneficial to both education and health. Educational outcomes such as improved grades, test scores, attendance, and student behavior have been linked with community involvement with schools (Sanders, 2018). Blank (2015) presented specific examples of academic improvements at Milwaukie (Oregon) High School linked to the implementation of a community involvement program that focused on education and health. After implementation, the school experienced increases in average daily attendance; improvements in reading, math, and writing proficiency; and an upgrade in the school's state rating from "Needs Improvement" to "Outstanding." The school's principal attributed the improvements to the coming together of school staff and community partners to support students. Beyond educational outcomes, authentic and mutually beneficial school-community collaborations have been identified as a positive factor for the support of health initiatives in schools. The Growing Well community schools' initiative in Cincinnati, Ohio, is an example of a district-wide collaboration in a large city school district. Through this program, increases have occurred in mental health services provided in individual schools and in the number of students receiving glasses, asthma screening, and dental screening (Blank, 2015).

There are numerous potential partners in communities that can provide volunteers, expertise, and financial and material resources. These partners include service and volunteer organizations such as the Rotary, Lions, and Kiwanis Clubs; the YMCA and YWCA; the Boys & Girls Clubs; Girl Scouts; faith-based organizations; the United Way; local businesses; libraries and museums; voluntary health agencies; hospitals and clinics; the local recreation department; the fire and police departments; media outlets; and sports franchises (Sanders, 2018). A community scan can identify individuals and organizations that have expertise, interests, and resources that can be helpful to schools and students.

Local colleges and universities are also potential partners. In a mutually beneficial partnership, colleges and universities can provide faculty members with expertise related to specific areas in education, school health, and evaluation and research. In addition, colleges and universities can provide opportunities for students in different grades to visit campus centers, museums, and other facilities. These visits can help students develop or increase interest in post–high school education opportunities. In turn, school administrators and teachers can provide presentations and engage in discussion with college and university faculty members and students to present "on-the-ground" perspectives and experiences from early childhood education and elementary, middle, and high school settings. One partnership between schools and universities are dual enrollment courses, which are offered for both high school and college credit. These courses may be already-existing courses in the school curriculum or courses that are codeveloped by school and college/university faculty members. These courses are offered for free or at a lesser cost than regular college courses and provide an introduction for students to college-level instruction. Research suggests that these courses increase the likelihood of high school students enrolling in college and completing a bachelor's degree (McMurtrie, 2017). Schools can also serve as sites for college students' applied experiences and internships and provide opportunities for collaborative practice and research activities among school administrators, teachers, and college/university faculty members. Local colleges and universities can also partner with schools to engage parents and students through the provision of information related to the college application, admission, and selection processes and the overall academic and social college experience. While some students and family members may have this awareness through a history of family members attending college, first-generation college parents and students may not have this insight.

A variety of benefits can result from school-community partnerships. As already noted, individuals and organizations in the community can provide financial support for school instructional resources and provide expertise to enhance teaching and learning in schools. Community partners can also provide sites for field trips that can enhance classroom experiences. Another important opportunity for community partnerships is involvement in decision-making. Both schools and community organizations use committees and task forces for decision-making and policy development. Community members can bring outside perspectives as members of school committees, while schools can provide a school staff or student perspective as members of community bodies. Opportunities also exist for school staff and students to interact with community members. Consideration can be given to students exhibiting at community art or health fairs. Another possibility is a book club where school staff, students, and individual community members read the same book and have periodic book discussions. Schools can also share facilities with community members. School gymnasiums can be used for community physical activity programs, and school classrooms can be used for community education classes. In the early 1990s, the author worked with a rural school district that had a focus on engaging community members in school activities. One activity involved the middle school hallways serving, at the end of the school day, as a winter walking site for interested teachers, administrators, parents, and family and community members. Another part of this effort involved a health resource room open to community members during the school day. The resource room not only contained current health materials (many donated by regional health organizations) for use by community members but also showcased the school heath education curriculum, including projects completed by students. These activities provided excellent opportunities for interaction among school staff and community members and demonstrated how the school was part of the community rather than a separate institution.

A specific approach to school-community partnerships is the community schools model. A community school represents a partnership between the school and other community resources. Its integrated approach to academics, services, supports, and opportunities is intended to promote student learning, stronger families, and healthier communities (California School Boards Association, n.d.). The services and supports can be coordinated and provided by the school, community health and social services agencies, civil rights organizations, faith-based organizations, food banks, colleges and universities, the business sector, and other community agencies and organizations. These services, often described as "wraparound" services, can include expanded learning activities for students, family, and community members; health and social services, sometimes through school-based clinics; legal assistance; and programs to support college admission, career preparation, and the attainment of citizenship (Blank & Villarreal, 2015; Weingarten, 2015). Four pillars of community schools are intended to provide support for teaching and learning: (1) integrated student supports, (2) expanded learning time and opportunities, (3) family and community engagement, and (4) collaborative leadership and practice (Maier et al., 2017). SBHCs, described earlier in this chapter, can play an important role in the implementation of the community schools model.

Research supports the community schools approach. Evaluation of the implementation of the community schools model showed improvements in math and reading standardized test scores in schools in Boston, Chicago, and Tulsa (Adams, 2019; Bryk et al., 2010; Walsh et al., 2014), while community schools models in Baltimore and Chicago demonstrated improved attendance rates and a decrease in chronic absenteeism (Bryk et al., 2010; Olson, 2014). A structured examination of 143 research studies based on the implementation of the community schools approach revealed important overall findings indicating that the community schools approach had a positive impact on school attendance, academic achievement, and high school graduation rates, as well as leading to a reduction in racial and economic achievement gaps. Regarding the cost-benefit analysis of implementation, the findings indicate a return of up to $15 in social value and economic benefits for every dollar spent on school-based services (Maier et al., 2017).

To provide the best teaching and learning opportunities and a meaningful education for students, schools and communities must support each other through equal partnerships. In order for these partnerships to thrive, careful consideration must be given to optimal planning, implementation, and evaluation. The following actions represent important considerations:

- Providing professional development for administrators, teachers, and other school staff members. Through these programs, school staff members can develop an understanding of the importance of community partnerships, important considerations for community engagement, and examples of partnership activities (Sanders, 2018).
- Promoting the understanding among all partners that the education of children and youth is a shared responsibility of families, schools, and the community. All representatives should have an awareness of the potential benefits of the partnership and examples of possible activities. The role of both the school and community should be considered when developing polices, processes, and activities in both sectors.
- Helping community partners become familiar with the school mission, philosophy, and core values and understand the lifelong reciprocal relationship between education and health.
- Creating an awareness of the impact of social injustices on chil-

dren's health and school success. It should be recognized by all that social justice is an important education and public health priority.

- Ensuring that community partners represent all segments of the community and that the individuals involved reflect the population of the community.
- Demonstrating that collaborative decision-making, transparency, and two-way communication are hallmarks of community partnership activities.
- Evaluating the processes and impact of the partnership. Sanders (2018) identifies reflection among partners as an important activity to review evaluation results and consider the implications for future programming.

A variety of opportunities exist for schools to partner with individuals and various types of organizations in the community. If planned, implemented, and evaluated in a deliberate, thoughtful, inclusive manner, students, schools, and the community can benefit. Because of this potential, community involvement should be viewed by schools not as an "extra" but instead as an "essential" component.

The Community: An Overarching Concept

Where students live has an impact on both their health status and their access to quality schools. Community support for schools represents community support for its children. Conversely, quality schools contribute to the strength of the community. As indicated in figure 6.1, the entire WSCC model is enclosed within the community. The space between the community and the school should be viewed not as a walled border but as an open two-way passage with continual traffic.

At the center of the WSCC model is a focus on the child. For the WSCC model to maximize its potential in impacting children, communities need to support their schools, and schools need to support communities. Mutual support will generate mutual benefits. Unfortunately, schools are sometimes viewed as a separate entity within the community for which its members and organizations have little input and responsibility. Just as unfortunate, schools sometimes do not visualize the potential of community members and organizations as partners, nor do they always see the community role in school decision-making, in school activities, and as providers of support and resources. Building a strong partnership between schools and communities requires a recognition of the essential nature of the partnership, ongoing communication, transparency, and commitment to the challenges and issues within both sectors, as well as a recognition of assets and needs that the partners bring to the relationship.

Schools represent a reflection of the community and a factor in its future. Families want to live in communities with good schools that provide students with a meaningful education. School quality is a factor in decisions made by prospective home buyers and by businesses considering locations for their work. It is also a factor in the determination of property values. Students in a school represent future community members, professionals, decision-makers, and neighbors. Students will be among those who sustain the positive qualities of a community and address its challenges and issues.

The community represents a resource for schools. Students are more likely to succeed academically when living in safe, socially just communities in which all residents have access to living-wage jobs, affordable housing, accessible public transportation, and a business community committed to social justice, quality education, and health for all residents. In addition, opportunities should be accessible for community members of all ages and abilities to engage in healthy leisure and meaningful growth and learning opportunities.

Schools and communities need to recognize mutual goals and interests and the potential impact of an active, two-way partnership. Schools should not just be physical structures that are located in communities, and communities should not be only a location for schools and a source of a tax-based revenue stream. A commitment and investment from one sector to the other is a commitment to and investment in both sectors. All students and all other stakeholders benefit from an active, two-way community-school partnership.

The WSCC model provides a framework for schools and the community to advance academic achievement and health for all children and youth. The purpose of this chapter is to provide background information and direction related to the implementation of WSCC. Schools and communities can also access excellent resources related to WSCC planning, implementation, and evaluation from CDC Healthy Schools and ASCD. Two special issues of the *Journal of School Health* from the American School Health Association (November 2015 and December 2020) provide additional WSCC insights from leaders in education and school health and perspectives derived from actual implementation of the model.

The WSCC model has the potential of engaging community members and school staff in action and decision-making, resulting in schools and communities that support and implement coordinated activities that not only increase the likelihood of health and academic success for students but also lead to improved school and community life in the present and the future. To be most effective, advocates and social movement leaders must be familiar with WSCC in order to describe the schematic of the model; its rationale; related policies, processes, and practices; and its potential for making a positive difference in students' health and learning.

CHAPTER 7

Moving Forward

Mobilizing a Social Movement

Our communities and the individuals living within them are dying of illnesses
we know how to prevent, that have their roots in our communities, and cannot be
effectively treated by any one group alone.   MICHENER ET AL. (2019)

BOTH RESEARCH and real-world experiences clearly demonstrate the complexity of the many factors that affect access for
children and youth to quality education, academic success, and
overall well-being. Social injustices such as racism and other forms of
systemic discrimination, inequity, poverty, homelessness, access to living-
wage jobs, substandard housing, inadequate public transportation, lack
of community resources, and overall lack of opportunity affect both education and health. Achieving academic success provides students with
a pathway to high school graduation, the attainment of higher levels of
education, and better adult health outcomes. The relationship between
education and health is reciprocal. Healthy students are more likely to
be academically successful, and academically successful students are
more likely to attain higher levels of education and experience better
health as adults. Academic achievement and the attainment of higher
levels of education require the coordinated engagement of schools, students' families, and community members and organizations.

The ultimate goal of education is for students to succeed academically
in order to live a life of well-being and fulfillment. While based on dif-

ferent strategies, the goal of public health and medicine is for individuals and communities to have equal access to good health in order to thrive throughout the various stages of life. Thus, as emphasized in chapter 1, equal access to good schools that address students' health and educational needs through a safe, socially just, supportive environment and the implementation of quality instruction that leads to higher levels of education attainment is a relevant goal for education, medicine, and public health. This goal is more likely to become a reality if the education, medical, and public heath sectors, along with other sectors within the community, such as various governmental and nongovernmental agencies, the business community, faith-based organizations, local colleges and universities, parents and family members, and student and youth leaders, engage together in a focused movement to support communities in the provision of equal access to quality education and health for all children and youth.

The importance of multisector efforts has been recognized within the education, medical, and public health professions. Kolbe (2019) has emphasized the potential of collaboration among education, public health, medicine, nursing, and other sectors in improving health, education, and economic outcomes. Within the medical sector, it has been acknowledged that many actions that improve patients' health take place not in a clinic or hospital but in the community. This recognition has provided the impetus for increased efforts to promote a partnership between the medical and public health sectors (McGinnis, 2016). Koo et al. (2016) note the importance of this partnership: "We posit that public health and health care, which have traditionally been divided and worked in parallel, can work together along with other partners to reduce the burden of clinical illness and improve the health and well-being of our country" (p. 4).

The American Academy of Pediatrics et al. (2012), in its policy statement *Community Pediatrics: Navigating the Intersection of Medicine, Public Health, and Social Determinants of Children's Health*, describes community pediatrics as "expanding the pediatrician's focus from one child to the well-being of all children in the community" (p. 624). The policy statement emphasizes collaboration with both the public health and education sectors by recommending that "pediatricians should work together with public health departments, school districts, child welfare agencies, community and children's hospitals, and colleagues in related professions to identify and decrease barriers to the health and well-being of children in the communities they serve" (p. 626). Furthermore, the policy statement suggests that pediatricians interact with community members to improve early education and childcare facilities, school-based health services, family support and resource centers, youth programs, recreation venues, and transportation systems. The American Academy of Family Physicians (2020), in their position statement *Integration of Primary Care and Public Health*, encourages family physicians to be leaders in the communities they serve and work with public health professionals to address social determinants of health and inequities in power, money, and resources. A second document, titled *The Physician Advocate Advancing Policies That Support Health Equity* (American Academy of Family Physicians, 2018), suggests that, when engaging in community advocacy, family physicians consider working not only with family medicine and health care partners but also with partners from other areas such as education, civil rights, business, religion, nonprofits, and families in the community. The American College of Physicians (n.d.) has also affirmed its commitment to public health, stating that the organization's mission includes "advocating for responsible positions on public policy relating to health care for the good of our patients and the public. We take evidence-based positions on a range of public health issues, from climate change to prescription drug pricing to smoking cessation to reducing firearms-related injuries and deaths to substance-use disorder to immigration" (para. 2).

Both the public health and education communities have also recognized the importance of cross-sector partnerships to address students' health and promote the likelihood of academic success. Kolbe et al. (2015) describe education and health partnerships as "an essential means to concomitantly improve both education outcomes and health outcomes in the 21st century" (p. 767). Commenting on a partnership between the Dakota County (Minnesota) Public Health Department and the West St. Paul–Mendota Heights School District, one of the school district administrative leaders stated, "Any district that works with public health will be a better district" (National Association of Chronic Disease Directors, 2017, p. 9). One example of this type of partnership is a collaboration between ASCD, a prominent national education organization, and the Centers for Disease Control and Prevention (CDC) in the development and ongoing promotion of the Whole School, Whole Community, Whole Child (WSCC) model. The focus of this model is on student health and academic success. Background on the development of this model and detailed information about the model itself are presented in chapter 6. Another example of collaboration between the education and public health sectors is the National Association of Chronic Disease Directors' report *Local Health Department and School Partnerships: Working Together to Build Healthier Schools.* The document provides two case studies of partnerships between local health departments and local schools and school districts in support of the implementation of components of the WSCC model. The case studies also demonstrate how the schools and school districts gained support from community agencies (National Association of Chronic Disease Directors, 2017).

Social Justice, Education, and Health: The Need for a Social Movement

Only a broad social movement has the power and vision to mobilize the forces that can transform educational and health systems to better achieve health and educational equity.   RUGLIS & FREUDENBERG (2010)

As emphasized throughout this book, enhancing social justice, improving education, and promoting health present a complex, multifaceted challenge. Because of this complexity, a community-wide, well-planned, sustained social movement is necessary to meet this challenge. The purpose of this chapter is to provide direction for educators, family physicians, pediatricians, and public health professionals to serve as conveners, leaders, and ongoing partners in a multisector coalition at the local level. The focus of the coalition will be advocacy intended to initiate and sustain policies, processes, and practices that promote and maintain a socially just, health-enhancing family, community, and school environment, resulting in equal access and equitable support for quality early childhood and elementary, middle, and high school education and experiences for all children. It is important to emphasize that while the education, medical, and public health sectors can take on the responsibility to initiate and engage in early leadership, immediately upon the first thoughts of organizing, other key individuals and community partners should be invited to participate. Organizations outside of the education, medicine, and public health sectors can bring complementary perspectives, skills, and resources to support and improve communities and schools (Kolbe et al., 2015).

DeSalvo et al. (2017) describe Public Health 3.0 as a new era of public health practice. At the core of Public Health 3.0 is the idea that local communities will be leaders in taking public health to the next level. This focus on community leadership in promoting public health should be reflected in the composition and actions of an education–public health–social justice coalition. Chang et al. (2020) reinforce this broad-based involvement, recommending that community members' voices be present throughout the planning, implementation, and evaluation efforts. No segment of the community should be overlooked. It is also important to not overlook those individuals within the community who are most affected by challenging local issues. Lack of these perspectives could lead to actions that do not reflect and address the real needs and issues of community members (Chang et al., 2020).

A coalition is described as a formal alliance of organizations and individuals that is formed to work toward a common goal (Butterfoss, 2013). A social movement represents a collective effort by a network of individuals and groups, including coalitions, with the intent to affect laws, policies, practices, and changes in culture. An education–health–social justice coalition may advocate as an individual organization or may collaborate with other organizations that are not members of the coalition. Van Dyke and Amos (2017) identify coalitions as a key factor in the success of social movements because of their ability to pool resources and mobilize large numbers of individuals. Collective efforts that emanate from a multisector social movement are likely to experience better results than the efforts of a single organization. Almeida (2019), in reference to social movements, states, "The collective mobilization of people creates a powerful human resource that can be used for a range of purposes" (p. 1). Research documents not only the impact of coalitions on the success of social movements but also the lack of success due to the absence of effective coalitions (Van Dyke & Amos, 2017).

The model presented in this chapter depicts a coalition that addresses issues that affect access to quality education for all children and youth. The coalition efforts, individually or collectively with other organizations, can be a component of a social movement on the local level addressing community and school issues related to social justice (restorative justice–based school discipline, social justice–oriented teaching, racism and inequity within the community), education (access to quality early childhood education, parent and family engagement, instruction that actively engages students in meaningful teaching and learning), and public health (access to physical activity in the school and community, school food services, inequity in health-promoting resources). There are also broader social forces at the state and national levels that have an impact on social justice–education–health issues that affect access to quality education on the local level. For example, at the local level, a community coalition can be focused on a school's efforts to implement a K–12 health education curriculum including sexuality education, while also being involved in a broader social action effort that is engaging multiple organizations in actively advocating against attempts by state-level officials to restrict schools' ability to address sexual orientation and gender identity in health education curricula. What is of key importance is the recognition by the local community coalition that the broader social issues can have an impact at the local level. Examples of related local and state/national actions are presented in table 7.1.

The following steps present a sequential approach toward the formation and eventual mobilization of individuals and organizations through a community-based coalition. The education–health–social justice coalition should focus on the interdependent relationships among education, health, and social justice; include broad community representation and engagement; establish and maintain knowledge of the community;

TABLE 7.1. Coalition Advocacy: Focal Point

Local	State and national
Working with the local school district on enhancement and infusion of critical thinking and students' analysis of current events in appropriate subjects within the K–12 curriculum	Collaborating with other organizations in the state in opposition to a proposed state ban on selected topics, instructional resources, and teaching methods in school curricula deemed to be controversial and in conflict with state values
Supporting early childhood education programs in the local community in their efforts to offer instruction and provide staffing that meet the early childhood program standards	Advocating with other coalitions and organizations to influence the state's US congressional delegation to support a proposed bill that would cover the cost of early childhood education for all children ages 3 and older
Advocating for the local school district to have all middle and high school health education courses taught by teachers with their primary professional preparation, certification, and interest in health education rather than assigning the courses to physical education teachers	Consulting with the state board of education and state department of education for the reinstatement of separate teacher standards for health education and physical education rather than the recent implementation of one set of standards for both disciplines

develop a clear mission and core values; and engage in actions that are driven by a specific, objective-based plan. The overall process for coalition formation, planning, implementation, and evaluation is presented in figure 7.1.

Making the Connection: Initial Discussions

An idea is not a movement but if it can be connected to relevant issues and nurtured through shared interest, an idea could fuel a movement.

MILDRED THOMPSON, quoted in Institute of Medicine (2014)

Coalitions and social movements do not happen on their own. People must act! One person or a small group of individuals who believe in the importance of social justice and quality education for all can initiate action by reaching out to others. While the emphasis in this chapter is

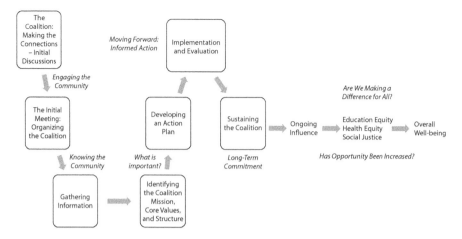

Figure 7.1. Coalition Formation and Action: Mobilizing a Social Movement

placed on the role of educators, physicians, and public health professionals in serving as the initiators or early champions of an education–health–social justice social movement, individuals outside of these professions can also be players in the initiation. Educators, public health professionals, and physicians are suggested as important early leaders in the formation of a coalition for this movement because of their common overarching professional goal (overall quality of life), expertise, and community networks. In addition, research shows high levels of community trust and respect for physicians and public health professionals (Wood & Grumback, 2019). Regarding physicians, while the focus of this social movement should be of interest to all physicians, family physicians, internal medicine physicians, and pediatricians have been identified for initial coalition leadership because of the nature of their professional practice. Their work involves interaction with a representative cross section of the population and addresses a range of health issues. In addition, their professional organizations, the American Academy of Family Physicians, the American College of Physicians, and the American Academy of Pediatrics, have recognized multisector, community-based action as important to their members' work (American Academy of Family Physicians, 2020; American College of Physicians, n.d.; Kuo et al., 2018).

TABLE 7.2. Potential Education–Medicine–Public Health Coalition Members (Community Level)

Teachers and School Administrators
School Representatives of 10 WSCC Model Components
Student Representatives
Family Practice Physicians and Pediatricians
Other Physicians and Health Care Providers
    Physician Specialists
    Dentists
    Nurses
Public Health Professionals
    Local or State Departments of Public Health
    Voluntary Health Agencies (American Cancer Society, American Heart Association, American Diabetes Association, American Lung Association)
Nongovernmental Health Organization Representatives
Representatives of Social Service Agencies
College/University Faculty Members in Education, Public Health, Medicine, Social Services
Leaders/Representative of Faith Community
Members of the Business Community
Leaders/Representatives of Neighborhood Organizations
Parks and Recreation Professionals
Representatives from Local Government
    City/Town Council
    Law Enforcement
    Housing
    Transportation
    Labor/Workforce Development

To move the coalition forward, the conveners must connect and engage in discussion with other individuals who may have personal or professional interest in promoting an education–health–social justice agenda for schools and the local community. This connection might take place when one person or a small group connects with other individuals within their profession or in another profession, or when outreach is made to individual stakeholders within the community. Examples of possible representatives from various organizations for outreach are presented in table 7.2.

Regardless of the nature of the initial connection, the focus of this interpersonal communication should be on information sharing and the recruitment of individuals to participate in an organizational meeting for the formation of the coalition. The discussion can focus on the lifelong reciprocal relationship that exists between health, academic success, and education attainment (see chap. 1). However, the discussion should go further. The following steps present a framework for these interactions (the book chapters noted in parentheses include background information related to the corresponding discussion topic):

1. Describe the reciprocal relationship that exists between health and academic success throughout a person's life. Highlight the basic idea that healthy kids are more likely to be successful academically and attain higher levels of education, and adults who attain higher levels of education are more likely to experience better adult health outcomes (see chap. 1).

2. Present the impact of social injustices on both education and health (see chaps. 2 and 5).

3. Emphasize that the goals of educators, public health professionals, and physicians overlap—all three professions want individuals to develop the knowledge and skills needed to thrive as adults and contribute to their own well-being, the well-being of others, and the well-being of the overall community. However, to impact a community and schools, community-wide representation is needed. The intent of this multisectoral, community-wide partnership is to mobilize a coalition that acts on the local level and serves as a partner in a social movement intended to enable all children, youth, and adults to live in socially just, safe, supportive communities and have equal access to a quality early childhood and elementary, middle, and high school education that provides preparation for a healthy, fulfilling life at the individual, family, and community levels.

Beyond these three focal points, the discussion can also address overall thoughts regarding the participants' current knowledge on local community and school issues; perceptions of barriers and supporting factors related to quality education, health, and overall well-being in the community; and the potential role of educators, public health professionals, and physicians in serving as leaders in a local coalition and community-wide social movement. The important "ask" of the interaction will be ascertaining individuals' interest and willingness to be involved in planning and convening a meeting to form a coalition. After this meeting, those willing to move forward will schedule a meeting to begin planning the organization of a coalition.

Moving toward a Coalition: The Organizational Meeting

Unfortunately, our nation's limited support and sectoral approach to education and health care have often prevented us from realizing the benefits of this reciprocal relationship, thus missing an important opportunity to improve school achievement, promote health, and reduce socioeconomic and racial/ethnic disparities in health and education. RUGLIS & FREUDENBERG (2010)

Once interested participants have stepped forward, expanding the group and planning the organizational meeting are the next steps. This process can begin by identifying potential meeting participants. One step will be further outreach to educators, local family practice physicians and pediatricians, public health professionals, representatives of local education organizations, and other potential participants listed in table 7.2. A resource developed through a partnership between the de Beaumont Foundation, the CDC, and Duke Community and Family Medicine titled *The Practical Playbook II—Building Multisector Partnerships That Work* identifies numerous multisector collaborations formed to promote community health. While coalition membership typically includes organizations, individual community members can also be important members of coalitions. These individuals may not necessarily be recognized for their affiliation with an organization but may be recognized by community members as informal leaders with an understanding of the pulse of the community or may be individual volunteers with a personal commitment to education, health, and social justice. It is important that the process is invitational, clearly demonstrates inclusivity, and ensures that all segments of the population and all areas of the overall community have representation.

In addition to identifying the potential participants for the organizational meeting, a time and location must be identified. Most important is the meeting agenda. Below is a suggested agenda that presents background information on the reciprocal relationship between education and health, provides an opportunity for active engagement of all participants, and sets the stage for moving forward. Another important part of the planning for the meeting is the identification of a facilitator or several facilitators to open and close the meeting and facilitate the open discussions. In addition, other group members will need to present information related to the topics discussed throughout this book.

Suggested Meeting Agenda
- Overview of the education-health reciprocal relationship. (See chap. 1.)
- Open discussion: What does it mean to be educated and healthy? What do you see as the goals of schools? (See chaps. 1, 5, and 6.)
- Factors that affect academic achievement and health: equity, social justice, early childhood, school connectedness, absenteeism, and graduation. (See chaps. 2, 3, and 4.)
- Factors present in schools that promote education and health. (See chaps. 5 and 6.)
- Open discussion: (1) Thoughts on the education-health relationship? (2) Thoughts on the quality of local schools? (3) Perceptions of barriers and supporting factors related to quality education, health, and overall well-being in the community? (4) Potential role of a local community coalition to address education and health at the local level? (5) Broad-based social issues at the state and national levels that affect access to quality education and health for children and youth?
- Moving forward: What are next steps? Who is in? Who is interested in helping to plan next steps? Who is willing to serve as a group coordinator or co-coordinator?

Following this meeting, a commitment should be sought from organizations for participation as coalition members. Once the membership has been determined, the new coalition is ready to move forward to two important tasks: information gathering and formalizing the mission, core values, and structure of the coalition.

Information Gathering

Public decisions affect the lives of millions of people in deep and lasting ways. For this reason it is essential that these decisions be based on accurate information and solid analysis, not assumptions or half-truths.

JIM SCHULTZ, quoted in Snyder & Iton (2020)

Once the first group of individuals and organizations who will engage in the coalition has been identified, the coalition needs to be formalized and prepared to move forward. Being informed is essential. One important early step is the gathering and analysis of information about the local schools and the assets, needs, and issues within the community. Information-gathering actions can include the review of relevant school and community policies; interviews with key school and community leaders; meetings with students, as well as their parents and family members, in the local schools; and open meetings with community members. The purposes of information gathering with school representatives include learning about the core values of the school system, approaches to teaching and learning, the overall school environment, and school accomplishments and challenges. The interactions with students, parents, and community members should focus on their perceptions of what is important in education, how the local community supports school-age children, community and school social justice issues, and local community and school challenges. The information gathering should focus not only on needs and issues but also on community and school assets. Examples of questions to guide this effort are presented in table 7.3.

This information-gathering phase may take considerable time. It is important that the coalition affirm its existence through periodic meetings during this phase. As this information is gathered, coalition meetings should be scheduled to review and discuss findings.

TABLE 7.3. Examples of Information-Gathering Questions

School
What is the school's mission? What are important core values?
How are students actively engaged in learning?
In what ways is learning assessed?
What extracurricular activities are available to all students?
How is students' health promoted?
What is the level of parent and family engagement in the school?
What are the positive and negative aspects of the school environment?
What are the school's most important assets for students and families?
What are the school's major challenges?

Community
What are the positive aspects of growing up in the community experienced by
children and youth?
What are the challenges faced by children and youth growing up in the community?
What are adults' perceptions of the schools in the community?
As a parent or supportive family member, what helps you or serves as a barrier to
you in supporting your child's education? As a community member, what helps
you or serves as a barrier to you in supporting local schools?

Identifying the Mission, Core Values, and Structure

Multisectoral partnerships are complex but rewarding and can lead to significant
and durable change. As public health transforms into a 21st century model,
communities will need to work together to create innovative and sustained
organizational structures that include agencies or organizations across multiple
sectors and with a shared vision. AUERBACH & DESALVO (2019)

Once the school and community information has been gathered and
analyzed, the coalition members will be more informed and prepared
to make decisions that are related to the organization's future direction
and action. So that the coalition is organized for decision-making and
action, a formal structure and function need to be addressed. Important to the direction of the coalition will be the development of a mission
statement and core values. A mission statement is a brief description
of the purpose of a program (McKenzie et al., 2017). It should define
success for the group or organization (Serpas et al., 2016). Because of
the broad-based nature of the coalition's focus (education, health, social
justice) and the diverse nature of the organizations represented in the
coalition, the development of core values is also recommended. Core

TABLE 7.4. Sample Coalition Mission and Core Values

Mission Statement
The mission of the Overline Coalition is to engage in broad-based advocacy and support so that all students live and learn in a safe, supportive, socially just, and health-promoting environment and have equal access to quality early childhood, elementary, middle, and high schools that offer meaningful teaching and learning. All children and youth should have the opportunity to develop and apply the knowledge and skills needed now and in the future to promote well-being, contribute to society, and live meaningful lives.

Core Values
Equity
Social Justice
Broad-Based School, Family, and Community Engagement
Advocacy
Support
Health, Safety, and Well-Being

---

values represent essential principles that are not compromised at any point in the organization's work. The principles are related to the coalition's mission and present a clear representation to all stakeholders of what is essential to the organization's existence. The mission statement and core values should reflect the input provided by the school and community stakeholders and provide direction to the coalition's action planning and overall work. All organizations included in the coalition and individual members should be engaged in the development of both the mission statement and core values. A hypothetical example of a coalition mission statement and concomitant core values is presented in table 7.4.

Leadership is essential to optimal functioning of coalitions. Whether through a formal or informal process, the coalition membership should select a chair or cochairs. Important responsibilities of the chair or cochairs include finalizing the agenda, facilitating coalition meetings, providing leadership in the delegation and monitoring of coalition activities and tasks, providing leadership during discussion or debates on coalition issues, and, when needed, being a personal representative for the coalition at meetings and events. Leadership terms should be set for a specific time period, often one year, with consecutive terms allowed (Butterfoss, 2009).

Because of the broad focus on an education–health–social justice coalition, a structure and process should be in place that keeps members informed of school and community accomplishments, issues, and actions. One method for maintaining this communication is through members serving as coalition liaisons. The liaisons can be responsible for providing coalition members with updates related to specific school and community topic areas. Liaisons should be representative of as many of the coalition organizations as possible. In order to increase organizational representation and decrease individual member workload, two individuals can serve as liaisons for each topic area. The liaisons would be responsible for monitoring actions and issues related to an assigned area. Examples of topic areas for liaisons include the following:

- Local governmental issues, policies, or laws that affect education and health
- Local school board activities
- Community/school social justice issues (equity, racism and other systemic discrimination, school discipline policies)
- Community opportunity issues (employment, transportation, access to healthy food and physical activity)
- State, national, and global issues (education, health, social justice)
- School curriculum and instruction issues
- Coordinated approach to teaching, learning, and health (WSCC model)
- Student engagement, accomplishments, and issues
- Early childhood programs (includes early childhood education)

As noted throughout this book, an education–health–social justice coalition must be focused on a variety of issues that affect schools and the ability of families, community members, and organizations to maximize access to and the quality of education for children and youth. Many of these issues are affected by education, health, and social justice-related policies. The importance of policies has been recognized by the public health profession through its "Health in All Policies" campaign. Health in All Policies has been defined as a "collaborative approach to improving health that incorporates health considerations into decision-making in all sectors and policy areas" (Rudolph et al., 2013, p. 135). Expanding this approach to a coalition effort, education, health, and social justice would be considered in all sectors and policies. Implementing this approach for education–health–social justice coalitions would involve informing policy makers of the interdependent relationship of these three areas; engaging decision-makers in consideration of the positive or negative education, health, and social justice impacts of a potential policy; and clearly communicating the coalition's position related to the policy.

Developing an Action Plan

Building bridges between public health, primary care, the school district, and other community organizations began with recognizing a common problem, making a cooperative decision to merge expertise and resources, and determining shared interventions.   SERPAS ET AL. (2016)

With the development of a mission statement, the identification of core values, the analysis of community and school information, and a structure in place, the development of an action plan is the next step in moving the coalition forward. The first step in the development of the action plan is the identification of goals and objectives. The goals and objectives should be informed by the school and community analysis and related directly to the organization's mission and core values. Goals represent more general outcomes, while objectives are more specific and lead to the attainment of goals. In most cases there are multiple objectives linked to a goal. The specificity of objectives is illustrated by using verbs that denote actions that can be measured or observed.

The goals and objectives provide the direction for coalition activities. Actions can be identified that will lead to the accomplishment of each of the objectives. While any action plan should be appropriately challenging and address immediate community and school issues, Johnson (2016) recommends that some less challenging "early wins" be included in a new organization's action plan. It is suggested that "early wins" build optimism, momentum, and multisector relationships as the movement continues. With a nascent coalition, early actions and objectives may be focused more on establishing relationships, further information gathering, and educating others about the organization and its mission. Follow-up action plans will be more focused on supportive and change-related actions. These actions might include advocating for changes in school or community policy or practice; addressing social justice issues such as the need for more diverse faculty, poverty, and inequity; providing diverse representation on community or school committees; organizing public forums on education, health, and social justice issues; using traditional and social media for education and advocacy; endorsing or identifying candidates for elected office; mobilizing voters; and engaging in social movement actions related to state, national, and global issues. These state and national issues may be addressed by the coalition individually or in partnership with other organizations as part of a state or national social movement.

An evaluation protocol should be established for all action plans during the planning phase. Michener et al. (2016) have identified several outcomes of evaluation:

- Determining successes that resulted from the implementation of actions.
- Identifying what actions worked well and which ones did not and why.
- Assessing the strength of the partnership.
- Documenting what has been accomplished within the community and schools.

One aspect of the evaluation should focus on process. This aspect should address members' perception of the process, including information such as satisfaction with communication within the committee, level of involvement with committee planning and implementation of activities, and the organization and scheduling of the meetings. Process evaluation should be conducted throughout the duration of the program. In addition, impact evaluation should be conducted that is based on the attainment of goals and objectives. As noted, objectives should define specific outcomes that can be measured or observed. Basically, impact evaluation determines whether or not the coalition is accomplishing the intent of the action plan.

Advocacy Considerations

Racism and other forms of discrimination, inequity, power and powerlessness, corporate agendas, political interests, and misinformation are among a variety of factors that create a lack of equal opportunity and affect education and health. These factors are seldom changed in a consequential manner through individual action. Advocates must inform, mobilize, and act to promote equal access to meaningful education for all children and youth and overall well-being for all community members.   BIRCH (n.d.)

Many coalition actions will focus on advocacy. Fisher and Hancher-Rauch (2022) describe advocacy as "action in support of a cause" (p. 148). Advocacy actions may focus on community and school policy changes, social justice issues, support for candidates for an elected office, and opposition or support for local, state, or federal legislation. These actions may involve interactions with elected community officials, school board members, school administrators, teachers, social service and private sector representatives, community members, parents, and students. The interactions may be planned or incidental, occur with one person or a group, and take place during a public or private meeting or through traditional or social media. The following considerations are presented to provide direction for coalition and social movement advocacy:

- Stress the basic message of the movement: healthy children are more likely to be successful in school, successful students who achieve higher levels of education are more likely to be healthier as adults, and social injustices affect both education and health.
- Good schools (early childhood through high school) and well-educated students benefit the entire community now and in the future.
- Social injustice negatively affects the community now and in the future.

- Focus on who needs to be influenced by the advocacy message: Who are the decision-makers? Who and what can influence the decision-makers?
- What are the best methods to present the advocacy message?
- Decision-makers and community members respond to different types of messages. Use both data and stories—some will respond best to data, others to stories, and some to both.
- Anticipate and be prepared for difficult questions. Prior to any advocacy effort, identify anticipated questions and develop appropriate responses.

Sustaining the Coalition and the Social Movement

But whatever we do, we need to work directly with those closest to the problems—teachers, principals, students, families and community leaders—to build a movement that is focused on preparing most or all students for the world that they live in, that promotes lasting change. It will not be simple and will take a commitment of many years and require leadership in the community.

ADAPTED FROM SCHOALES (2019)

Initiating a coalition and developing an action plan to address education, health, and social justice is a monumental first step in moving toward important change. The broad-based focus of social change is not a one-time or short-term effort, but rather an effort that is ongoing. Almeida (2019) has indicated that the broader the goals and collective action of the mobilization, the longer the time that is needed for the effort to be considered a movement. Note also that the community education and social context is not static. Best practices in education and health change over time, new issues surface, existing issues persist, personnel in organizations change, and community and school elections create changes in leadership and philosophy. Not only do changes occur that affect the community, but changes can also occur within the organizations that are coalition members. Because of this constant change, adjustments in goals, objectives, and actions are often necessary to maintain a vibrant coalition over time.

Because of the fluidity of community and school factors, an important step in sustaining coalition action is a regularly scheduled review and subsequent revisions of a coalition action plan. While the review process is conducted by coalition members, it can also be informed by open review meetings or online postings that can engage community and school stakeholders. This review can focus on actions and accomplishments and provide input on next steps.

Based on the review process, action plan revisions can include addressing new issues that require new goals, objectives, and actions; adjustments for changes in ongoing issues; and the elimination of issues that are no longer pertinent to the social movement. Another ongoing consideration is increasing the number of organizations in the coalition. There may be new organizations in the community that can contribute, organizations that have been overlooked, or organizations that are pertinent to new issues being addressed. While not needed as frequently as the regular reviews of the action plan, periodic reviews of the coalition mission and core values can also provide a check on the relevancy of the organization.

Sustainability can be a challenge for coalitions and movements. Being valued and supported by stakeholders, having a capacity to work together to address the mission, and upholding a vision for future activities are hallmarks of sustainability (Minyard et al., 2016). The following checkpoints are presented for consideration to maximize the success and sustainability of the coalition and the overall movement:

- Articulate a clear mission and core values.
- Know the community. Understand and respect the natural, social, cultural, and historic values of the community and its members (Foreman & Chappelle, 2019).
- Be invitational. Value the perceptions of all members of the community and all students. Make sure that the views of the community members and students who might be typically overlooked or not represented are elicited and considered (Norris & Hill, 2019).
- Promote inclusivity within the coalition—be intentional. Provide

all members and organizations an opportunity for engagement in coalition activities and dialogue (Issel & Wells, 2018).

- Demonstrate ongoing, meaningful communication both within the coalition and with external stakeholders (Minyard et al., 2016)
- Building and maintaining relationships is essential—between members of the coalition, between the coalition and community and education organizations, and between the coalition and members of the community (Van Dyke & Amos, 2017).
- Understand how social injustices such as history, power, and privilege affect both education and health. Individually and collectively, demonstrate a commitment toward anti-racism, equity, and social justice (Khalifa, 2018; Love, 2019).
- Create and maintain an environment in which stakeholders understand that the social movement issues have an impact on them (Almeida, 2019). Emphasize that current students are future neighbors, community workers, and leaders. Help the personal become political (Freudenberg, 2014).
- Plan activities based on an action plan rather than on a project-by-project approach (Butterfoss, 2009).
- Make decisions on issues using consensus rather than voting (Butterfoss, 2009).
- Use a variety of tactics to attain goals and objectives (Almeida, 2019).
- Use various forms of communication within the coalition and with outside decision-makers and stakeholders, including both traditional and social media (Fisher & Hancher-Rauch, 2022).
- Develop positive relationships with local media (Butterfoss, 2009).
- Stay up to date—keep up with the latest information, trends, and issues in the community, in the local school or schools, in education at the state and national levels, and in health and well-being.
- Conduct productive coalition meetings (Butterfoss, 2009). Prepare a summary of the important decisions and discussions (Michener & Castrucci, 2016).

- Conduct ongoing process and impact evaluation (Butterfoss, 2009).
- Showcase coalition and movement accomplishments to members and all stakeholders.

Sustainability should be thought of as an ongoing consideration for coalitions and movements. Following best practices, achieving successes, and showcasing progress will increase the likelihood of institutionalization and sustainability.

An important underpinning of this book is that educators, public health professionals, and physicians have the expertise and professional presence to provide leadership to initiate coalitions and engage in social movements that present, over time, a strong community voice for social justice and quality education for all children and their families. Echoing Ruglis and Freudenberg (2010), it is the intent that this book promote a "revitalized social movement for healthy schools" that results in a force that can move communities and schools "to advance a vision that can mobilize the diverse constituencies needed to change policies and practices" (pp. 1565–66).

Throughout the book, education and health are presented as important interdependent outcomes of students' school experience. Educators know that students are more likely to be successful if they are healthy and live in a supportive, socially just home and community environment. Physicians understand that where their patients live, learn, work, and play, as well as the social factors faced in their everyday lives, have an overwhelming influence on their health. Public health professionals recognize the importance of education, social justice, and the engagement of community members in the promotion of individual and community health. It is hoped that this book will encourage educators, physicians, public health professionals, and community members to lead and collaboratively engage in an ongoing social movement that results in continual monitoring, advocacy, and community support so that all children and youth have equal access to a meaningful education and, along with their family members, have the opportunity to live in socially just communities. These outcomes should lead to children and youth who are healthy, have academic and health-enhancing skills, exhibit a commitment to equity and social justice, and are prepared to not only thrive in their own lives but also be informed and engaged as community members and contribute to the overall well-being of others.

Education, Health, and Social Justice Organizations

The Afterschool Alliance. The mission of the Alliance is to ensure that all youth have access to affordable, quality afterschool programs by engaging public will to increase public and private investment in afterschool program initiatives at the national, state, and local levels. Encouraging sustainable investments, inspiring holistic youth development, supporting equitable access, and empowering community action are the core values related to the organization's work. The Alliance's efforts include serving as a resource and voice for affordable afterschool and summer programs. http://www.afterschoolalliance.org/aboutUs.cfm

Alliance for Early Success. The Alliance for Early Success works to put vulnerable young children on a path to success. As an alliance of state, national, and funding partners, our goal is to advance state policies that lead to improved health, learning, and economic outcomes for young children, starting at birth and continuing through age 8. The Alliance creates and enhances partnerships by bringing leaders together with the goal of achieving results faster and better than anyone could do alone. https://earlysuccess.org/about-us

Alliance for Excellence in Education (ALL4Ed). The mission of ALL4Ed is to promote high school transformation to make it possible for every child to graduate prepared for postsecondary learning and success in life. All4Ed strives to improve low-performing high schools while simultaneously supporting high expectations, innovation, and school system redesign. The work focuses on ensuring that all students enjoy a high school experience that allows them to identify and build on passions, strengths, and interests while receiving the comprehensive support they need to develop the academic knowledge and deeper learning skills necessary for success in postsecondary education, training, a career, and life. https://all4ed.org

The American Academy of Family Physicians (AAFP) Center for Diversity and Health Equity. The AAFP Center for Diversity and Health Equity addresses social determinants of health through The EveryONE Project. The project focuses on addressing social determinants of health by
- providing AAFP members with education and information about health equity;
- identifying and developing clinical tools and resources to address patients' social needs;
- supporting research and policy development;

- advocating for policies that encourage health equity;
- encouraging workforce diversity; and
- serving as a resource center for AAFP members.

https://www.aafp.org/family-physician/patient-care/the-everyone-project/aafp
-center-for-diversity-and-health-equity.html

American School Health Association. The mission of the American School Health Association is to transform all schools into places where every student learns and thrives. The American School Health Association envisions healthy students who learn and achieve in safe and healthy environments nurtured by caring adults functioning within coordinated school and community support systems. The Association is a multidisciplinary organization of administrators, counselors, dietitians, nutritionists, health educators, physical educators, psychologists, school health coordinators, school nurses, school physicians, and social workers.
http://www.ashaweb.org/about/

America's Promise Alliance. America's Promise Alliance is devoted to helping to create the conditions for success for all young people. The work of the Alliance is powered by the belief that all children are capable of learning and thriving and that every individual, institution, and sector shares the responsibility to help young people succeed.
https://www.americaspromise.org

ASCD. ASCD empowers educators to achieve excellence in learning, teaching, and leading so that every child is healthy, safe, engaged, supported, and challenged. The membership includes superintendents, principals, teachers, and advocates from all over the world. The ASCD community also includes affiliate organizations. ASCD is committed to helping educators enhance their crafts and enhance their roles by providing high-quality, research-based resources and support in the development of highly effective learning systems. Supporting the whole child is at the core of the ASCD mission. ASCD works to ensure that each student is healthy, safe, engaged, supported, and challenged.
http://www.ascd.org/about-ascd.aspx

Attendance Works. The mission of Attendance Works is to promote equal opportunities to learn and advance student success by reducing chronic absence. The organization's aspirations are to (1) build public awareness and political will to partner with students and families to address the challenges that prevent them from participating in learning; (2) encourage proven and innovative practices to take a data-driven approach to partnering with students and families to improve attendance and engagement; (3) facilitate peer learning among schools, districts, and states; and (4) advance policies (local, state, and federal) that improve attendance and reduce chronic attendance by making data systems more transparent, providing equitable access to resources and removing barriers to getting to school.
https://www.attendanceworks.org/mission/

Center on the Developing Child—Harvard University. The mission of the Center on the Developing Child is to drive science-based innovation that achieves breakthrough outcomes for children facing adversity. Founded in 2006, the Center catalyzes local, national, and international innovation in policy and practice focused on children and families. The Center designs, tests, and implements these ideas in collaboration with a broad network of research, practice, policy, community, and philanthropic leaders in order to identify transformational impacts on lifelong learning, behavior, and both physical and mental health.
https://developingchild.harvard.edu

Chiefs for Change. Chiefs for Change is a national organization whose members are current and former leaders of state and district education systems. The organization believes that every child must have access to an excellent education, fully prepared teachers who are provided with support to do their jobs well, high-quality instructional materials, and reliable and affordable pathways to college and meaningful careers. To attain these outcomes, the organization collectively advocates for policies and practices that have an impact on students' school experiences and works to develop future school leaders.
https://www.chiefsforchange.org/

Child Trends. Child Trends is a research organization focused exclusively on improving the lives of children and youth, especially those who are most vulnerable. The organization works to ensure that all kids thrive by conducting independent research and partnering with practitioners and policy makers to apply that knowledge. Child Trends believes that programs and policies that serve children are most effective when they are informed by data and evidence and grounded in deep knowledge of child and youth development.
https://www.childtrends.org/about-us

Communities in Schools. Working directly in 2,300 schools in 25 states and the District of Columbia, Communities in Schools builds relationships that empower students to stay in school and succeed in life. The school-based staff partners with teachers to identify challenges students face in class or at home and coordinate with community partners to bring outside resources inside schools.
https://www.communitiesinschools.org/about-us/

Council for a Strong America. The Council for a Strong America engages law enforcement, military, business, faith, and sports leaders who promote evidence-based policies and programs that enable kids to be healthy, well educated, and prepared for productive lives.
https://www.strongnation.org/

The Education Trust. The Education Trust is a national nonprofit that works to close opportunity gaps that disproportionately affect students of color and students from low-income families. Through research and advocacy, Ed Trust supports efforts that expand excellence and equity in education from preschool through college, increase

college access and completion particularly for historically underserved students, engage diverse communities dedicated to education equity, and increase political and public will to act on equity issues.
https://edtrust.org/who-we-are/

EveryDay Labs. EveryDay Labs, formerly known as InClassToday, works to improve student outcomes through the power of behavioral science. The organization partners with districts to reduce absenteeism. To date, the program has served students across more than 2,000 schools, preventing more than 400,000 absences, equating to over 150 million minutes of instructional time.
https://everydaylabs.com

Everyone Graduates Center (EGC)—Johns Hopkins University. The mission of EGC is to develop and disseminate the know-how required to enable all students to graduate from high school prepared for college, career, and civic life. Through a systematic and comprehensive approach, EGC combines analysis of the causes, location, and consequences of the nation's dropout crisis with the development of tools and models designed to keep all students on the path to high school graduation and capacity-building efforts to enable states, communities, school districts, and schools to provide all their students with the supports they need to succeed and the capacity to sustain them.
http://www.every1graduates.org

Facing History and Ourselves. Facing History and Ourselves uses lessons of history to challenge teachers and their students to stand up to bigotry and hate. Facing History's resources and trainings address topics including racism, anti-Semitism, and prejudice. The resources are designed to help students connect choices made in the past to those they will confront in their own lives. Independent research studies show that experience in a Facing History classroom motivates students to become upstanders in their communities, whether by challenging negative stereotypes at the dinner table, standing up to a bully in their neighborhood, or registering to vote when they are eligible.
https://www.facinghistory.org/about-us

Foundation for Child Development. The Foundation's mission is to use research to ensure that all young children benefit from early learning experiences that affirm their individual, family, and community assets; fortify them against harmful consequences arising from poverty, racism, prejudice, and discrimination; and strengthen their developmental potential. The Foundation supports policies, practices, and relevant research to understand young children, particularly our priority populations, and to understand the complex, individual and interacting systems that impact them. The Foundation believes that families, schools, nonprofit organizations, businesses, and government at all levels share complementary responsibilities in supporting policies and practices that promote children's well-being.
https://www.fcd-us.org/

Gay, Lesbian & Straight Education Network (GLSEN). GLSEN conducts extensive and original research to inform evidence-based solutions for K–12 education with a focus on LGBTQ students and those with marginalized identities. The organization has authored developmentally appropriate resources for educators to use throughout their school community. GLSEN also advises on, advocates for, and researches comprehensive policies designed to protect LGBTQ students and students of marginalized identities. The organization coordinates a network of 43 chapters in 30 states across the nation. These efforts are designed to empower students to affect change by supporting student-led efforts to positively impact their own schools and local communities and have thousands of registered Gay-Straight Alliances nationwide. https://www.glsen.org/about-us

Gay-Straight Alliance Network. Gay-straight alliances, or GSAs for short, are student-run organizations that unite LGBTQ+ and allied youth to build community and organize around issues impacting them in their schools and communities. GSAs have evolved beyond their traditional role of serving as safe spaces for LGBTQ+ youth in middle schools and high schools and have emerged as vehicles for deep social change related to racial, gender, and educational justice. https://gsanetwork.org/what-is-a-gsa/

Kaiser Permanente "Thriving Schools." Thriving Schools works to support schools to become beacons of health in communities. Two mutually reinforcing programmatic areas with Thriving Schools are Healthy Eating Active Living (HEAL) and Resilience in School Environments (RISE). The HEAL initiative supports schools and districts in developing solutions to support their nutritional and physical activity needs, while the RISE initiative supports school staff, teachers, districts, and the community in addressing the underlying factors of stress in schools and developing strategies and practices that foster more positive school environments. The Thriving Schools' vision is that every community can count on their school as a champion for good health that enables great learning. https://thrivingschools.kaiserpermanente.org

Learning Policy Institute. The Learning Policy Institute conducts and communicates independent research to improve education policy and practice. Working with policy makers, researchers, educators, community groups, and others, the Institute seeks to advance evidence-based policies that support empowerment and equitable learning for every child. The Institute connects policy makers and stakeholders at the local, state, and federal levels with the evidence, ideas, and actions needed to strengthen the education system from preschool through college and career readiness. https://learningpolicyinstitute.org/about

National Association for the Education of Young Children (NAEYC). NAEYC promotes high-quality early learning for all children, from birth through age 8, by connecting practice, policy, and research. The organization advances a diverse,

dynamic early childhood profession and supports all who care for, educate, and work on behalf of young children.
https://www.naeyc.org/

National Association of Latino Elected and Appointed Officials Fund (NALEO). The NALEO Educational Fund is a nonpartisan organization that facilitates full Latino participation in the American political process, from citizenship to public service. Founded in 1981, the NALEO Educational Fund uses integrated strategies that include increasing the effectiveness of Latino policy makers, mobilizing the Latino community to engage in civic life, and promoting policies that advance Latino political engagement. The NALEO Educational Fund provides national leadership on key issues that affect Latino participation in our political process, including immigration and naturalization, voting rights, election reform, the Census, and the appointment of qualified Latinos to top executive and judicial positions.
https://naleo.org/about/

National Black Child Development Institute (NBCDI). For more than 40 years, NBCDI has been at the forefront of engaging leaders, policy makers, professionals, and parents regarding critical and timely issues that directly impact Black children and their families. NBCDI delivers culturally relevant resources that respond to the unique strengths and needs of Black children around issues such as early childhood education, health, child welfare, literacy, and family engagement. With the support of affiliate networks in communities across the country, NBCDI is committed to its mission "to improve and advance the quality of life for Black children and their families through education and advocacy."
https://www.nbcdi.org/who-we-are

National Center for Children in Poverty (NCCP). NCCP conducts research and translates the findings into actionable recommendations to improve the lives and futures of low-income children and their families. NCCP delves into issues that contribute to child poverty to make meaningful change that reduces the number of families experiencing hardship. Founded in 1989 as a division of the Mailman School of Public Health at Columbia University, NCCP is a nonpartisan, public interest research organization.
http://www.nccp.org/about.html

National Center for Homeless Education (NCHE). Funded by the US Department of Education, NCHE operates the department's technical assistance center for the federal Education for Homeless Children and Youth (EHCY) program. In this role, NCHE works with schools, service providers, parents, and other interested stakeholders to ensure that children and youth experiencing homelessness can enroll and succeed in school.
https://nche.ed.gov

National Center for Restorative Justice. The organization works toward a world in which justice is equitable and compassionate through working with those that serve youth. The work is focused on five restorative priorities that can be implemented in schools, juvenile facilities, and families: conflict awareness, engage all stakeholders, empower author and victim, value empathy, and increase empathy. The restorative practices seek to build relationship, trust, and understanding through the leveraging of conflict. These practices foster youth capacity for not only educational and relational success but also self-reflective accountable citizenship. http://www.nationalcenterforrestorativejustice.com

National Center for Safe Routes to School. The National Center for Safe Routes to School promotes safe walking and biking. It provides ways for communities to get started and offers information available to make the future they envision a reality. The National Center coordinates Walk to School Day and Bike to School Day to help communities create the momentum needed for lasting change. The Center uses research-based evidence to highlight what works and translates this research into education, professional development tools, and training to provide communities the technical support needed to make community-enhancing decisions. http://www.saferoutesinfo.org

National Center on Early Childhood and Wellness (NCECHW). NCECHW advances best practices for linking health and early childhood education systems, health care professionals, and families. The organization's goal is to maximize resources for developing comprehensive and coordinated health and wellness services within early childhood education settings. The Center's work includes, but is not limited to, providing support on topics such as medical and dental home access, health promotion and disease prevention, emergency preparedness and environmental safety, trauma and toxic stress, screening, and nutrition. The Center promotes effective practices and professional development within programs serving high-risk, low-income children from birth to age 5, as well as pregnant women and expectant families. NCECHW is responsive to the unique needs of children who are dual language learners, in foster care, and experiencing homelessness, as well as children in Tribal early childhood programs and Migrant and Seasonal Head Start (MSHS) programs. https://eclkc.ohs.acf.hhs.gov/about-us/article/national-center-early-childhood -health-wellness-ncechw

The National Child Traumatic Stress Network (NCTSN). The NCTSN was created by Congress in 2000 as part of the Children's Health Act to raise the standard of care and increase access to services for children and families who experience or witness traumatic events. This unique network of frontline providers, family members, researchers, and national partners is committed to changing the course of children's lives by improving their care and moving scientific gains quickly into practice across the United States. The NCTSN is administered by the Substance Abuse and Mental Health Services Administration (SAMHSA) and coordinated by the UCLA–Duke University National Center for Child Traumatic Stress (NCCTS). https://www.nctsn.org

National Commission on Social, Emotional, and Academic Development. The Aspen Institute's National Commission on Social, Emotional, and Academic Development works to unite leaders to re-envision what constitutes success in our schools. With the help of teachers, parents, and students in communities across the country, the Commission explores how schools can fully integrate social, emotional, and academic development to support the whole student. https://www.aspeninstitute.org/programs/national-commission-on-social-emotional-and-academic-development/

National Dropout Prevention Center. The mission of the National Dropout Prevention Center is to increase graduation rates through research and evidence-based solutions. Since inception, the National Dropout Prevention Center has worked to improve opportunities for all young people to fully develop the academic, social, work, and healthy life skills needed to graduate from high school and lead productive lives. The center promotes awareness of successful programs and policies related to dropout prevention. http://dropoutprevention.org/who-we-are/our-mission/

National Head Start Association (NHSA). NHSA is a nonprofit organization committed to the belief that every child, regardless of circumstances at birth, has the ability to succeed in life. NHSA is the voice for more than 1 million children, 245,000 staff, and 1,600 Head Start grantees in the United States. Since 1974, NHSA has worked for policy changes that ensure that all at-risk children have access to the Head Start model of support for the whole child, the family, and the community. https://nhsa.org/

National Home Visiting Resource Center (NHVRC). The NHVRC goal is to support sound decisions in policy and practice to help children and families thrive. Early childhood home visiting is a service delivery strategy that matches expectant parents and parents of young children with a designated support person—typically a trained nurse, social worker, or early childhood specialist. Services are voluntary and provided in the family's home or another location of the family's choice. https://nhvrc.org/about-the-nhvrc/

National Institute for Early Education Research (NIEER). NIEER works to improve the learning and development of young children by producing and communicating knowledge to transform policy and practice. The organization collaborates with a network of local, state, national, and international leaders to design, conduct, and disseminate rigorous research, evaluation, and policy analysis. NIEER also helps prepare the next generation of leaders and researchers in early education. https://nieer.org/

NewSchools Venture Fund. NewSchools supports the efforts of teams of educators and innovators who are making a positive difference in public education. As a national nonprofit, NewSchools focuses on impact in four areas: innovative public schools, both district and charter; learning solutions that reinvent the student experience; organizations that advance Black and Latino leadership in education; and early-stage ideas outside its other investment areas that advance racial equity. https://www.newschools.org

Perception Institute. Perception Institute is a consortium of researchers, advocates, and strategists who translate cutting-edge mind science research on race, gender, ethnic, and other identities intended to reduce bias and discrimination and promote belonging. The work is done in education, health care, media, workplace, law enforcement, and civil justice sectors. https://perception.org/about-us/

Rales Center for the Integration of Health and Education. The Rales Center for the Integration of Health and Education works to fundamentally reimagine school health to improve student health and well-being and reduce health and educational inequality. The Rales Center's approach to school health is informed by the CDC's Whole School, Whole Community, Whole Child (WSCC) model. The Rales model provides comprehensive, preventive, and acute care; proactive screening and population health programs; chronic disease management; and family advocacy, alongside student and teacher wellness programming, socioemotional skills development, and linkages to mental health care. The Rales team aims to provide a safe, affirming, and supportive environment that can serve as a pathway to engagement with needed resources for many families. https://ralescenter.hopkinschildrens.org

School-Based Health Alliance (SBHA). The SBHA describes itself as "The National Voice for School-Based Health Care." In this role, the SBHA establishes and advocates for national policy priorities; promotes high-quality clinical practices and standards; supports data collection and reporting, evaluation, and research; and provides training, technical assistance, and consultation. An important focus of the organization's work is on the promotion and support of school-based health centers. https://www.sbh4all.org/wp-content/uploads/2021/04/SBHA_OnePager_4.21.pdf

Southern Education Foundation (SEF). The SEF is committed to advancing education policies and practices that elevate learning for low-income students and students of color in the southern states. The SEF analyzes and amplifies promising ideas through research, government affairs, civic engagement, leadership development, and strategic initiatives. To accomplish the SEF goals, the organization engages in a range of partnerships and coalitions. https://southerneducation.org/

Southern Poverty Law Center (SPLC). The SPLC is dedicated to fighting hate and bigotry and to seeking justice for the most vulnerable members of our society. Using litigation, education, and other forms of advocacy, the SPLC promotes the ideals of equal justice and equal opportunity. SPLC lawsuits have toppled institutional racism and stamped out remnants of Jim Crow segregation; destroyed some of the nation's most violent white supremacist groups; and protected the civil rights of children, women, the disabled, immigrants and migrant workers, the LGBTQ community, prisoners, and many others who faced discrimination, abuse, or exploitation. One SPLC resource is Learning for Justice. This resource provides practitioners who work with children from kindergarten through high school with materials to supplement the curriculum, inform practice, and create civil and inclusive school communities where children and youth are respected, valued, and welcome participants. https://www.splcenter.org/about

Student Experience Research Network (SERN). SERN, formerly the Mindset Scholars Network, advances the research, relationships, and capacity that is needed to support and enhance an education system in which every student is respected and valued. The organization's work focuses not only on respectful interpersonal interactions in school but also on practices, policies, and norms that communicate to every student that they are valued as a person and a thinker. https://studentexperiencenetwork.org/

T.E.A.C.H. Early Childhood® National Center. The T.E.A.C.H. Early Childhood® National Center develops, implements, and sustains programs and strategies to ensure the long-term success of children in school and in life. The Center provides leadership in the early childhood education field to states across the country and to policy makers on the critical importance and value of an educated, well-paid, and stable early childhood workforce to ensure the long-term success of children in school and in life. The T.E.A.C.H vision is for every child in an early childhood setting to have a teacher who is well educated and well compensated, as well as for every early childhood teacher to have access to affordable college education, workforce supports, and continuing professional development on a pathway to valued, sustained employment.
https://teachecnationalcenter.org/about-the-center/

Teaching for Change. Through drawing direct connections to real-world issues, Teaching for Change encourages teachers and students to question and rethink the world within and outside of schools; build a more equitable, multicultural society; and become active global citizens. The organization serves teachers, other school staff members, and parents and family members through the provision of professional development and publications and direction for parent organizing programs. Teaching for Change also curates SocialJusticBooks.org to promote multicultural and social justice books for children, as well as articles and books for educators. https://www.teachingforchange.org/

Too Small to Fail—Clinton Foundation. Too Small to Fail aims to help parents, communities, and businesses take specific actions to improve the health and well-being of children from birth to age 5 so that more of America's children are prepared

for success. Too Small to Fail's public awareness and action campaign raises awareness among parents and caregivers about the critical importance of talking, reading, and singing and provides them with tools to engage in these language-rich interactions.
https://www.clintonfoundation.org/programs/education-health-equity/too-small -fail/

Trans Student Educational Resources. Trans Student Educational Resources is a youth-led organization dedicated to transforming the educational environment for trans and gender-nonconforming students through advocacy and empowerment. In addition to a focus on creating a more trans-friendly education system, the organization educates the public and teaches trans activists how to be effective organizers. The organization believes that justice for trans and gender-nonconforming youth is contingent on an intersectional framework of activism.
https://transstudent.org/about/

Trans Youth Family Allies (TYFA). TYFA works to empower children and families by partnering with educators, service providers, and communities to develop supportive environments in which gender may be expressed and respected. TYFA's work intends to create a society free of suicide and violence in which all children are respected and celebrated. TYFA works to educate schools, health care professionals, daycare centers, courts and legal representatives, child welfare agencies, and communities; eliminate harassment, oppression, and violence; and form alliances with organizations and individuals.
http://www.imatyfa.org/about-us.html

The UCLA Center for Healthier Children, Families and Communities. The Center for Healthier Children, Families, and Communities was established at UCLA in 1995 to address some of the most challenging health and social problems facing children and families. Its mission is to improve society's ability to provide children with the best opportunities for health, well-being, and the chance to assume productive roles within families and communities.
https://ph.ucla.edu/research/centers/center-healthier-children-families-and -communities

University of Chicago Consortium on School Research. The University of Chicago Consortium conducts research of high technical quality to inform and assess policy and practice in the Chicago Public Schools. The Consortium seeks to expand communication among researchers, policy makers, and practitioners and build capacity for school reform by identifying what matters for student success and school improvement, creating critical indicators to chart progress, and conducting theory-driven evaluation to identify how programs and policies are working.
https://consortium.uchicago.edu/about

Welcoming Schools. The Human Rights Campaign Foundation's Welcoming Schools is a professional development program providing training and resources to elementary school educators. The training and resources focus on embracing families, creating LGBTQ- and gender-inclusive schools, preventing bias-based bullying, and supporting transgender and nonbinary students. https://welcomingschools.org/about

Preface

Institute of Medicine. (2015). *Exploring opportunities for collaboration between health and education to improve population health: Workshop summary.* National Academies Press. https://doi.org/10.17226/18979

Kelly, M. J., & Weitzen, S. (2010). The association of lifetime education with the prevalence of myocardial infarction: An analysis of the 2006 behavioral risk factor surveillance system. *Journal of Community Health, 35*(1), 76–80. https://doi.org/10.1007/s10900-009-9189-x

Marmot, M. (2015). *The health gap: The challenge of an unequal world.* Bloomsbury Press.

Zajacova, A., & Lawrence, E. M. (2018). The relationship between education and health: Reducing disparities through a contextual approach. *Annual Review of Public Health, 39*, 273–289. https://doi.org/10.1146/annurev-publhealth-031816-044628

Zimmerman, E. B., Woolf, S. H., & Haley, A. (2015). Understanding the relationship between education and health: A review of the evidence and an examination of community perspectives. In R. M. Kaplan, M. L. Spittel, & D. H. David (Eds.), *Population health: Behavioral and social science insights* (pp. 347–84). Agency for Health-Care Research and Quality & Office of Behavioral and Social Sciences Research, National Institutes of Health.

Chapter 1. Health and Education

AASA, The School Superintendents Association. (2019, July). Belief and position statement: Community collaborative and partnerships for education. https://www.aasa.org/uploadedFiles/About/AASA_Bylaws/Belief-Position-Statements.pdf

Abeles V. (2015). *Beyond measure: Rescuing an overscheduled, overtested, underestimated generation.* Simon & Schuster.

American Academy of Family Physicians. (2020). *Integration of primary care and public health.* https://www.aafp.org/about/policies/all/integration-primary-care.html

American College of Physicians. (n.d.). *Public health.* https://www.acponline.org/advocacy/where-we-stand/public-health

American Medical Association. (2001). *Declaration of professional responsibility: Medicine's social contract with humanity.* https://www.ama-assn.org/system/files/2020-03/declaration-professional-responsibility-english.pdf

American Public Health Association. (n.d.). *About CSHE.* http://www.schoolbasedhealthcare.org/About-CSHE

American School Health Association. (2018). *ASHA position statement: The Every Student Succeeds Act: Implications for K–12 health education and physical education.* http://www.ashaweb.org/wp-content/uploads/2018/12/ASHA-Position-Paper-ESSA-December2018Revision.pdf

Arah, O. A. (2009). On the relationship between individual and population health. *Medicine, Health Care and Philosophy, 12*(3), 235–244. https://doi.org/10.1007/s11019-008-9173-8

ASCD. (2015). *Statement for the integration of health and education.* https://files.ascd.org/staticfiles/ascd/pdf/siteASCD/wholechild/Statement-for-the-Integration-of-Health-and-Education_English.pdf

Ayers, W. (2004). *Teaching toward freedom: Moral commitment and ethical action in the classroom.* Beacon Press.

Barr, D. A. (2019). *Health disparities in the United States: Social class, race, ethnicity, and the social determinants of health* (3rd ed.). Johns Hopkins University Press.

Basch, C. E. (2011). Executive summary: Healthier students are better learners. *Journal of School Health, 81*(10), 591–592. https://doi.org/10.1111/j.1746-1561.2011.00631.x

Birch, D. A., & Videto, D. M. (Eds.). (2015). *Promoting health and academic success: The whole school, whole community, whole child approach.* Human Kinetics.

Bircher, J., & Kuruvilla, S. (2014). Defining health by addressing individual, social, and environmental determinants: New opportunities for health care and public health. *Journal of Public Health Policy, 35*(3), 363–386.

Bradley, B. J., & Greene, A. C. (2013). Do health and education agencies in the United States share responsibility for academic achievement and health? A review of 25 years of evidence about the relationship of adolescents' academic achievement and health behaviors. *Journal of Adolescent Health, 52*(5), 523–532. https://doi.org/10.1016/j.jadohealth.2013.01.008

Brown, D. C., Hummer, R. A., & Hayward, M. D. (2014). The importance of spousal education for the self-rated health of married adults in the United States. *Population research and policy review, 33*(1), 127–151. https://doi.org/10.1007/s11113-013-9305-6

Cabrera, J. C., Rodriguez, M. C., Karl, S. R., & Chavez, C. (2018). In what ways do health behaviors impact academic performance, educational aspirations, and commitment to learning? [Paper presentation]. American Educational Research Association (AERA) Conference 2018, New York, NY.

Centers for Disease Control and Prevention. (2014). *Health and academic achievement.* US Department of Health and Human Services. https://www.cdc.gov/healthyyouth/health_and_academics/pdf/health-academic-achievement.pdf

Centers for Disease Control and Prevention. (2020). *Youth risk behavior surveillance system (YRBSS).* US Department of Health and Human Services. https://www.cdc.gov/healthyyouth/data/yrbs/index.htm

Centers for Disease Control and Prevention. (2021a). *Alcohol behaviors and academic grades.* US Department of Health and Human Services. https://www.cdc.gov/healthyschools/health_and_academics/alcohol_use.htm

Centers for Disease Control and Prevention. (2021b). *Dietary behaviors and academic*

grades. US Department of Health and Human Services. https://www.cdc.gov
/healthyschools/health_and_academics/health_academics_dietary.htm

Centers for Disease Control and Prevention. (2021c). *Health and academics.* US Department of Health and Human Services. https://www.cdc.gov/healthyschools
/health_and_academics/index.htm

Centers for Disease Control and Prevention. (2021d). *Other health behaviors and academic grades.* US Department of Health and Human Services. https://www.cdc
.gov/healthyschools/health_and_academics/other_health_behaviors.htm

Centers for Disease Control and Prevention. (2021e). *Physical activity and sedentary behaviors and academic grades.* US Department of Health and Human Services.
https://www.cdc.gov/healthyschools/health_and_academics/physical-activity
-and-sedentary-behaviors-and-academic-grades.htm

Centers for Disease Control and Prevention. (2021f). *Tobacco product use behaviors and academic grades.* US Department of Health and Human Services. https://www
.cdc.gov/healthyschools/health_and_academics/tobacco_product_use.htm

The Colorado Education Initiative. (2015). *Connecting health and learning: Health is vital for student success: An overview of relevant research.* http://www.coloradoed
initiative.org/wp-content/uploads/2015/02/MakingtheCaseFF.pdf

Commission on the Reorganization of Secondary Education. (1918). *Cardinal principles of secondary education.* Department of the Interior, Bureau of Education.

Daniel, H., Bornstein, S. S., Kane, G. C., & Health and Public Policy Committee of the American College of Physicians. (2018). Addressing social determinants to improve patient care and promote health equity: An American College of Physicians position paper. *Annals of Internal Medicine, 168*(8), 577–578. https://doi
.org/10.7326/M17-2441

DeSalvo, K. B., Wang, Y. C., Harris, A., Auerbach, J., Koo, D., & O'Carroll, P. (2017). Peer reviewed: Public Health 3.0: A call to action for public health to meet the challenges of the 21st century. *Preventing chronic disease, 14,* 170017. https://doi
.org/10.5888/pcd14.170017

Dilley, J. (2009). *Research review: School-based health interventions and academic achievement.* Washington State Department of Health. https://www.doh.wa.gov/Portals
/1/Documents/8300/130-083-HealthAcademic-en-L.pdf

Educational Policies Commission, National Education Association of the United States, & American Association of School Administrators. (1938). *The purposes of education in American democracy.* National Education Association.

Educational Policies Commission of the National Education Association & American Association of School Administrators. (1961). *The central purpose of American education.* National Education Association.

Egerter, S., Braveman, P., Sadegh-Nobari, T., Grossman-Kahn, R., & Dekker, M. (2011, April 1). *Education and health.* Robert Wood Johnson Foundation. https://www
.rwjf.org/en/library/research/2011/05/education-matters-for-health.html

Eide, E. R., & Showalter, M. H. (2011). Estimating the relation between health and education: What do we know and what do we need to know? *Economics of Education Review, 30*(5), 778–791. https://doi.org/10.1016/j.econedurev.2011.03.009

Fineberg, H. V. (2011). Public health and medicine: Where the twain shall meet. *American Journal of Preventative Medicine, 41*(4), S149–S151. https://doi.org/10.1016/j.amepre.2011.07.013

Freudenberg, N., & Ruglis, J. (2007). Reframing school dropout as a public health issue. *Preventing Chronic Disease, 4*(4), 1–11. http://www.cdc.gov/pcd/issues/2007/oct/07_0063.htm

Galea, S., Tracy, M., Hoggatt, K. J., DiMaggio, C., & Karpati, A. (2011). Estimated deaths attributable to social factors in the United States. *American Journal of Public Health, 101*(8), 1456–1465. https://doi.org/10.2105/AJPH.2010.300086

Hahn, R. A., & Truman, B. I. (2015). Education improves public health and promotes health equity. *International Journal of Health Services, 45*(4), 657–678. https://doi.org/10.1177/0020731415585986

Hales, D. (2017). *An invitation to health: The power of now.* Cengage Learning.

Herbert, B. (2014). *Losing our way: An intimate portrait of a troubled America.* Anchor Books.

Hollander-Rodriguez, J., & DeVoe, J. (2018). Family medicine's task in population health: Defining it and owning it. *Family Medicine, 50*(9), 659–661. https://doi.org/10.22454/FamMed.2018.868771

Hummer, R. A., & Hernandez, E. M. (2013). The effect of educational attainment on adult mortality in the United States. *Population Bulletin, 68*(1), 1–16.

Institute of Medicine. (2012). *Primary Care and Public Health: Exploring Integration to Improve Public Health.* National Academies Press. https://doi.org/10.17226/13381

Institute of Medicine. (2015). *Exploring opportunities for collaboration between health and education to improve population health: Workshop summary.* National Academies Press. https://doi.org/10.17226/18979

Jarris, P. E., & Sellars, K. (2016). The value of integration: Public health, primary care, and beyond. In J. L. Michener, D. Koo, B. C. Castrucci, & J. B. Sprague (Eds.), *The practical playbook: Public health and primary care together* (pp. 28–32). Oxford University Press.

Kegler, M. C., Wolff, T., Christens, B. D., Butterfoss, F. D., Francisco, V. T., & Orleans, T. (2019). Strengthening our collaborative approaches for advancing equity and justice. *Health Education and Behavior, 46*(S1), S5–S8. https://doi.org/10.1177/1090198119871188

Kelly, M. J., & Weitzen, S. (2010). The association of lifetime education with the prevalence of myocardial infarction: An analysis of the 2006 behavioral risk factor surveillance system. *Journal of Community Health, 35*(1), 76–80. https://doi.org/10.1007/s10900-009-9189-x

Khairat, S., Zou, B., & Adler-Milstein, J. (2022). Factors and reasons associated with low COVID-19 vaccine uptake among highly hesitant communities in the US. *American Journal of Infection Control, 50*(3), 262–267.

Klein, A. (2019a). Answering your ESSA questions. *Education Week, 38*(27), 20–21.

Klein, A. (2019b). States, districts tackle the tough work of making ESSA a reality. *Education Week, 38*(27), 4–6.

Kolbe, L. J. (2019). School health as a strategy to improve both public health and education. *Annual Review of Public Health*, 40, 443–468. https://doi.org/10.1146/annurev-publhealth-040218-043727

Kolbe, L. J., Allensworth, D. D., Potts-Datema, W., & White, D. R. (2015). What have we learned from collaborative partnerships to concomitantly improve both education and health? *Journal of School Health*, 85(11), 766–774. https://doi.org/10.1111/josh.12312

Kuo, A. A., Thomas, P. A., Chilton, L. A., & Mascola, L. (2018). Pediatricians and public health: Optimizing the health and well-being of the nation's children. *Pediatrics*, 141(2), e20173848. https://doi.org/10.1542/peds.2017-3848

Marmot, M. (2015). *The health gap: The challenge of an unequal world*. Bloomsbury Press.

Mattson, G., & Remley, K. (2019). Shaping the next generation of providers. In J. L. Michener, B. C., Castrucci, D. W. Bradley, E. L. Hunter, C. W. Thomas, C. Patterson, & E. Corcoran (Eds.), *The practical playbook II: Building multisector partnerships that work* (pp. 457–464). Oxford University Press.

McGill, N. (2016). Education attainment linked to health throughout lifespan: Exploring social determinants of health. *The Nation's Health*, 46(6), 1–19. https://www.thenationshealth.org/content/46/6/1.3

Michener, J. L., Castrucci, B. C., Bradley, D. W., Hunter, E. L., & Thomas, C. W. (2019). Overview: The accelerating movement of partnerships for health. In J. L. Michener, B. C., Castrucci, D. W. Bradley, E. L. Hunter, C. W. Thomas, C. Patterson, & E. Corcoran (Eds.), *The practical playbook II: Building multisector partnerships that work* (pp. 3–6). Oxford University Press.

Mirowsky, J & Ross, C. E. (2003). *Education, social status, and health*. Transaction Publishers. https://doi.org/10.4324/9781351328081

Montez, J. K., Hayward, M. D., Brown, D. C., & Hummer, R. A. (2009). Why is the educational gradient of mortality steeper for men? *Journals of Gerontology Series B: Psychological Sciences and Social Sciences*, 64(5), 625–634.

National Association of Chronic Disease Directors. (2017a). *Local health departments and school partnerships: Working together with schools*. https://chronicdisease.org/local-health-department-and-school-partnerships-working-together-to-build/

National Association of Chronic Disease Directors. (2017b). *The whole school, whole community, whole child model: A guide to implementation*. https://chronicdisease.org/the-whole-school-whole-community-whole-child-model-a-guide-to-implementation/

Pachter, L. M., Lieberman, L., Bloom, S. L., & Fein, J. A. (2017). Developing a community-wide initiative to address childhood adversity and toxic stress: A case study of the Philadelphia ACE task force. *Academic Pediatrics*, 17(7), S130–S135. https://doi.org/10.1016/j.acap.2017.04.012

Plough, A. L. (2015). Building a culture of health: A critical role for public health services and systems research. *American Journal of Public Health*, 105(S2), S150–S152. https://doi.org/10.2105/AJPH.2014.302410

Ravitch, D. (2014). *Reign of error: The hoax of the privatization movement and the danger to America's public schools*. Vintage Books.

Robert Wood Johnson Foundation. (2016, September). *The relationship between school attendance and health.* https://www.rwjf.org/en/library/research/2016/09/the-relationship-between-school-attendance-and-health.html

Satcher, D., Kaczorowski, J., & Topa, D. (2005). The expanding role of the pediatrician in improving child health in the 21st century. *Pediatrics, 115*(4), 1124–1128. https://doi.org/10.1542/peds.2004-2825C

Schneider, J. (2017). *Beyond test scores: A better way to measure school quality.* Harvard University Press.

Serpas, S., Khaokham, C., Hillidge, S., & Watson, V. (2016). San Diego, California, promotes health weight to improve community health. In J. L. Michener, D. Koo, B. C. Castrucci, & J. B. Sprague (Eds.), *The practical playbook: Public health and primary care together* (pp. 313–328). Oxford University Press.

Silberberg, M., & Castrucci, B. C. (2016). Addressing social determinants of health. In J. L. Michener, D. Koo, B. C. Castrucci, & J. B. Sprague, (Eds.), *The practical playbook: Public health and primary care together* (pp. 151–161). Oxford University Press.

Slade, S. (2015). The whole child initiative. In D. A. Birch & D. M. Videto (Eds.), *Promoting health and academic success* (pp. 53–63). Human Kinetics.

Sleeter, C. E. (Ed.). (2007). *Facing accountability in education: Democracy and equity at risk.* Teachers College Press.

Valles, S. A. (2018). *Philosophy of population health: Philosophy for a new public health era.* Routledge.

Valois, R. F., Slade, S., & Ashford, E. (2011). *The Healthy School Communities model: Aligning health and education in the school setting.* Association for Supervision and Curriculum Development. http://www.ascd.org/ASCD/pdf/siteASCD/publications/Aligning-Health-Education.pdf

Witt, C. M., Chiaramonte, D., Berman, S., Chesney, M. A., Kaplan, G. A., Stange, K. C., Woolf, S. H., & Berman, B. M. (2017). Defining health in a comprehensive context: A new definition of integrative health. *American Journal of Preventive Medicine, 53*(1), 134–137. https://doi.org/10.1016/j.amepre.2016.11.029

Woolf, S. H., Johnson, R. E., Phillips, R. L., Jr., & Philipsen, M. (2007). Giving everyone the health of the educated: An examination of whether social change would save more lives than medical advances. *American Journal of Public Health, 97*(4), 679–683. https://doi.org/10.2105/AJPH.2005.084848

World Health Organization. (1948). *Constitution of the World Health Organization.* World Health Organization Basic Documents.

Zajacova, A., & Lawrence, E. M. (2018). The relationship between education and health: Reducing disparities through a contextual approach. *Annual Review of Public Health, 39,* 273–289. https://doi.org/10.1146/annurev-publhealth-031816-044628

Zimmerman, E., & Woolf, S. H. (2014, June 5). Understanding the relationship between education and health [Discussion paper]. *National Academy of Sciences.*

Zimmerman, E. B., Woolf, S. H., & Haley, A. (2015). Understanding the relationship between education and health: A review of the evidence and an examination of community perspectives. In R. M. Kaplan, M. L. Spittel, & D. H. David (Eds.),

Population health: Behavioral and social science insights (pp. 347–84). Agency for Health-Care Research and Quality & Office of Behavioral and Social Sciences Research, National Institutes of Health.

Chapter 2. Education and Health Disparities

Alexander, M. (2010). *The new Jim Crow: Mass incarceration in the age of colorblindness.* New Press.

Allensworth, D., Lewallen, T. C., Stevenson, B., & Katz, S. (2011). Peer reviewed: Addressing the needs of the whole child: What public health can do to answer the education sector's call for a stronger partnership. *Preventing Chronic Disease, 8*(2). http://www.cdc.gov/pcd/issues/2011/mar/10_0014.htm

Annie E. Casey Foundation. (2014). *Race equity and inclusion action guide: Embracing racial equity: 7 steps to advance and embed race equity and inclusion with your organization.* https://www.aecf.org/resources/race-equity-and-inclusion-action-guide

Annie E. Casey Foundation. (2016). *A shared sentence: The devastating toll of incarceration on kids, families and communities.* [Policy Report]. https://assets.aecf.org/m/resourcedoc/aecf-asharedsentence-2016.pdf

Annie E. Casey Foundation. (2019). *Fourth-graders who scored below proficient reading by English language learner status on the United States.* https://datacenter.kidscount.org/data/tables/5197-fourth-graders-who-scored-below-proficient-reading-by-english-language-learner-status#detailed/1/any/false/1729,871,573/1320,1321/11681

Banks, J. A. (2018). Foreword. In P. C. Gorski, *Reaching and teaching students in poverty: Strategies for erasing the opportunity gap* (pp. xi–xvii). Teachers College Press.

Barr, D. A. (2019). *Health disparities in the United States: Social class, race, ethnicity and the social determinants of health* (3rd ed). Johns Hopkins University Press.

Basile, K. C., Clayton, H. B., Rostad, W. L., & Leemis, R. W. (2020). Sexual violence victimization of youth and health risk behaviors. *American Journal of Preventive Medicine, 58*(4), 570–579. https://doi.org/10.1016/j.amepre.2019.11.020

Bazelon, E. (2019, April 7). If prisons don't work, what will? *The New York Times.* https://www.nytimes.com/2019/04/05/opinion/mass-incarceration-sentencing-reform.html

Benson, T. A., Fiarman, S. E., & Singleton, G. E. (2020). *Unconscious bias in schools: A developmental approach to exploring race and racism* (Rev. ed.). Harvard Education Press.

Berliner, D. (2013). Effects of inequality and poverty vs. teachers and schooling on America's youth. *Teachers College Record, 115*(12).

Berliner, D. C., Glass, G. V., Cisneros, J., Diaz, V. H., Dunn, L., Griffin, E. N., Hanson, J., Holloway-Libell, J., Joanou, J. P., Kulkarni, R., Lish, R., Mazza, B. S., Meens, D. E., Paufler, N. A., Pfleger, R., Shea, J. D., Stigler, M. L., Symonds, S., Thomas, M. H., . . . Wiley, K. (2014). *50 myths and lies that threaten America's public schools: The real crisis in education.* Teachers College Press.

Bovell-Ammon, A., Ettinger de Cuba, S., Coleman, S., Ahmad, N., Black, M. M., Frank,

D. A., Ochoa, E., & Cutts, D. B. (2019). Trends in food insecurity and SNAP participation among immigrant families of US-born young children. *Children, 6*(4), 55. https://doi.org/10.3390/children6040055

Breny, J. M. (2020). Continuing the journey toward health equity: Becoming antiracist in health promotion research and practice. *Health Education and Behavior, 47*(5), 665–670. https://doi.org/10.1177/1090198120954393

Budiman, A. (2020, August 20). *Key findings about U.S. immigrants.* PEW Research Center. https://www.pewresearch.org/fact-tank/2020/08/20/key-findings-about-u-s-immigrants/

Cardichon, J., Darling-Hammond, L., Yang, M., Scott, C., Shields, P. M., & Burns, D. (2020). *Inequitable opportunity to learn: Student access to certified and experienced teachers.* Learning Policy Institute.

Cardoza, K. (2019). Teaching migrant children. *Education Week, 38*(29), 12–16.

Carter, J. (2016, August 8). *Measuring the impact of poverty in education.* Higher Ed Dive. https://www.highereddive.com/news/measuring-the-impact-of-poverty-in-education/423321/

Case, A. F. (2019). Seeing and supporting immigrant teens. *Educational Leadership, 76*(8), 40–45.

Centers for Disease Control and Prevention. (2021). *Infant Mortality.* US Department of Health and Human Services. https://www.cdc.gov/reproductivehealth/maternalinfanthealth/infantmortality.htm

Centers for Disease Control and Prevention. (2022). *Health equity.* US Department of Health and Human Services. https://www.cdc.gov/healthequity/index.html

Children's Defense Fund. (2021). *The state of America's children: Youth justice.* https://www.childrensdefense.org/state-of-americas-children/soac-2021-youth-justice/

Coller, R. J., & Kuo, A. A. (2016). Social determinants of child health. In A. A. Kuo, R. J. Coller, S. Stewart-Brown, & M. Blair (Eds.), *Child health: A population perspective.* Oxford University Press.

Crosnoe, R., & Turley, R. N. L. (2011). K–12 educational outcomes of immigrant youth. *The Future of Children, 21*(1), 129–152.

Darling-Hammond, L. (2010). *The flat world and education: How America's commitment to equity will determine our future.* Teachers College Press.

Dorsainvil, M. (2021). The Biden administration's immigration policies and the impact on school health—a commentary. *Journal of School Health, 91*(7), 523–525. https://doi.org/10.1111/josh.13027

Dugan, J. (2021). Beware of equity traps and tropes. *Educational Leadership, 78*(6), 35–40.

Eager, J. (2019). Supporting students' intersecting identities. *Educational Leadership, 76*(8), 58.

Fernald, A., Marchman, V. A., & Weisleder, A. (2013). SES differences in language processing skill and vocabulary are evident at 18 months. *Developmental Science, 16*(2), 234–248. https://doi.org/10.1111/desc.12019

Fishman, S. H. (2020). Educational mobility among the children of Asian American immigrants. *American Journal of Sociology, 126*(2), 260–317. https://doi.org/10.1086/711231

Foreman, J., Jr. (2017). *Locking up our own: Crime and punishment in black America.* Farrar, Straus & Giroux.

Galea, S. (2018). *Healthier: Fifty thoughts on the foundations of population health.* Oxford University Press.

Garg, N., & Volerman, A. (2021). A national analysis of state policies on lesbian, gay, bisexual, transgender, and questioning/queer inclusive sex education. *Journal of School Health, 91*(2), 164–175. https://doi.org/10.1111/josh.12987

Gerson, M. (2018, December 18). Caring about prisoners helps us all. *Tuscaloosa News, 199*(352).

Ghandnoosh, N., Stammen, E., & Muhitch, K. (2021, February). *Parents in prison.* The Sentencing Project. https://www.sentencingproject.org/wp-content/uploads/2021/11/Parents-in-Prison.pdf

Gifford, E. J., Kozecke, L. E., Golonka, M., Hill, S. N., Costello, E. J., Shanahan, L., & Copeland, W. E. (2019). Association of parental incarceration with psychiatric and functional outcomes of young adults. *JAMA Network Open, 2*(8), e1910005–e1910005. https://www.doi.org/10.1001/jamanetworkopen.2019.10005

Goodwin, J. (2018). Viewpoint. *Homelessness and Education,* 3–4. http://dropoutprevention.org/wp-content/uploads/2018/12/ndpc_newsletter_winter2018.pdf

Gorski, P. C. (2017, December 9). *Basic principles for equity literacy.* Equity Literacy Institute, EdChange Initiative. https://www.austinisd.org/sites/default/files/dept/equity-office/docs/Equity%20Literacy%20Principles.pdf

Gorski, P. C. (2018). *Reaching and teaching students in poverty: Strategies for erasing the opportunity gap.* Teachers College Press.

Gramlich, J. (2021). *America's incarceration rate falls to lowest level since 1995.* Pew Research Center. https://policycommons.net/artifacts/1808148/americas-incarceration-rate-falls-to-lowest-level-since-1995/2542938/

Greytak, E. A., Kosciw, J. G., Villenas, C., & Giga, N. M. (2016). *From teasing to torment: School climate revisited. A survey of US secondary school students and teachers.* GLSEN. https://www.glsen.org/sites/default/files/2019-12/From_Teasing_to_Tormet_Revised_2016.pdf

Haberman, M. (1991). The pedagogy of poverty versus good teaching. *Phi Delta Kappan, 73*(4), 290–294. https://doi.org/10.1177/003172171009200223

Hall, P. (2019). The instructional leader's most difficult job. *Educational Leadership, 76*(6), 12–17.

Hart, B., & Risley, T. R. (1995). *Meaningful differences in the everyday experience of young American children.* Paul H. Brookes Publishing.

Herbert, B. (2014). *Losing our way: An intimate portrait of a troubled America.* Doubleday.

Huynh-Hohnbaum, A. L., Bussell, T., & Gi, L. E. E. (2015). Incarcerated mothers and fathers: How their absences disrupt children's high school graduation. *International Journal of Psychology and Educational Studies, 2*(2), 1–11. https://doi.org/10.17220/ijpes.2015.02.001

Ingersoll, R., Merrill, L., & Stuckey, D. (2018). The changing face of teaching. *Educational Leadership, 75*(8), 44–49.

Institute of Medicine. (2015). *Exploring opportunities for collaboration between health and education to improve population health: Workshop summary.* National Academies Press. https://doi.org/10.17226/18979

Ivey-Stephenson, A. Z., Demissie, Z., Crosby, A. E., Stone, D. M., Gaylor, E., Wilkins, N., Lowry, R., & Brown, M. (2020). Suicidal ideation and behaviors among high school students—Youth Risk Behavior Survey, United States, 2019. *Morbidity and Mortality Weekly Reports Supplements, 69*(1), 47–55. https://doi.org/10.15585/mmwr.su6901a6

Johns, M. M., Lowry, R., Haderxhanaj, L. T., Rasberry, C. N., Robin, L., Scales, L., Stone, D., & Suarez, N. A. (2019). Trends in violence victimization and suicide risk by sexual identity among high school students—Youth Risk Behavior Survey, United States, 2015–2019. *Morbidity and Mortality Weekly Reports Supplements, 69*(1), 19–27. https://doi.org/10.15585/mmwr.su6901a3

Jones, C. (2016). Pondering the meaning of life: "And how are the children?" *The Nation's Health, 46*(9), 3.

Jones, C. P., Jones, C. Y., Perry, G. S., Barclay, G., & Jones, C. A. (2009). Addressing the social determinants of children's health: A cliff analogy. *Journal of Health Care for the Poor and Underserved, 20*(4), 1–12. https://doi.org/10.1353/hpu.0.0228

Kang-Brown, J., Montagnet, C., & Heiss, J. (2021). *People in jail and prison in spring 2021.* Vera Institute of Justice. https://www.vera.org/downloads/publications/people-in-jail-and-prison-in-spring-2021.pdf

Khalifa, M. (2018). *Culturally responsive school leadership.* Harvard Education Press.

Klein, D. E., & Lima, J. M. (2021). The prison industrial complex as a commercial determinant of health. *American Journal of Public Health, 111*(10), 1750–1752. https://doi.org/10.2105/AJPH.2021.306467

Kosciw, J. G., Clark, C. M., Truong, N. L., & Zongrone, A. D. (2020). *The 2019 national school climate survey: The experiences of lesbian, gay, bisexual, transgender, and queer youth in our nation's schools.* GLSEN. https://www.glsen.org/research/2019-national-school-climate-survey

Kugler, M. D. (2018). Current developments in immigration law: The debate surrounding "birth tourism." *Georgetown Immigration Law Journal, 32*(3), 321–327.

Lehner, P. (2017). Money doesn't ensure equity. *Education Week, 36*(33), 20.

Love, B. L. (2019a, June 12). The "spirit murdering" of black and brown children. *Education Week, 38*(35), 38.

Love, B. L. (2019b). *We want to do more than survive: Abolitionist teaching and the pursuit of educational freedom.* Beacon Press.

Love, B. L. (2021). Empty promises of equity: Whether white people are ready or not, policies have to change. *Education Week, 40*(18), 25.

Milner, H. R., IV. (2015). *Rac(e)ing to class: Confronting poverty and race in schools' classrooms.* Fourth Printing.

Morsy, L., & Rothstein, R. (2016, December 15). *Mass incarceration and children's outcomes: Criminal justice policy is education policy.* Economic Policy Institute. https://www.epi.org/publication/mass-incarceration-and-childrens-outcomes/

Murchison, G., Adkins, D., Conard, L. A., Ehrensaft, D., Elliott, T., Hawkins, L. A.,

Lopez, X., Newby, H., Ng, H., Vetters, R., & Wolf-Gould, C. (2016). *Supporting and caring for transgender children*. Human Rights Campaign, American Academy of Pediatrics, & American College of Osteopathic Pediatricians. http://hrc.im/supportingtranschildren

National Academies of Sciences, Engineering, and Medicine. (2017). *Communities in action: Pathways to health equity* (A. Baciu, Y. Negussie, & A. Geller, Eds.). National Academies Press. https://doi.org/10.17226/24624

National Academies of Sciences, Engineering, and Medicine. (2019). *A roadmap to reducing child poverty*. National Academies Press.

National Association for the Education of Young Children. (2019, April). *Advancing equity in early childhood education* [Position statement]. https://www.naeyc.org/sites/default/files/globally-shared/downloads/PDFs/resources/positionstatements/advancingequitypositionstatement.pdf

National Center for Education Statistics. (2019, February). *Indicator 15: Retention, suspension, and expulsion*. https://nces.ed.gov/programs/raceindicators/indicator_rda.asp

National Center for Education Statistics. (2021a, February). *Rates of high school completion and bachelor's degree attainment among persons age 25 and over, by race/ethnicity and sex: Selected years, 1910 through 2020*. https://nces.ed.gov/programs/digest/d20/tables/dt20_104.10.asp

National Center for Education Statistics. (2021b, May). *Public high school graduation rates*. Department of Education, Institute of Education Sciences. https://nces.ed.gov/programs/coe/indicator/coi

National Center for Education Statistics. (2022, May). *English learners in public schools*. Department of Education, Institute of Education Sciences. https://nces.ed.gov/programs/coe/indicator/cgf/english-learners

National Center for Homeless Education. (2021). *Student homelessness in America: Years 2017–18 and 2019–20*. University of North Carolina at Greensboro. https://nche.ed.gov/wp-content/uploads/2021/12/Student-Homelessness-in-America-2021.pdf

The Nation's Report Card. (n.d.-a). *NAEP report card: 2019 NAEP mathematics assessment*. https://www.nationsreportcard.gov/highlights/mathematics/2019/

The Nation's Report Card. (n.d.-b). *NAEP report card: 2019 NAEP reading assessment*. https://www.nationsreportcard.gov/highlights/reading/2019/

Navarro, V. (2009). What we mean by social determinants of health. *International Journal of Health Services, 39*(3), 423–441. https://doi.org/10.2190/HS.39.3.a

Ndugga, N., & Artiga, S. (2021, May 11). *Disparities in health and health care: 5 key questions and answers*. KFF. https://www.kff.org/racial-equity-and-health-policy/issue-brief/disparities-in-health-and-health-care-5-key-question-and-answers/

Neuman, S. B., & Celano, D. C. (2012). Worlds apart: One city, two libraries, and ten years of watching inequality grow. *American Educator, 36*(3), 13–19. http://files.eric.ed.gov/fulltext/EJ986677.pdf

Oberg, C. (2018). The rights of children on the move and the Budapest Declaration. *Children, 5*(5), 61. https://doi.org/10.3390/children5050061

Office of Disease Prevention and Health Promotion. (n.d.). Social determinants of health. *Healthy People 2030*. US Department of Health and Human Services. https://health.gov/healthypeople/objectives-and-data/social-determinants -health

Office of Disease Prevention and Health Promotion. (2021). How does Healthy People 2030 define health disparities and health equity? *Healthy People 2030*. US Department of Health and Human Services. https://health.gov/our-work/healthy -people/healthy-people-2030/questions-answers#q9

Office of Minority Health. (2021). *Profile: Black/African Americans*. US Department of Health and Human Services. https://www.minorityhealth.hhs.gov/omh/browse .aspx?lvl=3&lvlid=61

Orr, A., Baum, J., Brown, J., Gill, E., Kahn, E., & Salem, A. (2015). *Schools in transition: A guide for supporting transgender students in K–12 schools*. Human Rights Campaign Foundation. https://www.hrc.org/resources/schools-in-transition -a-guide-for-supporting-transgender-students-in-k-12-s

Patrick, K., Socol, A. R., & Morgan, I. (2020, January 9). *Inequities in advanced coursework: What's driving them and what leaders can do*. The Education Trust. https:// edtrust.org/resource/inequities-in-advanced-coursework/

Phelan, L. W., & Teitel, L. (2019, February 26). *Beyond diversity to equitable, inclusive schools*. D.C. Policy Center. https://www.dcpolicycenter.org/publications/beyond -diversity-to-equitable-inclusive-schools/

Porta, C. M., Singer, E., Mehus, C. J., Gower, A. L., Saewyc, E., Fredkove, W., & Eisenberg, M. E. (2017). LGBTQ youth's views on gay-straight alliances: Building community, providing gateways, and representing safety and support. *Journal of School Health, 87*(7), 489–497. https://doi.org/10.1111/josh.12517

Poteat, V. P. (2017). Gay-straight alliances: Promoting student resilience and safer school climates. *American Educator, 40*(4), 10–14.

Potochnick, S. (2018). The academic adaptation of immigrant students with interrupted schooling. *American Educational Research Journal, 55*(4), 859–892. https://doi .org/10.3102/0002831218761026

Ravitch, D. (2014). *Reign of error: The hoax of the privatization movement and the danger to America's public schools*. Vintage Books.

Root & Rebound, & #cut50. (2019). *First step to second chances: A guide for people leaving federal prison under the first step act*. https://www.thedreamcorps.org /wp-content/uploads/2019/11/First-Step-to-Second-Chances-Guide.pdf

Runyan, A. (2018). What is intersectionality and why is it important? *Academe, 104*(6), 10–14.

Sadowski, M. (2017). More than a safe space: How schools can enable LGBTQ students to thrive. *American Educator, 40*(4), 4–9.

Samuels, C. A. (2019, October 22). The challenging, often isolating work of school district chief equity officers. *Education Week*. https://www.edweek.org/leadership /the-challenging-often-isolating-work-of-school-district-chief-equity-officers /2019/10

Schaeffer, K. (2021, December 15). *U.S. public school students often go to schools where at least half of their peers are the same race or ethnicity.* PEW Research Center. https://www.pewresearch.org/fact-tank/2021/12/15/u-s-public-school-students -often-go-to-schools-where-at-least-half-of-their-peers-are-the-same-race-or -ethnicity/

Shattuck, D. G., Willging, C. E., & Green, A. E. (2020). Applying a structural-competency framework to the implementation of strategies to reduce disparities for sexual and gender minority youth. *Journal of School Health, 90*(12), 1030–1037. https://doi.org/10.1111/josh.12964

Shlafer, R. J., Reedy, T., & Davis, L. (2017). School-based outcomes among youth with incarcerated parents: Differences by school setting. *Journal of School Health, 87*(9), 687–695. https://doi.org/10.1111/josh.12539

Simmons, D. (2020). Confronting inequity/the trauma we don't see. *Educational Leadership, 77*(8), 88–89.

Southern Education Foundation. (n.d.). *Who we are.* https://southerneducation.org /who-we-are/

Stoltzfus, K. (2019). What schools can do for immigrant students, *Education Update, 6*(11), 2–3.

Suárez-Orozco, M. & Suárez-Orozco, C. (2015). Children of immigration. *Phi Delta Kappan, 97*(4), 8–14. https://kappanonline.org/children-of-immigration/

Szucs, L. E., Lowry, R., Fasula, A. M., Pampati, S., Copen, C. E., Hussaini, K. S., Kachur, R. E., Koumans, E. H., & Steiner, R. J. (2020). Condom and contraceptive use among sexually active high school students—Youth Risk Behavior Survey, United States, 2019. *Morbidity and Mortality Weekly Reports Supplements, 69*(1), 11–18. https://doi.org/10.15585/mmwr.su6901a2

Toomey, R. B., Syvertsen, A. K., & Shramko, M. (2018). Transgender adolescent suicide behavior. *Pediatrics, 142*(4), e20174218. https://doi.org/10.1542/peds.2017-4218

Turney, K., & Goodsell, R. (2018). Parental incarceration and children's wellbeing. *The Future of Children, 28*(1), 147–164. https://www.jstor.org/stable/26641551

Turney, K., & Haskins, A. R. (2014). Falling behind? Children's early grade retention after paternal incarceration. *Sociology of Education, 87*(4), 241–258. https://doi .org/10.1177/0038040714547086

UNICEF Innocenti. (2020). *Worlds of influence: Understanding what shapes child wellbeing in rich countries.* Innocenti Report Card 16, UNICEF Office of Research, Innocenti, Florence. https://www.unicef-irc.org/publications/pdf/Report-Card -16-Worlds-of-Influence-child-wellbeing.pdf

US Department of Justice. (2020, January 15). *Department of justice announces enhancements to the risk assessment system and updates on First Step Act implementation.* https://www.justice.gov/opa/pr/department-justice-announces-enhancements -risk-assessment-system-and-updates-first-step-act

Varlas, L. (2017, September). Lessons from Little Rock. *ASCD Education Update, 59*(9), 1, 4–5.

Vera Institute of Justice. (n.d.). *Ending mass incarceration.* https://www.vera.org/ending -mass-incarceration

Viadero, D. (2020). Am I part of the race problem? *Education Week, 40*(6), 8–10.

Wakefield, S., & Wildeman, C. (2014). *Children of the prison boom: Mass incarceration and the future of the American inequality.* Oxford University Press.

Wilson-Simmons, R., Jiang, Y., & Aratani, Y. (2017). *Strong at the broken places: The resiliency of low-income parents.* National Center for Children in Poverty, Columbia University Mailman School of Public Health. https://files.eric.ed .gov/fulltext/ED574450.pdf

Yates, S. Q. (2018, October 17). How Trump can turn around his criminal-justice failures. *Washington Post*, A17.

Yellman, M. A., Bryan, L., Sauber-Schatz, E. K., & Brener, N. (2020). Transportation risk behaviors among high school students—Youth Risk Behavior Survey, United States, 2019. *Morbidity and Mortality Weekly Reports Supplements, 69*(1), 77–83. https://doi.org/10.15585/mmwr.su6901a9

Youth.gov. (n.d.). *Youth involved with the juvenile justice system.* https://youth.gov/youth -topics/juvenile-justice/youth-involved-juvenile-justice-system

Zill, N. (2020, July 8). *How do the children of immigrant parents perform in school?* Institute for Family Studies. https://ifstudies.org/blog/how-do-the-children-of -immigrant-parents-perform-in-school

Chapter 3. Early Childhood

Alabama Partnership for Children. (n.d.). *Pre-K skills for school readiness.* https:// alabamapartnershipforchildren.org/wp-content/uploads/2016/12/PreK_Skills _2013.pdf

Bassok, D., Finch, J. E., Lee, R., Reardon, S. F., & Waldfogel, J. (2016). Socioeconomic gaps in early childhood experiences: 1998 to 2010. *Aera Open, 2*(3), 1–22. https:// doi.org/10.1177/2332858416653924

Bauer, L., & Schanzenback, D. (2016). The long-term impact of the Head Start program. *The Hamilton Project.*

Bellis, M. A., Hughes, K., Ford, K., Rodriguez, G. R., Sethi, D., & Passmore, J. (2019). Life course health consequences and associated annual costs of adverse child-hood experiences across Europe and North America: A systematic review and meta-analysis. *The Lancet Public Health, 4*(10), e517–e528. https://doi.org/10.1016 /S2468-2667(19)30145-8

Bergen, D., Lee, L., DiCarlo, C., & Burnett, G. (2020). *Enhancing brain development in infants and young children: Strategies for caregivers and educators.* Teachers College Press.

Bethell, C. D., Simpson, L. A., & Solloway, M. R. (2017). Child well-being and adverse childhood experiences in the United States. *Academic Pediatrics, 17*(7), S1–S3. https://doi.org/10.1016/j.acap.2017.06.011

Better Beginnings. (2017). *Kindergarten readiness indicator checklist for parents.* Arkan-sas Department of Human Services. https://www.nwachildcare.org/uploads/5/2 /6/7/52673417/kric_9_28_17.pdf

Biglan, A., Van Ryzin, M. J., & Hawkins, J. D. (2017). Evolving a more nurturing society to prevent adverse childhood experiences. *Academic Pediatrics, 17*(7), S150–S157. https://doi.org/10.1016/j.acap.2017.04.002

Bruner, C. (2017). ACE, place, race, and poverty: Building hope for children. *Academic Pediatrics, 17*(7), S123–S129. https://doi.org/10.1016/j.acap.2017.05.009

Campbell, F. A., Pungello, E. P., Burchinal, M., Kainz, K., Pan, Y., Wasik, B. H., Barbarin, O. A., Sparling, J. J., & Ramey, C. T. (2012). Adult outcomes as a function of an early childhood educational program: An Abecedarian Project follow-up. *Developmental Psychology, 48*(4), 1033–1043. https://doi.org/10.1037/a0026644

Center on the Developing Child. (n.d.). *What is epigenetics? And how does it relate to child development?* Harvard University. https://46y5eh11fhgw3ve3ytpwxt9r -wpengine.netdna-ssl.com/wpcontent/uploads/2019/02/EpigeneticsInfographic _FINAL.pdf

Child and Adolescent Health Measurement Initiative. (n.d.-a). *2018–2019 National Survey of Children's Health (NSCH) data query.* Data Resource Center for Child and Adolescent Health, US Department of Health and Human Services, Health Resources and Services Administration (HRSA), and Maternal and Child Health Bureau (MCHB). https://www.childhealthdata.org/browse/survey/allstates?q =7915

Child and Adolescent Health Measurement Initiative. (n.d.-b). *2018–2019 National Survey of Children's Health (NSCH) data query.* Data Resource Center for Child and Adolescent Health, US Department of Health and Human Services, Health Resources and Services Administration (HRSA), and Maternal and Child Health Bureau (MCHB). https://www.childhealthdata.org/browse/survey/results?q =7915&r=1

Child and Adolescent Health Measurement Initiative. (n.d.-c). *2018–2019 National Survey of Children's Health (NSCH) data query.* Data Resource Center for Child and Adolescent Health, US Department of Health and Human Services, Health Resources and Services Administration (HRSA), and Maternal and Child Health Bureau (MCHB). https://www.childhealthdata.org/browse/survey/results?q=7915 &r=1&g=787

Child and Adolescent Health Measurement Initiative. (n.d.-d). *2018–2019 National Survey of Children's Health (NSCH) data query.* Data Resource Center for Child and Adolescent Health, US Department of Health and Human Services, Health Resources and Services Administration (HRSA), and Maternal and Child Health Bureau (MCHB). https://www.childhealthdata.org/browse/survey/results?q=7915 &r=1&g=795

Child and Family Research Partnership. (2015, July). *The top 5 benefits of home visiting programs.* The University of Texas and Lyndon B. Johnson School of Public Affairs. https://childandfamilyresearch.utexas.edu/sites/default/files/201506 _5Benefits_HomeVisitingPrograms.pdf

Crosnoe, R., Banazzo, C., & Wu, N. (2015). *Healthy learners: A whole child approach to reducing disparities in early education.* Teachers College Press.

D'Angiulli, A., Herdman, A., Stapells, D., & Hertzman, C. (2008). Children's event-related potentials of auditory selective attention vary with their socioeconomic status. *Neuropsychology, 22*(3), 293. https://doi.org/10.1037/0894-4105.22.3.293

Darling-Hammond, L., & Cook-Harvey, C. M. (2018). *Educating the whole child:*

Improving school climate to support student success. Learning Policy Institute. https://learningpolicyinstitute.org/product/educating-whole-child

Davis, M., Costigan, T., & Schubert, K. (2017). Promoting lifelong health and well-being: Staying the course to promote health and prevent the effects of adverse childhood and community experiences. *Academic Pediatrics, 17*(7), S4–S6. https://doi.org/10.1016/j.acap.2016.12.002

Elango, S., García, J. L., Heckman, J. J., & Hojman, A. (2016). Early childhood education. In R. A. Moffit (Ed.), *Economics of means-tested transfer programs in the United States* (Vol. 2, pp. 235–297). University of Chicago Press.

Ellis, W. R., & Dietz, W. H. (2017). A new framework for addressing adverse childhood and community experiences: The building community resilience model. *Academic Pediatrics, 17*(7), S86–S93. https://doi.org/10.1016/j.acap.2016.12.011

Felitti, V. J., Anda, R. F., Nordenberg, D., Williamson, D. F., Spitz, A. M., Edwards, V., & Marks, J. S. (1998). Relationship of childhood abuse and household dysfunction to many of the leading causes of death in adults: The Adverse Childhood Experiences (ACE) study. *American Journal of Preventive Medicine, 14*(4), 245–258. https://doi.org/10.1016/S0749-3797(98)00017-8

Fernald, A., Marchman, V. A., & Weisleder, A. (2013). SES differences in language processing skill and vocabulary are evident at 18 months. *Developmental Science, 16*(2), 234–248. https://doi.org/10.1111/desc.12019

Friedman-Krauss, A., Bernstein, S., & Barnett, S. W. (2019). *Early childhood education: Three pathways to better health. Preschool policy update.* National Institute for Early Education Research. http://nieer.org/wp-content/uploads/2018/12/NIEER-Policy-Update_Health_2019.pdf

Friedman-Krauss, A. H., Barnett, W. S., Garver, K. A., Hodges, K. S., Weisenfeld, G. G., & Gardiner, B. A. (2021). *The state of preschool 2020: State preschool yearbook.* The National Institute for Early Education Research & Rutgers Graduate School of Education. https://nieer.org/wp-content/uploads/2021/08/YB2020_Full_Report_080521.pdf

García, J. L., Heckman, J. J., Leaf, D. E., & Prados, M. J. (2016). *The life-cycle benefits of an influential early childhood program* (No. w22993). National Bureau of Economic Research.

Geller, A. (2021). Youth-police contact: Burdens and inequities in an adverse childhood experience, 2014–2017. *American Journal of Public Health, 111*(7), 1300–1308. https://doi.org/10.2105/AJPH.2021.306259

Golinkoff, R. M., Hoff, E., Rowe, M. L., Tamis-LeMonda, C. S., & Hirsh-Pasek, K. (2019). Language matters: Denying the existence of the 30-million-word gap has serious consequences. *Child Development, 90*(3), 985–992. https://doi.org/10.1111/cdev.13128

Hahn, R. A., Barnett, W. S., Knopf, J. A., Truman, B. I., Johnson, R. L., Fielding, J. E., Muntaner, C., Jones, C. P., Fullilove, M. T., Hunt, P. C., & Community Preventive Services Task Force. (2016). Early childhood education to promote health equity: A community guide systematic review. *Journal of Public Health Management and Practice, 22*(5), E1–E8. https://doi.org/10.1097/PHH.0000000000000378

Harris, N. B., Marques, S. S., Oh, D., Bucci, M., & Cloutier, M. (2017). Prevent, screen, heal: Collective action to fight the toxic effects of early life adversity. *Academic Pediatrics, 17*(7), S14–S15. https://doi.org/10.1016/j.acap.2016.11.015

Healthychildren.org. (2019, July 22). Is your preschooler ready for kindergarten? The American Academy of Pediatrics. https://www.healthychildren.org/English /ages-stages/preschool/Pages/Is-Your-Child-Ready-for-School.aspx

Heckman, J. (2008, May). *Schools, skills, and synapses.* Discussion Paper Series No. 3515. https://docs.iza.org/dp3515.pdf

Heckman, J., Moon, S. H., Pinto, R., Savelyev, P., & Yavitz, A. (2010). The rate of return to the HighScope Perry Preschool Program. *Journal of Public Economics, 94*(1–2), 114–128. https://doi.org/10.1016/j.jpubeco.2009.11.001

Heckman, J. J., & Karapakula, G. (2019). *Intergenerational and intragenerational externalities of the Perry Preschool Project* (Working Paper No. 25889). National Bureau of Economic Research. https://www.nber.org/system/files/working _papers/w25889/w25889.pdf

Iasevoli, B. (2019, May 19). *How cities are convincing voters to pay higher taxes for public preschool.* The Hechinger Report. https://hechingerreport.org/how-cities-are -convincing-voters-to-pay-higher-taxes-for-public-preschool/

Jimenez, M. E., Wade, R., Lin, Y., Morrow, L. M., & Reichman, N. E. (2016). Adverse experiences in early childhood and kindergarten outcomes. *Pediatrics, 137*(2). https://doi.org/10.1542/peds.2015-1839

Kaiser Family Foundation. (2020, December 14). *Paid family and sick leave in the U.S.* https://www.kff.org/womens-health-policy/fact-sheet/paid-family-leave-and -sick-days-in-the-u-s/

Karoly, L. A., & Auger, A. (2016). *Informing investments in preschool quality and access in Cincinnati: Evidence of impacts and economic returns from national, state, and local preschool programs.* RAND Corporation. https://www.rand.org/content /dam/rand/pubs/research_reports/RR1400/RR1461/RAND_RR1461.pdf

Kay, N., & Pennucci, A. (2014). *Early childhood education for low-income students: A review of the evidence and benefit-cost analysis.* Washington State Institute for Public Policy.

Kim, P., Evans, G. W., Angstadt, M., Ho, S. S., Sripada, C. S., Swain, J. E., Liberzon, I., & Phan, K. L. (2013). Effects of childhood poverty and chronic stress on emotion regulatory brain function in adulthood. *Proceedings of the National Academy of Sciences, 110*(46), 18442–18447. https://doi.org/10.1073/pnas.1308240110

Kuo, A. A., Coller, R. J., Stewart-Brown, S., & Blair, M. (2016). *Child health: A population perspective.* Oxford University Press.

Lamy, C. E. (2013). How preschool fights poverty. *Educational Leadership, 70*(8), 32–36.

Lee, S. Y., Kim, R., Rodgers, J., & Subramanian, S. V. (2021). Treatment effect heterogeneity in the head start impact study: A systematic review of study characteristics and findings. *SSM—Population Health, 16*, 100916. https://doi.org/10.1016/j.ssmph .2021.100916

Montialoux, C. (2016). *Policy brief: Revisiting the impact of Head Start.* IRLE: Institute for Research on Labor and Employment. University of California, Berkeley.

Morgan, H. (2019). Why is it so hard to send my kid to a good preschool? The shocking truth about early education in America. *Voices of Reform: Educational Research to Inform and Reform, 2*(1), 59–72. http://dx.doi.org/10.32623/2.00006

The National Association for the Education of Young Children. (n.d.) *A high-quality program for your preschooler.* https://www.naeyc.org/our-work/families/high-quality-program-for-preschooler

The National Association for the Education of Young Children. (2019). *Advancing equity in early childhood education.* https://www.naeyc.org/resources/position-statements/equity

National Center for Education Statistics. (2021). *Enrollment rates of young children.* https://nces.ed.gov/programs/coe/indicator/cfa

National Conference of State Legislatures. (2021, August 8). *Adverse childhood experiences.* https://www.ncsl.org/research/health/adverse-childhood-experiences-aces.aspx

National Home Visiting Resource Center. (2019). *2019 home visiting yearbook.* James Bell Associates and the Urban Institute. https://nhvrc.org/yearbook/2019-yearbook/

National Research Council, Institute of Medicine, Committee on Integrating the Science of Early Childhood Development, Shonkoff, J. P., & Phillips, D. A. (Eds.). (2000). *From neurons to neighborhoods: The science of early childhood development.* National Academies Press. https://doi.org/10.17226/9824

The National Scientific Council on the Developing Child. (2007). *The science of early childhood development.* http://www.developingchild.net

Neuman, S. B. (2014). Content-rich instruction in preschool. *Educational Leadership, 72*(2), 36–40.

Nurse-Family Partnership. (2021). *Research trials and outcomes: The gold standard of evidence.* https://www.nursefamilypartnership.org/wp-content/uploads/2021/02/NFP-Research-Trials-and-Outcomes.pdf

Office of Head Start. (2020, November 3). *Head Start services.* US Department of Health and Human Services. https://www.acf.hhs.gov/ohs/about/head-start

Pachter, L. M., Lieberman, L., Bloom, S. L., & Fein, J. A. (2017). Developing a community-wide initiative to address childhood adversity and toxic stress: A case study of the Philadelphia ACE task force. *Academic Pediatrics, 17*(7), S130–S135. https://doi.org/10.1016/j.acap.2017.04.012

Putnam, R. (2015). *Our kids: The American dream in crisis.* Simon & Schuster.

The Raising of America. (2015). *Action toolkit.* California Newsreel. https://www.raisingofamerica.org/sites/default/files/ActionToolkit.pdf

Ravitch, D. (2014). *Reign of error: The hoax of the privatization movement and the danger to America's public schools.* Vintage Books.

Reardon, S. F., & Portilla, X. A. (2016). Recent trends in income, racial, and ethnic school readiness gaps at kindergarten entry. *Aera Open, 2*(3), 1–18. https://doi.org/10.1177/2332858416657343

Reynolds, A. J. (2017). When early-ed. investments pay off. *Education Week, 37*(5), 28.

Sandstrom, H. (2019). *Early childhood home visiting programs and health* (Health Policy Brief). Health Affairs. https://doi.org/10.1377/hpb20190321.382895

Soleimanpour, S., Geierstanger, S., & Brindis, C. D. (2017). Adverse childhood experiences and resilience: Addressing the unique needs of adolescents. *Academic Pediatrics, 17*(7), S108–S114. https://doi.org/10.1016/j.acap.2017.01.008

Supplee, L. (2016, October 25). *5 things to know about early childhood home visiting.* Child Trends. https://www.childtrends.org/publications/5-things-to-know -about-early-childhood-home-visiting

UCLA Center for Healthier Children, Families, and Communities. (n.d.-a). *About.* https://www.healthychild.ucla.edu/pages/about

UCLA Center for Healthier Children, Families, and Communities. (n.d.-b). *Systems innovation & improvement: Early Development Instrument (EDI).* https://www .healthychild.ucla.edu/pages/edi

UCLA Center for Healthier Children, Families, and Communities. (n.d.-c). *Systems innovation & improvement: Transforming early childhood community systems (TECCS).* https://www.healthychild.ucla.edu/pages/teccs

Venet, A. S., & Duane, A. (2021, May). Let's get critical. *Educational Leadership, 78*(8), 25–30.

Wechsler, M. E., Kirp, D. L., Ali, T. T., Gardner, M., Maier, A., Melnick, H., & Shields, P. M. (2018). *On the road to high-quality early learning: Changing children's lives.* Teachers College Press.

Woods-Jaeger, B. A., Cho, B., Sexton, C. C., Slagel, L., & Goggin, K. (2018). Promoting resilience: Breaking the intergenerational cycle of adverse childhood experiences. *Health Education and Behavior, 45*(5), 772–780. https://doi.org/10.1177/1090 19811775285

Chapter 4. High School Graduation

American Academy of Pediatrics Council on School Health. (2013). Policy statement: Role of the school physician. *Pediatrics, 131*(1), 178–182. https://doi.org/10.1542 /peds.2012-2995

American Public Health Association. (2019). *Integrating public health in schools to improve graduation.* http://schoolbasedhealthcare.org

American University. (2021, January 14). *Why is school attendance important? The effects of chronic absenteeism.* https://soeonline.american.edu/blog/importance -of-school-attendance

Arenson, M., Hudson, P. J., Lee, N., & Lai, B. (2019). The evidence on school-based health centers: A review. *Global Pediatric Health, 6,* 1–10. https://doi.org/10.1177 %2F2333794X19828745

Askeland, K. G., Haugland, S., Stormark, K. M., Bøe, T., & Hysing, M. (2015). Adolescent school absenteeism and service use in a population-based study. *BMC Public Health, 15*(1), 1–9. https://doi.org/10.1186/s12889-015-1978-9

Attendance Works. (n.d.). *Superintendents.* https://www.attendanceworks.org/take -action/educators/superintendents-call-to-action/

Attendance Works. (2015). *Establishing school-wide attendance incentives.* http://www
.attendanceworks.org/wordpress/wp-content/uploads/2015/07/Establishing
-School-wide-attendance-incentives-rev-7-14-15.pdf

Attendance Works & Everyone Graduates Center. (2021). *Using chronic absence to map
interrupted schooling, instructional loss and educational inequity: Insights from
school year 2017–18 data.* https://www.attendanceworks.org/wp-content/uploads
/2019/06/Attendance-Works-Using-Chronic-Absence-to-Map_020221.pdf

Atwell, M. N., Balfanz, R., Manspile, E., Byrnes, V., & Bridgeland, J. M. (2020). *Building
a grad nation: Progress and challenge in raising high school graduation rates.*
Civic and the Everyone Graduates Center at the School of Education at Johns
Hopkins University. https://files.eric.ed.gov/fulltext/ED610686.pdf

Balfanz, R., & Byrnes, V. (2012). The importance of being in school: A report on absenteeism in the nation's public schools. *The Education Digest, 78*(2), 4.

Balfanz, R., & Byrnes, V. (2013). *Meeting the challenge of combating chronic absenteeism:
Impact of the NYC mayor's interagency task force on chronic absenteeism and
school attendance and its implications for other cities.* https://countmeinmaine
.org/site/wp-content/uploads/2014/06/NYCChronicAbsenteeismImpactReport
_FINAL_11_19_2013.pdf

Baltimore Education Research Consortium. (2011). *Destination graduation: Sixth grade
early warning indicators for Baltimore City Schools.* Baltimore Education Research Consortium.

Balu, R., & Ehrlich, S. B. (2018). Making sense out of incentives: A framework for considering the design, use, and implementation of incentives to improve attendance.
Journal of Education for Students Placed at Risk (JESPAR), 23(1–2), 93–106. https://
doi.org/10.1080/10824669.2018.1438898

Bartanen, B. (2020). Principal quality and student attendance. *Educational Researcher,
49*(2), 101–113. https://doi.org/10.3102/0013189X19898702

Beem, A. A., Batlivala, C., & Norwood, A. A. (2019). School-based health centers as
the pediatric expanded medical home. *Journal of School Health, 89*(11), 934–937.
https://doi.org/10.1111/josh.12825

Bergman, P., & Chen, E. W. (2019). Leveraging parents through low-cost technology:
The impact on high frequency information on student achievement. *The Journal
of Human Resources, 56*(1), 125–158. https://doi.org/10.3368/jhr.56.1.1118-9837R1

Blum, R. W. (2005). A case for school connectedness. *Educational Leadership, 62*(7),
16–20.

Blum, R. W., & Libbey, H. P. (2004). School connectedness (executive summary). *Journal of School Health, 74*(7), 231–232.

Centers for Disease Control and Prevention. (2009a). *Fostering school connectedness:
Improving student health and academic achievement.* US Department of Health
and Human Services. https://stacks.cdc.gov/view/cdc/21066

Centers for Disease Control and Prevention. (2009b). *School connectedness: Strategies
for increasing protective factors among youth.* US Department of Health and
Human Services. https://stacks.cdc.gov/view/cdc/5767/

Centers for Disease Control and Prevention. (2018). *School connectedness.* US Department of Health and Human Services. https://www.cdc.gov/healthyyouth /protective/school_connectedness.htm#:~:text=Students%20who%20feel%20 connected%20to,and%20stay%20in%20school%20longer

Centers for Disease Control and Prevention. (2019). *School health services.* US Department of Health and Human Services. https://www.cdc.gov/healthyschools /schoolhealthservices.htm

Centers for Disease Control and Prevention. (2020). *Adolescent and school health: Adolescent connectedness.* US Department of Health and Human Services. https://www.cdc.gov/healthyyouth/protective/youth-connectedness-important -protective-factor-for-health-well-being.htm

Chang, H. N., & Romero, M. (2008). Present, engaged, and accounted for: The critical importance of addressing chronic absence in the early grades. Report. *National Center for Children in Poverty, 19*(1), 10–18.

Coelho, R., Fischer, S., McKnight, F., Matteson, S., & Schwartz, T. (2015). *The effects of early chronic absenteeism on third-grade academic achievement measures.* University of Wisconsin–Madison. https://www.attendanceworks.org/wp-content /uploads/2019/06/Effects-of-Early-Chronic-Absenteeism-on-Third-Grade -Academic-Achievement.pdf

Diplomas Now. (2017, February). *Findings from the first decade and what's next.* http:// diplomasnow.org/wp-content/uploads/2017/02/Diplomas-Now-Findings-from -the-First-Decade-and-What%E2%80%99s-Next.pdf

Erb-Downward, J., & Watt, P. (2018). *Missing school, missing a home: The link between chronic absenteeism, economic instability and homelessness in Michigan.* Poverty Solutions, University of Michigan. http://files.eric.ed.gov/fulltext/ED594019.pdf

Farrington, C. (2017). Foreword. In D. L. Feldman, A. T. Smith, & B. L. Waxman, *"Why we drop out": Understanding and disrupting student pathways to leaving school* (pp. vii–viii). Teachers College Press.

Feldman, D. L., Smith, A. T., & Waxman, B. L. (2017). *"Why we drop out": Understanding and disrupting student pathways to leaving school.* Teachers College Press.

Fisher, D., & Frey, N. (2019). "There was this teacher. . . ." *Educational Leadership, 76*(8), 82–83.

Fullan, M., Gardner, M., & Drummy, M. (2019). Going deeper. *Educational Leadership, 76*(8), 64–69.

Grinshteyn, E., & Tony Yang, Y. (2017). The association between electronic bullying and school absenteeism among high school students in the United States. *Journal of School Health, 87*(2), 142–149. https://doi.org/10.1111/josh.12476

Guryan, J., Christenson, S., Cureton, A., Lai, I., Ludwig, J., Schwarz, C., Shirey, E., & Turner, M. C. (2021). The effect of mentoring on school attendance and academic outcomes: A randomized evaluation of the Check & Connect Program. *Journal of Policy Analysis and Management, 40*(3), 841–882. https://doi.org/10.1002/pam .22264

Hall, H. R. (2019). What do black adolescents need from schools? *Educational Leadership, 76*(8), 52–57.

Hammond, C., Linton, D., Smink, J., & Drew, S. (2007). *Dropout risk factors and exem-*

plary programs. National Dropout Prevention Center, Communities in Schools, Inc.

Hardie, E. (2019). Giving teens a place at the table. *Educational Leadership, 76*(8), 18–23.

Johns, M. M., Poteat, V. P., Horn, S. S., & Kosciw, J. (2019). Strengthening our schools to promote resilience and health among LGBTQ youth: Emerging evidence and research priorities from the State of LGBTQ Youth Health and Wellbeing Symposium. *LGBT Health, 6*(4), 146–155. https://doi.org/10.1089/lgbt.2018.0109

Jordan, P. (2019, July). *Attendance playbook: Smart solutions for reducing chronic absenteeism*. FutureEd & Attendance Works. https://future-ed.org/wp-content/uploads/2019/07/Attendance-Playbook.pdf

Kearney, C. A. (2003). Bridging the gap among professionals who address youths with school absenteeism: Overview and suggestions for consensus. *Professional Psychology: Research and Practice, 34*(1), 57. https://doi.org/10.1037/0735-7028.34.1.57

Kearney, C. A., & Bensaheb, A. (2006). School absenteeism and school refusal behavior: A review and suggestions for school-based health professionals. *Journal of School Health, 76*(1), 3–7.

KidsData. (n.d.). *High school graduation*. Population Reference Bureau. https://www.kidsdata.org/research/21/high-school-graduation#related-research/18

Malika, N., Granillo, C., Irani, C., Montgomery, S., & Belliard, J. C. (2021). Chronic absenteeism: Risks and protective factors among low-income, minority children and adolescents. *Journal of School Health, 91*(12), 1046–1054. https://doi.org/10.1111/josh.13096

Martinez, A. K. (2016). *School attendance, chronic health conditions and leveraging data for improvement: Recommendations for state education and health departments to address student absenteeism*. National Association of Chronic Disease Directors. https://chronicdisease.org/resource/resmgr/school_health/nacdd_school_attendance_and_.pdf

McCabe, E. M., Davis, C., Mandy, L., & Wong, C. (2022). The role of school connectedness in supporting the health and well-being of youth: Recommendations for school nurses. *NASN school nurse, 37*(1), 42–47. https://doi.org/10.1177/1942602X211048481

McWhirter, E. H., Garcia, E. A., & Bines, D. (2018). Discrimination and other education barriers, school connectedness, and thoughts of dropping out among Latina/o students. *Journal of Career Development, 45*(4), 330–344. https://doi.org/10.1177/%2F0894845317696807

Mehta, J., & Fine, S. (2019). *In search of deeper learning: The quest to remake the American high school*. Harvard University Press.

Milner, H. R., IV. (2019). No more "waiting on 16." *Educational Leadership, 76*(5), 86–87.

National Center for Education Statistics. (2021). *Public high school graduation rates*. Department of Education, Institute of Education Sciences. https://nces.ed.gov/programs/coe/indicator/coi

Olson, L. S. (2014). *A first look at community schools in Baltimore*. Baltimore Education Research Consortium.

Orpinas, P., Raczynski, K., Hsieh, H. L., Nahapetyan, L., & Horne, A. M. (2018). Longitudinal examination of aggression and study skills from middle to high school: Implications for dropout prevention. *Journal of School Health, 88*(3), 246–252. https://doi.org/10.1111/josh.12602

Patnode, A. H., Gibbons, K., & Edmunds, R. (2018). *Attendance and chronic absenteeism: Literature review.* University of Minnesota, College of Education and Human Development, Center for Applied Research and Educational Improvement. http://www.floridarti.usf.edu/resources/format/pdf/Chronic%20Absenteeism%20Lit%20Review%202018.pdf

Quin, D. (2017). Longitudinal and contextual associations between teacher-student relationships and student engagement: A systematic review. *Review of Educational Research, 87*(2), 345–387. https://doi.org/10.3102/0034654316669434

Rogers, T., & Feller, A. (2018). *Supplementary materials for reducing student absences at scale by targeting parents' misbeliefs.* Nature Human Behavior. https://doi.org/10.1038/s41562-018-0328-1

Romero, C. (2018, October). *What we know about belonging from scientific research.* Mindset Scholars Network. https://studentexperiencenetwork.org/wp-content/uploads/2018/11/What-We-Know-About-Belonging.pdf

Smythe-Leistico, K., & Page, L. C. (2018). Connect-text: Leveraging text-message communication to mitigate chronic absenteeism and improve parental engagement in the earliest years of schooling. *Journal of Education for Students Placed at Risk (JESPAR), 23*(1–2), 139–152. https://doi.org/10.1080/10824669.2018.1434658

Sparks, S. D. (2019, March 12). Why teacher-student relationships matter. *Education Week, 38*(25). https://www.edweek.org/teaching-learning/why-teacher-student-relationships-matter/2019/03

Stanley, K. R., & Plucker, J. A. (2008). Improving high school graduation rates. *Education Policy Brief, 6*(7), 1–12.

Steiner, R. J., Sheremenko, G., Lesesne, C., Dittus, P. J., Sieving, R. E., & Ethier, K. A. (2019). Adolescent connectedness and adult health outcomes. *Pediatrics, 144*(1). https://doi.org/10.1542/peds.2018-3766

Superville, D. R. (2019, March 13). Students give frank advice on how to make school engaging. *Education Week, 38*(25), 3–5.

Teaching Tolerance. (2016). *Critical practices for anti-bias education.* Southern Poverty Law Center. https://www.learningforjustice.org/sites/default/files/2017-06/PDA%20Critical%20Practices_0.pdf

Tomek, S., Bolland, A. C., Hooper, L. M., Hitchcock, S., & Bolland, J. M. (2017). The impact of middle school connectedness on future high school outcomes in a black American sample. *Middle Grades Research Journal, 11*(1), 1–12.

Chapter 5. Quality Schools

Alvarez, B. (2021, September 21). *Teaching with an anti-racist lens.* National Education Association. https://www.nea.org/advocating-for-change/new-from-nea/teaching-anti-racist-lens

American Psychological Association Zero Tolerance Task Force. (2008). Are zero tolerance policies effective in the schools? An evidentiary review and recommendations. *The American Psychologist, 63*(9), 852–862.

Augustine, C. H., Engberg, J., Grimm, G. E., Lee, E., Wang, E. L., Christianson, K., & Joseph, A. A. (2018). *Can restorative practices improve school climate and curb suspensions? An evaluation of the impact of restorative practices in a mid-sized urban school district.* RAND Corporation.

Ayers, W. (2004). *Teaching toward freedom: Moral commitment and ethical action in the classroom.* Beacon Press.

Bacher-Hicks, A., Billings, S., Deming, D. (2021). Proving the school-to-prison pipeline: Stricter middle schools raise the risk of adult arrest. *Education Next, 21*(4), 52–57.

Baker, B. D. (2016). *Does money matter in education?* Albert Shanker Institute. http://files.eric.ed.gov/fulltext/ED563793.pdf

Barnum, M. (2019, August 13). *4 new studies bolster the case: More money for schools helps low-income students.* Chalkbeat. https://www.chalkbeat.org/2019/8/13/21055545/4-new-studies-bolster-the-case-more-money-for-schools-helps-low-income-students

Bartanen, B., & Grissom, J. A. (2019). *School principal race and the hiring and retention of racially diverse teachers* (EdWorking Paper No. 19-59). Annenberg Institute, Brown University. https://doi.org/10.26300/ny03-zw18

Berliner, D. C., & Glass, G. V. (2014). *50 myths & lies that threaten America's public schools: The real crisis in education.* Teachers College Press.

Bernhardt, V. L. (2015). Toward systemwide change. *Educational Leadership, 73*(3), 56–61.

Birch, D. A. (2021). Addressing social justice through school health education: Thoughts on an expanded focus. *Journal of School Health, 91*(6), 439–442. https://doi.org/10.111/josh.13017

Birch, D. A., Mitchell Q. P., & Priest, H. M. (2015). Components of the WSCC model. In D. A. Birch & D. M. Videto (Eds.), *Promoting health and academic success: The whole school, whole community, whole child approach* (pp. 29–50). Human Kinetics.

Black, D. W. (2016). Taking teacher quality seriously. *William and Mary Law Review, 57*(5), 1597–1669. https://scholarship.law.wm.edu/wmlr/vol57/iss5/2

Bondono, O., Cooper de Uribe, A., Hargreaves, A., Hee Stock, K., Johnson, J., Rosato, S., & Wolfe, J. (2021). What it really means to appreciate teachers. *Education Week, 40*(33), 16.

Brady, L., Fryberg, S., Markus, H. R., Griffiths, C., Yang, J., Rodriguez, P., & Mannen-Martinez, L. (2021). Teaching means talking about socially sensitive topics. *Education Week, 40*(23), 15–16.

Bryk, A. S., Sebring, P. B., Allensworth, E., Luppescu, S., & Easton, J. Q. (2010). *Organizing schools for improvement: Lessons from Chicago.* University of Chicago Press.

Burch, K. (2001). A tale of two citizens: Asking the Rodriguez question in the twenty-first century. *Education Studies, 32*(3), 264–278.

Cascio, E. U., & Reber, S. (2013). The poverty gap in school spending following the introduction of Title I. *American Economic Review, 103*(3), 423–427. https://doi.org/10.1257/aer.103.3.423

Collins, C. (2021). It was always about control. *Teaching Tolerance*, (66), 42–45.

Cookson, P. W., Jr. (2013). *Class rules: Exposing inequality in American high schools.* Teachers College Press.

Cope, S. (2019, November 5). The power of a wealthy PTA. *The Atlantic.* https://www .theatlantic.com/education/archive/2019/11/pta-fundraising-schools/601435/

Counts, J., Randall, K. N., Ryan, J. B., & Katsiyannis, A. (2018). School resource officers in public schools: A national review. *Education and Treatment of Children, 41*(4), 405–430. https://doi.org/10.1353/etc.2018.0023

Crosse, S., Gottfredson, D. C., Bauer, E. L., Tang, Z., Harmon, M. A., Hagen, C. A., & Greene, A. D. (2021). Are effects of school resource officers moderated by student race and ethnicity? *Crime and Delinquency, 68*(3), 1–28. https://doi.org/10.1177%2 F0011128721999346

Darling-Hammond, L. (2010). *The flat world and education: How America's commitment to equity will determine our future.* Teachers College Press.

Davenport, G. (2022). Adaptive leadership for school equity. *Educational Leadership, 79*(6), 22–25.

Edgenuity. (n.d.). *K–12 education federal funding.* https://www.edgenuity.com/resources /funding/

Education Commission of the States. (2019, August 5). *50-state comparison: K–12 funding.* https://www.ecs.org/50-state-comparison-k-12-funding/

Ellis, W. R. (2020). Healing communities to health school. *Educational Leadership, 18*(2), 52–57.

Fabelo, T., Thompson, M. D., Plotkin, M., Carmichael, D., Marchbanks, M. P., III, & Booth, E. A. (2011, July). *Breaking schools' rules: A statewide study of how school discipline relates to students' success and juvenile justice involvement* (NCJ No. 235311). https://www.ojp.gov/ncjrs/virtual-library/abstracts/breaking-schools -rules-statewide-study-how-school-discipline

Fisher, D., & Frey, N. (2019). Show & tell: A video column / getting started with restorative practices. *Educational Leadership, 77*(2), 84–85.

Flannery, M. E. (2015, January 5). *The school-to-prison pipeline: Time to shut it down.* National Education Association. https://www.nea.org/advocating-for-change /new-from-nea/school-prison-pipeline-time-shut-it-down

Fried, A. (2019). Don't do restorative justice unless you can do it right. *Education Week, 38*(36), 21.

Fronius, T., Darling-Hammond, S., Perrson, H., Guckenburg, S., Hurley, N., & Petrosino, A. (2019, March). *Restorative justice in U.S. schools: An updated research review.* WestEd Justice and Prevention Research Center. https://files.eric.ed.gov /fulltext/ED595733.pdf

Gabor, A. (2018). *After the education wars: How smart schools upend the business of reform.* New Press.

Gailer, J., Addis, S., & Dunlap, L. (2018). *Improving school outcomes for trauma-impacted students.* National Dropout Prevention Center & Successful Practices Network. http://dropoutprevention.org/wp-content/uploads/2018/10/Trauma -Skilled-Schools-Model-Final-I.pdf

Gay, G. (2000). *Culturally responsive teaching: Theory,.research, and practice.* Teachers College Press.

George, J. (2021). Critical race theory isn't a curriculum. It's a practice. *Education Week, 40*(34), 24.

Goldstein, D. (2017, April 9). Share PTA aid? Some parents would rather split up district. *The New York Times,* pp. 1, 18.

González, T. (2012). Keeping kids in schools: Restorative justice, punitive discipline, and the school to prison pipeline. *Journal of Law and Education, 41*(2), 281–335.

Gorski, P. C. (2018). *Reaching and teaching students in poverty: Strategies for erasing the opportunity gap* (2nd ed.). Teachers College Press.

Gorski, P. (2020). How trauma-informed are we, really? *Educational Leadership, 78*(2), 14–19.

Griggs, B. (2020). Finding the confidence to speak up. *Education Week, 40*(4), 19.

Grissom, J. A., Egalite, A. J., & Lindsay, C. A. (2021). *How principals affect students and schools: A systematic synthesis of two decades of research.* The Wallace Foundation. https://www.wallacefoundation.org/knowledge-center/Documents/How-Principals-Affect-Students-and-Schools.pdf

Haberman, M. (2000). Urban schools: Day camps or custodial centers? *Phi Delta Kappan, 82*(3), 203–208.

Hall, P. (2019). The instructional leader's most difficult job. *Educational Leadership, 76*(6), 12–17.

Heitzeg, N. A. (2009). Education or incarceration: Zero tolerance policies and the school to prison pipeline. In *Forum on Public Policy Online* (Vol. 2009, No. 2). Oxford Round Table.

Henderson, D. X., Walker, L., Barnes, R. R., Lunsford, A., Edwards, C., & Clark, C. (2019). A framework for race-related trauma in the public education system and implications on health for black youth. *Journal of School Health, 89*(11), 926–933. https://doi.org/10.1111/josh.12832

Hoover, S. A. (2019). Policy and practice for trauma-informed schools. *State Education Standard, 19*(1), 25–29. https://nasbe.nyc3.digitaloceanspaces.com/2019/01/Hoover_January-2019-Standard.pdf

Hopkins, B. (2003). *Just schools: A whole school approach to restorative justice.* Jessica Kingsley Publishers.

Howard, T. C. (2010). *Why race and culture matter in schools: Closing the achievement gap in American classrooms.* Teachers College Press.

Jackson, C. K., Johnson, R. C., & Persico, C. (2016). The effects of school spending on educational and economic outcomes: Evidence from school finance reforms. *The Quarterly Journal of Economics, 131*(1), 157–218. https://doi.org/10.1093/qje/qjv036

Justice Policy Institute. (2011, November). *Education under arrest: The case against police in schools.* https://justicepolicy.org/wp-content/uploads/justicepolicy/documents/educationunderarrest_fullreport.pdf

Khalifa, M. (2018). *Culturally responsive school leadership.* Harvard Education Press.

Keels, M. (2020, October). Building racial equity through trauma-responsive discipline. *Educational Leadership, 78*(2), 40–45, 51.

Kendi, I. X. (2019). *How to be anti-racist*. One World.

Lesley, B. A. (2018). *Weighing costs & benefits: Research on student weights and school finance*. Equity Center. https://www.equitycenter.org/sites/default/files/2018-10/Weighing_Costs_Benefits_10118_final_web_002.pdf

Lewontin, M. (2017). The path to least suspensions. *Education Update, 59*(3), 1, 4–5.

Lloyd, S. C., & Harwin, A. (2019). Ed-Finance researchers' "wish list." *Education Week, 38*(4), 9.

Love, B. L. (2019). *We want to do more than survive: Abolitionist teaching and the pursuit of educational freedom*. Beacon Press.

Mehta, J., Yurkofsky, M., & Frumin, K. (2022). Linking continuous improvement and adaptive leadership. *Educational Leadership, 79*(6), 36–41.

Milner, H. R., IV. (2018). Relationship-centered teaching: Addressing racial tensions in classrooms. *Kappa Delta Pi Record, 54*(2), 60–66. https://doi.org/10.1080/00228958.2018.1443646

Minahan, J. (2019). Trauma-informed teaching strategies. *Educational Leadership, 77*(2), 30–35.

Morgan, I., & Amerikaner, A. (2018). Funding gaps 2018: An analysis of school funding equity across the US and within each state. *Education Trust*.

Morris, E. W., & Perry, B. L. (2016). The punishment gap: School suspension and racial disparities in achievement. *Social Problems, 63*(1), 68–86. https://doi.org/10.1093/socpro/spv026

Morrison, B. E., & Vaandering, D. (2012). Restorative justice: Pedagogy, praxis, and discipline. *Journal of School Violence, 11*(2), 138–155. https://doi.org/10.1080/15388220.2011.653322

NAACP Legal Defense Fund. (n.d.). *Critical race theory: Frequently asked questions*. https://www.naacpldf.org/critical-race-theory-faq/

Nadeem, E., Floyd-Rodríguez, V., de la Torre, G., & Greswold, W. (2021). Trauma in schools: An examination of trauma screening and linkage to behavioral health care in school-based health centers. *Journal of School Health, 91*(5), 428–436. https://doi.org/10.1111/josh.13014

National Center for Education Statistics. (2022). *Public school revenue sources*. US Department of Education, Institute of Education Sciences. https://nces.ed.gov/programs/coe/indicator/cma

Noltemeyer, A. L., Ward, R. M., & Mcloughlin, C. (2015). Relationship between school suspension and student outcomes: A meta-analysis. *School Psychology Review, 44*(2), 224–240.

Northshore School District. (n.d.). *Our mission and work*. https://www.nsd.org/our-district/who-we-are/racial-educational-justice/our-work

Okonofua, J. A., Paunesku, D., & Walton, G. M. (2016). Brief intervention to encourage empathic discipline cuts suspension rates in half among adolescents. *Proceedings of the National Academy of Sciences, 113*(19), 5221–5226. https://doi.org/10.1073/pnas.1523698113

Pendharkar, E. (2021). Efforts to root out racism in schools would unravel under critical race theory bills. *Education Week, 40*(34), 8.

Pigott, C., Stearns, A. E., & Khey, D. N. (2018). School resource officers and the school to prison pipeline: Discovering trends of expulsions in public schools. *American Journal of Criminal Justice, 43*(1), 120–138. https://doi.org/10.1007/s12103-017-9412-8

Pitts, B. R. (2020). White teachers, mis-education, and the psycho-social lynching of black history. In L. J. King (Ed.), *Perspective of black histories in schools* (pp. 159–178). Information Age Publishing Inc.

Ravitch, D. (2010). *The death and life of the great American school system: How testing and choice are undermining education.* Basic Books.

Ravitch, D. (2014). *Reign of error: The hoax of the privatization movement and the danger to America's public schools.* Vintage Books.

Ravitch, D. (2015). Foreword: An alternate universe. In P. Sahlberg (Ed.), *Finnish 2.0 lessons: What can the world learn from educational change in Finland?* (2nd ed., pp. xi–xii). Teachers College Press.

Rimmer, J. (2016). Developing principals as equity-centered instructional leaders. In S. Petty (Ed.), *Equity-centered capacity building.* Equity Centered Capacity Building Network. https://capacitybuildingnetwork.org/table-of-contents/

Rumberger, R. W., & Losen, D. J. (2016). *The high cost of harsh discipline and its disparate impact.* Center for Civil Rights Remedies at The Civil Rights Project at UCLA. https://escholarship.org/uc/item/85m2m6sj

Rumsey, A., & Milsom, A. (2017). *Dropout prevention and trauma: Addressing a wide range of stressors that inhibit student success* [White paper]. National Dropout Prevention Center/Network. http://www.dropoutprevention.org/wp-content/uploads/2017/10/dropout-prevention-and-trauma-2017-10.pdf

Samuels, C. A. (2020, July 15). 6 ways district leaders can build racial equity. *Education Week, 39*(7). https://www.edweek.org/leadership/6-ways-district-leaders-can-build-racial-equity/2020/06

Sawchuk, S. (2021a). School resource officers (SROs) explained: Their duties, effectiveness, and more. *Education Week.* https://www.edweek.org/leadership/school-resource-officer-sro-duties-effectiveness

Sawchuk, S. (2021b). What is critical race theory and why is it under attack? *Education Week, 40*(34), 4–5.

Sawchuk, S., Schwartz, S., Pendharkar, E., & Najarro, I. (2021). Defunded, removed, and put in check: School police a year after George Floyd. *Education Week,* 40(36), 12–13.

Schneider, J. (2017). *Beyond test scores: A better way to measure school quality.* Harvard University Press.

Schwartz, S. (2021). Four states have placed legal limits on how teachers can discuss race. More may follow. *Education Week, 40*(34), 6.

Sheetz, M. & Senge, P. (2016). Systematic change and equity. In Petty, S. (Ed.), *Equity Centered Capacity Building.* Equity Centered Capacity Building Network. https://capacitybuildingnetwork.org/article3/

Simmons, D. (2020, October). Confronting inequity / healing black students' pain. *Educational Leadership, 78*(2), 80–81.

Skiba, R. J., Arredondo, M. I., & Williams, N. T. (2014). More than a metaphor: The contribution of exclusionary discipline to a school-to-prison pipeline. *Equity and Excellence in Education, 47*(4), 546–564. https://doi.org/10.1080/10665684.2014.958965

Skiba, R. J., & Rausch, M. K. (2006). Zero tolerance, suspension, and expulsion: Questions of equity and effectiveness. In C. M. Evertson & C. S. Weinstein (Eds.), *Handbook of classroom management: Research, practice, and contemporary issues* (pp. 1063–1089). Lawrence Erlbaum Associates Publishers.

Sleeter, C. E. (Ed.). (2007). *Facing accountability in education: Democracy and equity at risk.* Teachers College Press.

Sparks, S. D. (2021). 4 myths about suspensions that could hurt students in the long term. *Education Week, 41*(4), 7.

Stinchcomb, J. B., Bazemore, G., & Riestenberg, N. (2006). Beyond zero tolerance: Restoring justice in secondary schools. *Youth Violence and Juvenile Justice, 4*(2), 123–147. https://doi.org/10.1177/1541204006286287

Temkin, D., Harper, K., Stratford, B., Sacks, V., Rodriguez, Y., & Bartlett, J. D. (2020). Moving policy toward a whole school, whole community, whole child approach to support children who have experienced trauma. *Journal of School Health, 90*(12), 940–947. https://doi.org/10.1111/josh.12957

Tomlinson, C. A. (2020). Learning from kids who hurt. *Educational Leadership, 78*(2), 28–33.

Torres, C. (2019). The urgent need for anti-racist education. *Education Week, 39*(1), 22–23.

Turn and Talk. (2018). Q&A with Deborah Lowenberg Ball. *Educational Leadership, 75*(8), 10.

Tyler, T. R. (2006). Restorative justice and procedural justice: Dealing with rule breaking. *Journal of Social Issues, 62*(2), 307–326. https://doi.org/10.1111/j.1540-4560.2006.00452.x

Welsh, R. O. (2021). Why, really, are so many black kids suspended? *Education Week, 41*(3), 24.

Will, M., & Najarro, I. (2022, April 18). What is culturally responsive teaching? *Education Week.* https://www.edweek.org/teaching-learning/culturally-responsive-teaching-culturally-responsive-pedagogy/2022/04?M=4148212&UUID=7034bc92d6daebae410564e67dbf5473

Willoughby, B. (2012). *Responding to hate and bias at school: A guide for administrators, counselors and teachers.* Teaching Tolerance and Southern Poverty Law Center. http://files.eric.ed.gov/fulltext/ED541255.pdf

Zehr, H. (2002). *The little book of restorative justice.* Good Books.

Chapter 6. The Whole School, Whole Community, Whole Childhood Model

Adams, C. M. (2019). Sustaining full-service community schools: Lessons from the Tulsa area community schools initiative. *Journal of Education for Students Placed at Risk (JESPAR), 24*(3), 288–313. https://doi.org/10.1080/10824669.2019.1615924

Aldana, S. G., Merrill, R. M., Price, K., Hardy, A., & Hager, R. (2005). Financial impact of a comprehensive multisite workplace health promotion program. *Preventive Medicine, 40*(2), 131–137. https://doi.org/10.1016/j.ypmed.2004.05.008

Allensworth, D. (2015). Historical overview of coordinated school health. In D. A. Birch & D. M. Videto (Eds.), *Promoting health and academic success: The whole school, whole community, whole child approach* (pp. 13–28). Human Kinetics.

Allensworth, D. D. (1994). Understanding the focus for school health improvement. In D. D. Allensworth, C. W. Symons, & R. S. Olds (Eds.), *Healthy students 2000: An agenda for continuous improvement in America's schools* (pp. 1–8). American School Health Association.

Allensworth, D. D., & Kolbe, L. J. (1987). The comprehensive school health program: Exploring an expanded concept. *Journal of School Health, 57*(10), 409–12.

American School Counselor Association. (2020a). *Empirical research studies supporting the value of school counseling.* https://www.schoolcounselor.org/asca/media/asca/Careers-Roles/Effectiveness.pdf

American School Counselor Association. (2020b). *Information for administrators and district directors.* https://www.schoolcounselor.org/administrators

American School Counselor Association. (2020c). *The role of the school counselor.* https://www.schoolcounselor.org/getmedia/ee8b2e1b-d021-4575-982c-c84402cb2cd2/Role-Statement.pdf

Arenson, M., Hudson, P. J., Lee, N., & Lai, B. (2019). The evidence on school-based health centers: A review. *Global Pediatric Health, 6*, 1–10. https://doi.org/10.1177%2F1942602X19852749

ASCD. (n.d.-a). *The whole child initiative: Challenged.* https://library.ascd.org/m/1d2bd6cd7ba9a7a5/original/WC_Tenets_Challenged.pdf

ASCD. (n.d.-b). *The whole child initiative: Engaged.* https://library.ascd.org/m/4db133cfe30eb754/original/WC_Tenets_Engaged.pdf

ASCD. (n.d.-c). *The whole child initiative: Healthy.* https://library.ascd.org/m/5a9a355ad6e7bf6a/original/WC_Tenets_Healthy.pdf

ASCD. (n.d.-d). *The whole child initiative: Safe.* https://library.ascd.org/m/1181b74bb7d405e6/original/WC_Tenets_Safe.pdf

ASCD. (n.d.-e). *The whole child initiative: Supported.* https://library.ascd.org/m/549590d76f13c01e/original/WC_Tenets_Supported.pdf

ASCD. (2007). *The learning compact redefined: A call to action: A report of the commission on the whole child.* https://library.ascd.org/m/21e2f544234c3e97/original/WCC-Learning-Compact.pdf

ASCD. (2014). *Whole School, whole community, whole child: A collaborative approach to learning and health.* https://files.ascd.org/staticfiles/ascd/pdf/siteASCD/publications/wholechild/wscc-a-collaborative-approach.pdf

Belfield, C., Bowden, A. B., Klapp, A., Levin, H., Shand, R., & Zander, S. (2015). The economic value of social and emotional learning. *Journal of Benefit-Cost Analysis, 6*(3), 508–544. https://doi.org/10.1017/bca.2015.55

Beyers, J. M., Bates, J. E., Pettit, G. S., & Dodge, K. A. (2003). Neighborhood structure, parent processes, and the development of externalizing behaviors: A multilevel

analysis. *American Journal of Community Psychology, 31*, 35–53. https://doi.org
/10.1023/A:1023018502759

Birch, D. A. (2021). Addressing social justice through school health education: Thoughts
on an expanded focus. *Journal of School Health, 91*(6), 439–442. https://doi.org/10
.111/josh.13017

Birch, D. A., & Auld, M. E. (2019). Public health and school health education: Aligning
forces for change. *Health Promotion Practice, 20*(6), 818–823. https://doi.org/10
.1177/1524839919870184

Birch, D. A., Goekler, S., Auld, M. E., Lohrmann, D. K., & Lyde, A. (2019). Quality
assurance in teaching K–12 health education: Paving a new path forward. *Health
Promotion Practice, 20*(6), 845–857. https://doi.org/10.1177%2F1524839919868167

Birch, D. A., Mitchell Q. P., & Priest, H. M. (2015). Components of the WSCC Model.
In D. A. Birch & D. M. Videto (Eds.), *Promoting health and academic success:
The whole school, whole community, whole child approach* (pp. 29–50). Human
Kinetics.

Birch, D. A., & Videto, D. M. (2015). Whole school, whole community, whole child:
A new model for health and academic success. In D. A. Birch & D. M. Videto
(Eds.), *Promoting health and academic success: The whole school, whole commu-
nity, whole child approach* (pp. 3–11). Human Kinetics.

Blair, S. N., Smith, M., Collingwood, T. R., Reynolds, R., Prentice, M. C., & Sterling,
C. L. (1986). Health promotion for educators: Impact on absenteeism. *Preventive
Medicine, 15*(2), 166–175. https://doi.org/10.1016/0091-7435(86)90086-1

Blank, M. J. (2015). Building sustainable health and education partnerships: Stories from
local communities. *Journal of School Health, 85*(11), 810–816. https://doi.org/10
.1111/josh.12311

Blank, M. J., & Villarreal, L. (2015). Where it all comes together: How partnerships
connect communities and schools. *American Educator, 39*(3), 4. https://files.eric
.ed.gov/fulltext/EJ1076382.pdf

Blue Zones. (n.d.). *Walking school buses get kids moving, alert, and ready to learn.*
https://www.bluezones.com/2017/09/walking-school-buses-get-kids-moving
-alert-and-ready-to-learn/#

Bryk, A. S., Bender Sebring, P., Allensworth, E., Luppescu, S., & Easton, J. Q. (2010).
Organizing schools for improvement: Lessons from Chicago. University of Chicago
Press.

California School Boards Association. (n.d.). *Community schools.* https://www.csba.org
/en/GovernanceAndPolicyResources/ConditionsOfChildren/ParentFamCom
EngageandCollab/CommunitySchools

Carter, G. (2014, March). *Integrating coordinated school health and the whole child
initiative.* Symposium conducted at the Society for Public Health Education
Annual Conference, Baltimore, MD.

Castro, M., Expósito-Casas, E., López-Martín, E., Lizasoain, L., Navarro-Asencio, E.,
& Gaviria, J. L. (2015). Parental involvement on student academic achievement:
A meta-analysis. *Educational Research Review, 14*, 33–46. https://doi.org/10.1016
/j.edurev.2015.01.002

Center for Social and Emotional Education. (n.d.). *National school climate standards: Benchmarks to promote effective teaching, learning and comprehensive school improvement.* http://www.casciac.org/pdfs/school-climate-standards-csee.pdf

Centers for Disease Control and Prevention. (2017). *School health index: A self-assessment and planning guide.* US Department of Health and Human Services. https://www.cdc.gov/healthyschools/shi/pdf/Middle-High-Total-2017.pdf

Centers for Disease Control and Prevention. (2018). *Strategies for classroom physical activity in schools.* US Department of Health and Human Services. https://www.cdc.gov/healthyschools/physicalactivity/pdf/2019_04_25_Strategies-for-CPA_508tagged.pdf

Centers for Disease Control and Prevention. (2019a). *Characteristics of an effective health education curriculum.* US Department of Health and Human Services. https://www.cdc.gov/healthyschools/sher/characteristics/

Centers for Disease Control and Prevention. (2019b). *Health Education Curriculum Analysis Tool (HECAT).* US Department of Health and Human Services. https://www.cdc.gov/healthyyouth/hecat/

Centers for Disease Control and Prevention. (2019c). *School health services.* US Department of Health and Human Services. https://www.cdc.gov/healthyschools/schoolhealthservices.htm

Centers for Disease Control and Prevention. (2019d). *School meals.* US Department of Health and Human Services. https://www.cdc.gov/healthyschools/npao/schoolmeals.htm

Centers for Disease Control and Prevention. (2020). *Physical education.* US Department of Health and Human Services. https://www.cdc.gov/healthyschools/physicalactivity/physical-education.htm

Centers for Disease Control and Prevention. (2022). *Benefits of physical activity.* US Department of Health and Human Services. https://www.cdc.gov/physicalactivity/basics/pa-health/index.htm

Clofelter, C. T., Ladd, H. F., Vigdor, J. L. (2007). *Are teacher absences worth worrying about in the U.S.?* (NBER Working Paper No. 13648). National Bureau of Economic Research. https://www.nber.org/papers/w13648

Collaborative for Academic, Social, and Emotional Learning. (2020). *CASEL's SEL Framework: What are the core competence areas and where are they promoted?* https://casel.org/wp-content/uploads/2020/12/CASEL-SEL-Framework-11.2020.pdf

Community Preventive Services Task Force. (2016). School-based health centers to promote health equity: Recommendation of the Community Preventive Services Task Force. *American Journal of Preventive Medicine, 51*(1), 127–128. http://dx.doi.org/10.1016/j.amepre.2016.01.008

Council on School Health. (2012). School-based health centers and pediatric practice. *Pediatrics, 129*(1), 387–393. http://www.pediatrics.org/cgi/doi/10.1542/peds.2011-3443

County Health Rankings and Roadmaps. (2019, November 4). *Walking school buses.* University of Wisconsin Population Health Institute and Robert Wood Johnson

Foundation. https://www.countyhealthrankings.org/take-action-to-improve
-health/what-works-for-health/strategies/walking-school-buses

Daily, S. M., Mann, M. J., Lilly, C. L., Dyer, A. M., Smith, M. L., & Kristjansson, A. L.
(2020). School climate as an intervention to reduce academic failure and educate
the whole child: A longitudinal study. *Journal of School Health, 90*(3), 182–193.
https://doi.org/10.1111/josh.12863

Devore, C. D., Wheeler, L. S. M., & American Academy of Pediatrics Council on School
Health. (2013). Role of the school physician. *Pediatrics, 131*(1), 178–182. https://doi
.org/10.1542/peds.2012-2995

DeWitt, P., & Slade, S. (2014). *School climate change: How do I build a positive environment for learning?* ASCD.

Domina, T. (2005). Leveling the home advantage: Assessing the effectiveness of parental
involvement in elementary school. *Sociology of Education, 78*(3), 233–249. https://
doi.org/10.1177%2F003804070507800303

Durlak, J. A., Weissberg, R. P., Dymnicki, A. B., Taylor, R. D., & Schellinger, K. B. (2011).
The impact of enhancing students' social and emotional learning: A meta-
analysis of school-based universal interventions. *Child Development, 82*, 405–
432. https://doi.org/10.1111/j.1467-8624.2010.01564.x

Economic Research Center. (2020, October 1). *National school lunch program.* US
Department of Agriculture. https://www.ers.usda.gov/topics/food-nutrition
-assistance/child-nutrition-programs/national-school-lunch-program.aspx

Eitland, E., MacNaughton, P., Cedeno Laurent, M., Spengler, J., Bernstein, A., & Allen. J.
(2017, October 5). *School buildings and student success: How school buildings
influence student health, thinking and performance.* Healthy Buildings, Harvard
T. H. Chan School of Public Health. https://www.hsph.harvard.edu/c-change
/news/school-buildings-and-student-success/

El Nokali, N. E., Bachman, H. J., & Votruba-Drzal, E. (2010). Parent involvement and
children's academic and social development in elementary school. *Child Development, 81*, 988–1005. https://doi.org/10.1111/j.1467-8624.2010.01447.x

Epstein, J. L., Sanders, M. G., Sheldon, S. B., Simon, B. S., Salinas, K. C., Jansorn, N. R.,
Van Voorhis, F. L., Martin, C. S., Thomas, B. G., Greenfield, M. D., Hutchins,
D. J., & Williams, K. J. (2018). *School, family, and community partnerships: Your
handbook for action* (4th ed.). Corwin Press.

Farrey, T. (2020, June 22). *Why we're reimagining school sports in America.* Aspen Institute. https://www.aspeninstitute.org/blog-posts/why-were-reimagining-school
-sports-in-america/

Ferlazzo, L. (2011, May). Involvement or engagement? *Educational Leadership, 68*(8),
10–14.

Filardo, M., Vincent, J. M., Sung, P., & Stein, T. (2006). *Growth and disparity: A decade
of U.S. public school construction.* Building Educational Success Together. https://
files.eric.ed.gov/fulltext/ED498100.pdf

Gall, G., Pagano, M. E., Desmond, M. S., Perrin, J. M., & Murphy, J. M. (2000). Utility of
psychosocial screening at a school-based health center. *Journal of School Health,
70*(7), 292–298. https://doi.org/10.1111/j.1746-1561.2000.tb07254.x

Goodwin, S. C. (1993). Health and physical education—agonists or antagonists? *Journal of Physical Education, Recreation and Dance, 64*(7), 74–79. https://doi.org/10.1080/07303084.1993.10606791

Griffith, D., & Slade, S. (2018). A whole child umbrella. *Educational Leadership, 76*(2), 36–38.

Hartline-Grafton, H. (2016, January). *Research shows that the school nutrition standards improve the school nutrition environment and student outcomes.* Food Research and Action Center. https://frac.org/wp-content/uploads/school-nutrition-brief.pdf

Healthy Buildings program. (n.d.). *Schools for Health: Foundations for student success—how school buildings influence student health, thinking and performance.* Harvard T. H. Chan School of Public Health. https://forhealth.org/Harvard.Schools_For_Health.Foundations_for_Student_Success.pdf

Herbert, P. C., Lohrmann, D. K., & Hall, C. (2017). Targeting obesity through health promotion programs for school staff. *Strategies, 30*(1), 28–34. https://doi.org/10.1080/08924562.2016.1251867

Higgins, S., & Katsipataki, M. (2015). Evidence from meta-analysis about parental involvement in education which supports their children's learning. *Journal of Children's Services, 10*(3), 280–290. https://doi.org/10.1108/JCS-02-2015-0009

Hill, N. E., Castellino, D. R., Lansford, J. E., Nowlin, P., Dodge, K. A., Bates, J. E., & Pettit, G. S. (2004). Parent academic involvement as related to school behavior, achievement, and aspirations: Demographic variations across adolescence. *Child Development, 75*(5), 1491–1509. https://doi.org/10.1111/j.1467-8624.2004.00753.x

Hill, N. E., & Tyson, D. F. (2009). Parental involvement in middle school: A meta-analytic assessment of the strategies that promote achievement. *Developmental Psychology, 45*(3), 740–763. https://psycnet.apa.org/doi/10.1037/a0015362

Hodges, B. C., & Videto, D. M. (2015). Planning for WSCC. In D. A. Birch & D. M. Videto (Eds.), *Promoting health and academic success: The whole school, whole community, whole child approach* (pp. 29–50). Human Kinetics.

Holmes, B. W., Allison, M., Ancona, R., Attisha, E., Beers, N., De Pinto, C., Gorski, P., Kjolhede, C., Lerner, M., Weiss-Harrison, A., & Young, T. (2016). Role of the school nurse in providing school health services. *Pediatrics, 137*(6), e20160852. https://doi.org/10.1542/peds.2016-0852

Institute of Medicine. (2015). *Exploring opportunities for collaboration between health and education to improve population health: Workshop summary.* National Academies Press. https://doi.org/10.17226/18979

Jeynes, W. (2012). A meta-analysis of the efficacy of different types of parental involvement programs for urban students. *Urban Education, 47*(4), 706–742. https://doi.org/10.1177%2F0042085912445643

Jeynes, W. H. (2016). A meta-analysis: The relationship between parental involvement and African American school outcomes. *Journal of Black Studies, 47*(3), 195–216. https://doi.org/10.1177%2F0021934715623522

Jeynes, W. H. (2017). A meta-analysis: The relationship between parental involvement and Latino student outcomes. *Education and Urban Society, 49*(1), 4–28. https://doi.org/10.1177%2F0013124516630596

Joint Committee on National Health Education Standards. (2007). *Achieving excellence.* The American Cancer Society.

Jones, S., Brush, K., Bailey, R., Brion-Meisels, G., McIntyre, J., Kahn, J., Nelson, B., & Stickle, L. (2017, March). *Navigating SEL from the inside out.* Harvard Graduate School of Education & Wallace Foundation. https://www.wallacefoundation.org /knowledge-center/Documents/Navigating-Social-and-Emotional-Learning -from-the-Inside-Out.pdf

Jones, S. M., McGarrah, M. W., & Kahn, J. (2019). Social and emotional learning: A principled science of human development in context. *Educational Psychologist, 54*(3), 129–143. https://doi.org/10.1080/00461520.2019.1625776

Keeton, V., Soleimanpour, S., & Brindis, C. D. (2012). School-based health centers in an era of health care reform: Building on history. *Current Problems in Pediatric and Adolescent Health Care, 42*(6), 132–156. http://dx.doi.org/10.1016/j. cppeds.2012.03 .002

Kitzmiller, E. M., & Rodriguez, A. D. (2021, August 6). The link between educational inequality and infrastructure. *The Washington Post.* https://www.washington post.com/outlook/2021/08/06/school-buildings-black-neighborhoods-are -health-hazards-bad-learning/

Knopf, J. A., Finnie, R. K., Peng, Y., Hahn, R. A., Truman, B. I., Vernon-Smiley, M., Johnson, V. C., Johnson, R. L., Fielding J. E., Muntaner, C., Hunt, P. C., Jones, C. P., Fullilove, M. T., & Community Preventive Services Task Force. (2016). School-based health centers to advance health equity: A community guide systematic review. *American Journal of Preventive Medicine, 51*(1), 114–126. https:// doi.org/10.1016/j.amepre.2016.01.009

Kohl, H. W., III, & Cook, H. D. (Eds.). (2013). *Educating the student body: Taking physical activity and physical education to school.* National Academies Press.

Kolbe, L. J. (2019). School health as a strategy to improve both public health and education. *Annual Review of Public Health, 40,* 443–463. https://doi.org/10.1146 /annurev-publhealth-040218-043727

Kong, A. S., Burks, N., Conklin, C., Roldan, C., Skipper, B., Scott, S., Sussman, A. L., & Leggott, J. (2010). A pilot walking school bus program to prevent obesity in Hispanic elementary school children: Role of physician involvement with the school community. *Clinical Pediatrics, 49*(10), 989–991. https://doi.org/10.1177 /0009922810370364

Lewallen, T. C., Hunt, H., Potts-Datema, W., Zaza, S., & Giles, W. (2015). The whole school, whole community, whole child model: A new approach for improving educational attainment and healthy development for students. *Journal of School Health, 85*(11), 729–739. https://doi.org/10.1111/josh.12310

Lloyd, L. K., Schmidt, E. A., Swearingen, C. C., & Cavanaugh, A. C. (2019). Planning, development, and implementation of a university-led, low-cost employee wellness program in a preK–12th-grade public school district. *Journal of School Health, 89*(8), 669–679. https://doi.org/10.1111/josh.12791

Lofink, H., Kuebler, J., Juszczak, L., Schlitt, J., Even, M., Rosenberg, J., & White, I. (2013). *2010–2011 Census report of school-based health centers.* School-Based Health

Alliance. http://www.sbh4all.org/wp-content/uploads/2015/02/CensusReport
_2010-11CensusReport_7.13.pdf

Love, H. E., Schlitt, J., Soleimanpour, S., Panchal, N., & Behr, C. (2019). Twenty years of school-based health care growth and expansion. *Health Affairs, 38*(5), 755–764. https://doi.org/10.1377/hlthaff.2018.05472

Maier, A., Daniel, J., Oakes, J., & Lam, L. (2017, December). *Community schools as an effective school improvement strategy: A review of the evidence.* Learning Policy Institute.

Mann, M. J., & Lohrmann, D. K. (2019). Addressing challenges to the reliable, large-scale implementation of effective school health education. *Health Promotion Practice, 20*(6), 834–844. https://doi.org/10.1177%2F1524839919870196

Massey, W. V., Stellino, M. B., Mullen, S. P., Claassen, J., & Wilkison, M. (2018). Development of the Great Recess Framework—Observational Tool to measure contextual and behavioral components of elementary school recess. *BMC Public Health, 18*(1), 1–11. https://doi.org/10.1186/s12889-018-5295-y

Massey, W. V., Thalken, J., Szarabajko, A., Neilson, L., & Geldhof, J. (2021). Recess quality and social and behavioral health in elementary school students. *Journal of School Health, 91*(9), 730–740. https://doi.org/10.1111/josh.13065

McClanahan, R., & Weismuller, P. C. (2015). School nurses and care coordination for children with complex needs: An integrative review. *The Journal of School Nursing, 31*(1), 34–43. https://doi.org/10.11772F1059840514550484

McMurtrie, B. (2017). A springboard to college: How higher education is teaming up with high schools to encourage students to take the leap earlier. *The Chronicle of Higher Education, 63*(31), A8–A14.

McNall, M. A., Lichty, L. F., & Mavis, B. (2010). The impact of school-based health centers on the health outcomes of middle school and high school students. *American Journal of Public Health, 100*(9), 1604–1610. https://doi.org/10.2105 /AJPH.2009.183590

Merkel, C. (2013). How inequities in athletic funding in New Jersey public schools may be the key to underperformance. *Seton Hall Journal of Sports and Entertainment Law, 23*(2), 385–410.

Michael, S. L., Merlo, C. L., Basch, C. E., Wentzel, K. R., & Wechsler, H. (2015). Critical connections: Health and academics. *Journal of School Health, 85*(11), 740–758. https://doi.org/10.1111/josh.12309

Miller, R. (2008). *Tales of teacher absence: New research yields patterns that speak to policymakers.* Center for American Progress.

Moening, K., Lieberman, M., & Zimmerman, S. (2016). *Step by step: How to start a walking school bus at your school.* California Department of Public Health. https:// www.saferoutespartnership.org/sites/default/files/resource_files/step-by-step -walking-school-bus-2017.pdf

Mohl, B., & Patel, H. (2015). Rich-poor divide in high school sports. *Commonwealth Magazine, 20*(4), 32–37.

MSW@USC. (2019, February 4). *The role of school social workers.* University of Southern California. https://msw.usc.edu/mswusc-blog/what-is-a-school-social-worker/

Murray, R., Ramstetter, C., & American Academy of Pediatrics Council on School Health. (2013). The crucial role of recess in school. *Pediatrics, 131*(1), 183–188. https://doi.org/10.1542/peds.2012-2993

Murray, S. D., Hurley, J., & Ahmed, S. R. (2015). Supporting the whole child through coordinated policies, processes, and practices. *Journal of School Health, 85*(11), 795–801. https://doi.org/10.1111/josh.12306

National Association of Early Childhood Specialists in State Departments of Education. (2001). *Recess and the importance of play. A position statement on young children and recess.* http://files.eric.ed.gov/fulltext/ED463047.pdf

National Association of School Nurses. (2016). The role of the 21st century school nurse. *NASN School Nurse, 32*(1), 56–58.

National Association of School Nurses. (2017). *Definition of school nursing.* https://www.nasn.org/about-nasn/about

National Association of School Nurses. (2020). *School nurse workload: Staffing for safe care.* https://www.nasn.org/advocacy/professional-practice-documents/position-statements/ps-workload#:~:text=of%20School%20Nurses.,(2020).,Nurse%20Workload%20(Position%20Statement).&text=%E2%80%9CTo%20optimize%20student%20health%2C%20safety,all%20day%2C%20every%20day.%E2%80%9D

National Association of School Psychologists. (n.d.). *School psychologists.* [Infographic]. https://www.nasponline.org/assets/Documents/Resources%20and%20Publications/Resources/Who%20Are%20School%20Psychologists%20Infographic_2020.pdf

National Association of School Psychologists. (2015). *School psychologists: Improving student and school outcomes* [Research Summary]. https://www.nasponline.org/Documents/Research%20and%20Policy/Research%20Center/School_Psychologists-Improving_Student_Outcomes-Final.pdf

National Association of School Psychologists. (2020). *Who are school psychologists.* https://www.nasponline.org/about-school-psychology/who-are-school-psychologists

National Association of Social Workers. (2012). *NASW practice standards & guidelines.* https://www.socialworkers.org/Practice/Practice-Standards-Guidelines

National Center for Safe Routes to School (n.d.-a). *Deciding if a walking school bus is the right fit.* http://guide.saferoutesinfo.org/walking_school_bus/deciding_if_a_walking_school_bus_is_the_right_fit.cfm

National Center for Safe Routes to School. (n.d.-b). *Option 2: Reaching out to more children.* http://guide.saferoutesinfo.org/walking_school_bus/reaching_out_to_more_children.cfm

National Consensus for School Health Education. (2022). *National health education standards: Model guidance for curriculum and instruction* (3rd ed.). www.schoolhealtheducation.org

Office of Disease Prevention and Health Promotion. (n.d.). Physical activity. *Healthy People 2030.* US Department of Health and Human Services. https://health.gov/healthypeople/objectives-and-data/browse-objectives/physical-activity

Olson, L. S. (2014). *A first look at community schools in Baltimore.* Baltimore Education Research Consortium. http://baltimore-berc.org/wpcontent/uploads/2014/12/CommunitySchoolsReportDec2014.pdf

Osher, D., & Berg, J. (2017). *School climate and social and emotional learning: The integration of two approaches*. Edna Bennet Pierce Prevention Research Center, Pennsylvania State University.

Project Play. (n.d.). *Youth sports facts: Why youth sports matter*. Aspen Institute. https://www.aspenprojectplay.org/youth-sports-facts

Ran, T., Chattopadhyay, S. K., Hahn, R. A., & Community Preventive Services Task Force. (2016). Economic evaluation of school-based health centers: A community guide systematic review. *American Journal of Preventive Medicine, 51*(1), 129–138. https://doi.org/10.1016/j.amepre.2016.01.017

Rhode Island Department of Education. (2017). *Rhode Island's Every Student Succeeds Act state plan*. https://www2.ed.gov/admins/lead/account/stateplan17/riconsolidatedstateplanfinal.pdf

Sanders, M. G. (2018). School-community partnerships: The little extra that makes a big difference. In J. L. Epstein, M. G. Sanders, S. B. Sheldon, B. S. Simon, K. C. Salinas, N. R. Jansorn, F. L. Van Voorhis, C. S. Martin, B. G. Thomas, M. D. Greenfield, D. J. Hutchins, & K. J. Williams (Eds.), *School, family, and community partnerships: Your handbook for action* (4th ed., pp. 33–42). Corwin Press.

School-Based Health Alliance. (n.d.). *About school-based health care*. https://www.sbh4all.org/what-we-do/school-based-health-care/aboutsbhcs/

School Nutrition Association. (n.d.-a). *Nutrition standards for school meals*. https://schoolnutrition.org/wp-content/uploads/2022/06/Nutrition-Standards-for-School-Meals.pdf

School Nutrition Association. (n.d.-b). *Smart snacks in school*. https://schoolnutrition.org/wp-content/uploads/2022/06/Competitive-Foods-Fact-Sheet.pdf

School Nutrition Association. (2019). *Keys to excellence: Standards of practice for nutrition integrity*. https://schoolnutrition.org/wp-content/uploads/2022/09/Keys-to-Excellence-Standards.pdf

School Social Work Association of America. (n.d.-a). *Role of school social worker*. https://www.sswaa.org/school-social-work

School Social Work Association of America. (n.d.-b). *The role of a school social worker*. [Infographic]. https://aab82939-3e7b-497d-8f30a85373757e29.filesusr.com/ugd/426a18_003ab15a5e9246248dff98506e46654b.pdf

Schultz, N. S., Chui, K. K., Economos, C. D., Lichtenstein, A. H., Volpe, S. L., & Sacheck, J. M. (2019). A qualitative investigation of factors that influence school employee health behaviors: Implications for wellness programming. *Journal of School Health, 89*(11), 890–898. https://doi.org/10.1111/josh.12831

SHAPE America, American Heart Association, & Voices for Healthy Kids. (2016). *2016 shape of the nation: Status of physical education in the USA*. https://www.shapeamerica.org/uploads/pdfs/son/Shape-of-the-Nation-2016_web.pdf

SHAPE America—Society of Health and Physical Educators. (2010). *Opportunity to learn: Guidelines for elementary, middle & high school physical education: A side-by-side comparison*. https://www.shapeamerica.org/upload/Opportunity-to-Learn-Guidelines.pdf

SHAPE America—Society of Health and Physical Educators. (2015). *The essential components of physical education.* https://www.shapeamerica.org/upload/The EssentialComponentsOfPhysicalEducation.pdf

Sheldon, S. B. (2018). Improving student outcomes with school, family, and community partnerships: A research review. In J. L. Epstein, M. G. Sanders, S. B. Sheldon, B. S. Simon, K. C. Salinas, N. R. Jansorn, F. L. Van Voorhis, C. S. Martin, B. G. Thomas, M. D. Greenfield, D. J. Hutchins, & K. J. Williams (Eds.), *School, family, and community partnerships: Your handbook for action* (4th ed., pp. 43–62). Corwin Press.

Sheldon, S. B., & Epstein, J. L. (2002). Improving student behavior and school discipline with family and community involvement. *Education and urban society, 35*(1), 4–26. https://doi.org/10.1177%2F001312402237212

Shifrer, D., Pearson, J., Muller, C., & Wilkinson, L. (2015). College-going benefits of high school sports participation: Race and gender differences over three decades. *Youth and Society, 47*(3), 295–318. https://doi.org/10.1177/0044118X12461656

Simmons, D. (2019). How to be an antiracist educator. *ASCD Education Update, 61*(10).

Slade, S. (2015a). Building on the past and moving into the future. In D. A. Birch & D. M. Videto (Eds.), *Promoting health and academic success* (pp. 185–194). Human Kinetics.

Slade, S. (2015b). The whole child initiative. In D. A. Birch & D. M. Videto (Eds.), *Promoting health and academic success* (pp. 53–63). Human Kinetics.

Smith, L., Norgate, S. H., Cherrett, T., Davies, N., Winstanley, C., & Harding, M. (2015). Walking school buses as a form of active transportation for children—a review of the evidence. *Journal of School Health, 85*(3), 197–210. https://doi.org/10.1111/josh.12239

Smith, T. E., Sheridan, S. M., Kim, E. M., Park, S., & Beretvas, S. N. (2020). The effects of family-school partnership interventions on academic and social-emotional functioning: A meta-analysis exploring what works for whom. *Educational Psychology Review, 32*, 511–544. https://doi.org/10.1007/s10648-019-09509-w

Soleimanpour, S., & Geierstanger, S. (2014). *Documenting the link between school-based health centers & academic success: A guide for the field.* California School-Based Health Alliance. http://www.schoolhealthcenters.org/wp-content/uploads/2014/07/SBHCs-Academic-Success-CA-Alliance-2014.pdf

Strolin-Goltzman, J., Sisselman, A., Auerbach, C., Sharon, L., Spolter, S., & Corn, T. B. (2012). The moderating effect of school type on the relationship between school-based health centers and the learning environment. *Social Work in Public Health, 27*(7), 699–709. https://doi.org/10.1080/19371910903323815

Taub, A., Goekler, S., Auld, M. E., Birch, D. A., Muller, S., Wengert, D., & Allegrante, J. P. (2014). Accreditation of professional preparation programs for school health educators: The changing landscape. *Health Education and Behavior, 41*(4), 349–358. https://doi.org/10.1177/1090198114539686

Taylor, R. D., Oberle, E., Durlak, J. A., & Weissberg, R. P. (2017). Promoting positive youth development through school-based social and emotional learning interventions: A meta-analysis of follow-up effects. *Child Development, 88*(4), 1156–1171. https://doi.org/10.1111/cdev.12864

Temkin, D., Solomon, B. J., Katz, E., & Steed, H. (2019). Creating healthy schools: Students, educators, and policymakers name priorities. *State Education Standard*, *19*(1), 11–17.

Tomlinson, C. A. (2018). Dignity in the classroom. *Educational Leadership, 76*(2), 86–88.

US Department of Education & Office of Elementary and Secondary Education. (2019). *The role of districts in developing high-quality school emergency operations plans.* https://rems.ed.gov/docs/District_Guide_508C.pdf

US Department of Education, Office of Elementary and Secondary Education, & Office of Safe and Healthy Students. (2013). *Guide for developing high-quality school emergency operations.* https://rems.ed.gov/docs/School_Guide_508C.pdf

Valois, R. F. (2015). Evaluating WSCC. In D. A. Birch & D. M. Videto (Eds.). *Promoting health and academic success: The whole school, whole community, whole child approach* (pp. 165–182). Human Kinetics.

Van Cura, M. (2010). The relationship between school-based health centers, rates of early dismissal from school, and loss of seat time. *Journal of School Health, 80*(8), 371–377. https://doi.org/10.1111/j.1746-1561.2010.00516.x

Victoria State Government. (2022, March 29). *Active travel.* https://www.education.vic.gov.au/school/teachers/teachingresources/discipline/physed/Pages/activetravel.aspx

Videto, D. M., & Birch, D. A. (2015). Implementing WSCC. In D. A. Birch & D. M. Videto (Eds.), *Promoting health and academic success: The whole school, whole community, whole child approach* (pp. 149–164). Human Kinetics.

Videto, D. M., & Dake, J. A. (2019). Promoting health literacy through defining and measuring quality school health education. *Health Promotion Practice, 20*(6), 824–833. https://doi.org/10.1177/1524839919870194

Wallace, J., Covassin, T., Nogle, S., Gould, D., & Kovan, J. (2017). Concussion knowledge and reporting behavior differences between high school athletes at urban and suburban high schools. *Journal of School Health, 87*(9), 665–674. https://doi.org/10.1111/josh.12543

Walsh, M. E., Madaus, G. F., Raczek, A. E., Dearing, E., Foley, C., An, C., Lee-St. John, T. J., & Beaton, A. (2014). A new model for student support in high-poverty urban elementary schools: Effects on elementary and middle school academic outcomes. *American Educational Research Journal, 51*(4), 704–737. https://doi.org/10.3102/0002831214541669

Wang, L. Y., Vernon-Smiley, M., Gapinski, M. A., Desisto, M., Maughan, E., & Sheetz, A. (2014). Cost-benefit study of school nursing services. *JAMA Pediatrics, 168*(7), 642–648. https://doi:10.1001/jamapediatrics.2013.5441

Watson, A., Timperio, A., Brown, H., Best, K., & Hesketh, K. D. (2017). Effect of classroom-based physical activity interventions on academic and physical activity outcomes: A systematic review and meta-analysis. *International Journal of Behavioral Nutrition and Physical Activity, 14*(1), 114. https://doi.org/10.1186/s12966-017-0569-9

Webber, M. P., Carpiniello, K. E., Oruwariye, T., Lo, Y., Burton, W. B., & Appel, D. K. (2003). Burden of asthma in inner-city elementary schoolchildren: Do school-based health centers make a difference? *Archives of Pediatrics and Adolescent Medicine, 157*(2), 125–129. https://doi.org/10.1001/archpedi.157.2.125

Weingarten, R. (2015). Schools at the center of communities. *American Educator, 39*(3), 14.

Yoder, C. M. (2020). School nurses and student academic outcomes: An integrative review. *The Journal of School Nursing, 36*(1), 49–60. https://doi.org/10.1177/1059840518824397

Youth.gov. (n.d.). *Afterschool programs.* https://youth.gov/youth-topics/afterschool-programs

Chapter 7. Moving Forward

Almeida, P. (2019). *Social movements: The structure of collective mobilization.* University of California Press.

American Academy of Family Physicians. (2018). *The physician advocate: Advancing policies that support health equity.* https://www.aafp.org/dam/AAFP/documents/patient_care/everyone_project/physican-advocate.pdf

American Academy of Family Physicians. (2020). *Integration of primary care and public health.* https://www.aafp.org/about/policies/all/integration-primary-care.html

American Academy of Pediatrics Council on Community Pediatrics, Gorski, P. A., Kuo, A. A., Granado-Villar, D. C., Gitterman, B. A., Brown, J. M., Chilton, L. A., William, H. C., Gambon, T. B., Kraft, C. A., Paz-Soldan, G. J., & Zind, B. (2012). Community pediatrics: Navigating the intersection of medicine, public health, and social determinants of children's health. *Pediatrics, 131*(3), 623–628. https://doi.org/10.1542/peds.2012-3933

American College of Physicians. (n.d.). *Public health.* https://www.acponline.org/advocacy/where-we-stand/public-health

Auerbach, J., & DeSalvo, K. B. (2019). The practical playbook in action: Improving health through cross-sector partnerships. In J. L. Michener, B. C. Castrucci, D. W. Bradley, E. L. Hunter, C. W. Thomas, C. Patterson, & E. Corcoran (Eds.), *The practical playbook II: Building multisector partnerships that work* (pp. 15–22). Oxford University Press.

Butterfoss, F. D. (2009). Building and sustaining coalitions. In R. J. Bensley & J. Brookins-Fisher (Eds.), *Community health education methods: A practical guide* (3rd ed., pp. 299–332). Jones and Bartlett Publishers.

Butterfoss, F. D. (2013). *Ignite! Getting your community coalition fired up for change.* AuthorHouse.

Chang, D. I., Gertel-Rosenberg, A., Blackburn, K. B., & Taylor, B. (2020). *Preliminary findings on the role of health care in multi-sector networks for population health: Notes from the field.* Nemours Children's Health System, Nemours National Office of Policy & Prevention. https://www.movinghealthcareupstream.org/wp-content/uploads/2020/03/HealthCareRolesInPopulationHealthNetworks.pdf

DeSalvo, K. B., Wang, Y. C., Harris, A., Auerbach, J., Koo, D., & O'Carroll, P. (2017). Peer reviewed: Public Health 3.0: A call to action for public health to meet the challenges of the 21st century. *Preventing Chronic Disease, 14.* https://doi.org/10.5888/pcd14.170017

Fisher, J., & Hancher-Rauch, H. L. (2022). Advocacy. In C. Fertman & M. L. Grim (Eds.), *Health promotion programs: From theory to practice* (3rd ed., pp. 148–165). John Wiley & Sons Inc.

Foreman, K., & Chappelle, S. B. (2019). Insight from national experts: From the community-based organization sector. In J. L. Michener, B. C. Castrucci, D. W. Bradley, E. L. Hunter, C. W. Thomas, C. Patterson, & E. Corcoran (Eds.), *The practical playbook II: Building multisector partnerships that work* (pp. 23–34). Oxford University Press.

Freudenberg, N. (2014). *Lethal but legal: Corporations, consumption, and protecting public health*. Oxford University Press.

Institute of Medicine. (2014). *Supporting a movement for health and health equity: Lessons from social movements: Workshop summary*. The National Academies Press. https://www.ncbi.nlm.nih.gov/books/NBK268728/pdf/Bookshelf_NBK 268728.pdf

Issel, L. M., & Wells, R. (2018). *Health program planning and evaluation: A practical, systematic approach for community health* (4th ed.). Jones & Bartlett Learning.

Johnson, F. S. (2016). The role of early wins in long-term success. In J. L. Michener, D. Koo, B. C. Castrucci, & J. B. Sprague (Eds.), *The practical playbook: Public health and primary care together* (pp. 95–99). Oxford University Press.

Khalifa, M. (2018). *Culturally responsive school leadership*. Harvard Education Press.

Kolbe, L. J. (2019). School health as a strategy to improve both public health and education. *Annual Review of Public Health, 40*, 443–463. https://doi.org/10.1146 /annurev-publhealth-040218-043727

Kolbe, L. J., Allensworth, D. D., Potts-Datema, W., & White, D. R. (2015). What have we learned from collaborative partnerships to concomitantly improve both education and health? *Journal of School Health, 85*(11), 766–774. https://doi.org/10.1111 /josh.12312

Koo, D., Michener, J. L., Sprague, J. B., & Castrucci, B. C. (2016). Principles of partnerships between public health and primary care. In J. L. Michener, D. Koo, B. C. Castrucci, & J. B. Sprague (Eds.), *The practical playbook: Public health and primary care together* (pp. 3–12). Oxford University Press.

Kuo, A. A., Thomas, P. A., Chilton, L. A., Mascola, L., & American Academy of Pediatrics Council on Community Pediatrics, Section on Epidemiology, Public Health, and Evidence. (2018). Pediatricians and public health: Optimizing the health and well-being of the nation's children. *Pediatrics, 141*(2). https://doi.org /10.1542/peds.2017-3848

Love, B. L. (2019). *We want to do more than survive: Abolitionist teaching and the pursuit of educational freedom*. Beacon Press.

McGinnis, J. M. (2016). Foreword: The value of integration. In J. L. Michener, D. Koo, B. C. Castrucci, & J. B. Sprague (Eds.), *The practical playbook: Public health and primary care together* (pp. ix–x). Oxford University Press.

McKenzie, J. F., Neiger, B. L., & Thackeray, R. (2017). *Planning, implementing, and evaluating health promotion programs: A primer* (7th ed.). Pearson.

Michener, J. L., & Castrucci, B. C. (2016). Stages of partnerships between public health and primary care. In J. L. Michener, D. Koo, B. C. Castrucci, & J. B. Sprague (Eds.), *The practical playbook: Public health and primary care together* (pp. 43–65). Oxford University Press.

Michener, J. L., Castrucci, B. C., Bradley, D. W., Hunter, E. L., & Thomas, C. W. (2019). Overview: The accelerating movement of partnerships for health. In J. L. Michener, B. C. Castrucci, D. W. Bradley, E. L. Hunter, C. W. Thomas, C. Patterson, & E. Corcoran (Eds.), *The practical playbook II: Building multisector partnerships that work* (pp. 3–4). Oxford University Press.

Michener, J. L., Koo, D., Castrucci, B. C., & Sprague, J. B. (Eds.). (2016). *The practical playbook: Public health and primary care together.* Oxford University Press.

Minyard, K. J., Martinez, A. P., & Adimu, T. F. (2016). Positioned for sustainability. In J. L. Michener, D. Koo, B. C. Castrucci, & J. B. Sprague (Eds.), *The practical playbook: Public health and primary care together* (pp. 83–94). Oxford University Press.

National Association of Chronic Disease Directors. (2017). *Local health department and school partnerships: Working together to build healthier schools.* https://chronicdisease.org/resource/resmgr/school_health/nacdd_health_department_and_.pdf

Norris, T., & Hill, A. (2019). Building an agenda for population health from the grassroots up. In J. L. Michener, B. C. Castrucci, D. W. Bradley, E. L. Hunter, C. W. Thomas, C. Patterson, & E. Corcoran (Eds.), *The practical playbook II: Building multisector partnerships that work* (pp. 261–270). Oxford University Press.

Rudolph, L., Caplan, J., Ben-Moshe, K., & Dillon, L. (2013). *Health in all policies: A guide for state and local governments.* American Public Health Association, Public Health Institute. https://www.apha.org/-/media/Files/PDF/factsheets/Health_inAll_Policies_Guide_169pages.ashx

Ruglis, J., & Freudenberg, N. (2010). Toward a healthy high schools movement: Strategies for mobilizing public health for educational reform. *American Journal of Public Health, 100*(9), 1565–1570. https://doi.org/10.2105/AJPH.2009.186619

Schoales, V. (2019, May 1). The end of education reform. *Education Week, 38*(1), 24.

Serpas, S., Khaokham, C., Hillidge, S., & Watson, V. (2016). San Diego, California, promotes health weight to improve community health. In J. L. Michener, D. Koo, B. C. Castrucci, & J. B. Sprague (Eds.), *The practical playbook: Public health and primary care together* (pp. 313–328). Oxford University Press.

Snyder, H. M., & Iton, A. B. (2020). *Advocacy for public health policy change: An urgent imperative.* American Public Health Association.

Van Dyke, N., & Amos, B. (2017). Social movement coalitions: Formation, longevity, and success. *Sociology Compass, 11*(7), e12489. https://doi.org/10.1111/soc4.12489

Wood, J., & Grumback, K. (2019). The role of primary care in population and community health: Pragmatic approaches to integration. In J. L. Michener, B. C. Castrucci, D. W. Bradley, E. L. Hunter, C. W. Thomas, C. Patterson, & E. Corcoran (Eds.), *The practical playbook II: Building multisector partnerships that work* (pp. 101–108). Oxford University Press.